Disclaimer: This textbook is not intended to provide, and disclaims any suggestion that it does provide, medical advice of any nature. The information made available through this textbook should not be used in place of seeking professional opinions by licensed practitioners. Only licensed medical professionals may offer medical advice, diagnosis and recommendations for treatment of medical conditions. You assume full responsibility for appropriate use of the information available through this textbook.

As Medicine is an ever-changing science, with new research and clinical experience, changes in treatment and techniques are required. The author(s) has (have) checked with sources believed to be reliable in effort to provide information that is complete and generally in accord with standards accepted at the time of publication. The opinions expressed in this work represent those of the author(s) and, in view of the possibility of human error or changes in medical science, neither the author(s), RAEducation.com LLC, nor any other party who has been involved in the preparation or publication of this work warrants that the information contained herein is in every respect accurate or complete and they are not responsible for any errors or omissions or for the results obtained from the use of such information. Readers and viewers are encouraged to confirm the information contained herein with other sources.

©2018  RAEducation.com LLC.
André P. Boezaart MD, PhD, with artwork by Mary K. Bryson
Published by RAEducation.com LLC
Produced by Kristine Lyle, Printers Workshop, Kalona, IA
First Edition published in 2004, Second Edition published in 2017
ISBN: 978-1-948083-06-5

# André P. Boezaart

MBChB, MPraxMed, DA(CMSA), FFA(CMSA), MMed(Anesth), PhD

Professor of Anesthesiology and Orthopaedic Surgery

Chief of Division of Acute and Peri-operative Pain Medicine

Chief of Acute Pain Service

University of Florida College of Medicine, Gainesville, Florida, USA

**Co-Authors:**

Paul E. Bigeleisen, MD; Donald S. Bohannon, MD; Svedlana V. Chembrovich, MD;

David A. Edwards, MD, PhD; Barys V. Ihnatsenka, MD;

Johan P. Reyneke, BChD, MChD, FMFMOS(CMSA), PhD

Cameron R. Smith, MD, PhD; Linda Le-Wendling, MD; Yury Zasimovich, MD

**Artwork by:**

Mary K. Bryson, MAMS, CMI

Bryson Biomedical Illustration

Langhorne, Pennsylvania

Educational electronic and printed media for the website
RAEducation.com owned by RAEducation.com LLC.

Please visit www.RAEducation.com

for video tutorials on this and other topics

# Preface

As educators, we are often asked by colleagues to teach them how to do a certain nerve block. If, however, the colleague truly understands where the nerve lives (the macroanatomy), what it lives in (the microanatomy), and how to find the nerve (the sono- and functional anatomy), s/he already knows how to do the block; all s/he needs to learn are a few finer set-up and technical nuances.

Students also ask how can they be as effective with their single-injection and continuous nerve blocks as the masters, and how they can be assured not to lose their skills if they don't regularly practice or perform the blocks. The answer to these two questions is exactly the same as that of the first question.

Advanced anatomical knowledge satisfies the 2nd and 3rd basic requirements for successful Acute and Perioperative Pain Medicine:

1. Correct and meticulous indications
2. Correct nerve
3. Correct technique
4. Correct equipment
5. Correct recipient of the block

This 3rd Edition of "The Primer" is an extension of the 1st and 2nd Editions; the 1st of which did not include microanatomy and sonoanatomy, and the 2nd of which was revised for better clarity. Because of the glowing interest in the pterygopalatine block for vascular headaches such as migraine, cluster headache and postdural puncture headache, a comprehensive discussion of the macro- micro- sono-, and surface anatomy of the pterygopalatine ganglion was also included. It, however, remains only a Primer, and further study will be required for full proficiency – a quest that should never be satisfied. The book is designed so that viewing the figures, reading their legends, and watching the dynamic sono- and functional anatomy video tutorials on the RAEducation.com website, should give the student an adequate working knowledge to effectively perform most, if not all, high-yield nerve blocks. They should certainly provide enough anatomy knowledge to answer all AMA Board questions on RA and APM Anatomy – including micro and sonoanatomy.

The content of this book should be regarded as the absolute minimum of anatomical knowledge required. Students are strongly advised and encouraged to seek deeper knowledge from the multitude of great anatomical textbooks available. "Must Know Anatomy for Regional Anesthesia and Acute Pain Medicine" has been specifically written to fill this potential gap. Throughout this book there are URL references to video tutorials, lecture videos, and lectures in pdf format. Clicking on, or copying any URL in the pages that follow, will take you to these further educational material that is created as part of this book for those interested in a deeper study of the subject.

And␣ré P. Boezaart, 2018

# Co-Authors

## André P. Boezaart,
MBChB, MPraxMed, DA(CMSA), FFA(CMSA) MMed(Anesth), PhD
Professor of Anesthesiology and Orthopaedic Surgery
Departments of Anesthesiology and Orthopaedic Surgery and Rehabilitation
Chief, Division of Acute and Perioperative Pain Medicine; Chief, Acute Pain Service
University of Florida College of Medicine, Gainesville, Florida, USA

## Paul E. Bigeleisen, MD
Professor of Anesthesiology, Department of Anesthesiology
University of Maryland, Baltimore, Maryland, USA

## Donald S. Bohannon, MD
Associate Professor of Anesthesiology, Department of Anesthesiology
Division of Acute and Perioperative Pain Medicine
University of Florida College of Medicine, Gainesville, Florida, USA

## Svedlana V. Chembrovich, MD
Fellow Physician, Department of Anesthesiology
Division of Acute and Perioperative Pain Medicine
University of Florida College of Medicine, Gainesville Florida, USA

## David A. Edwards, MD, PhD
Associate Professor, Department of Anesthesiology
Vanderbilt University Medical Center, Nashville, Tennessee, USA

## Barys V. Ihnatsenka, MD
Associate Professor of Anesthesiology, Department of Anesthesiology
Division of Acute and Perioperative Pain Medicine
University of Florida College of Medicine, Gainesville, Florida, USA

## Linda Le-Wendling, MD
Associate Professor of Anesthesiology, Department of Anesthesiology
Division of Acute and Perioperative Pain Medicine
University of Florida College of Medicine, Gainesville, Florida, USA

## Johan P. Reyneke, BChD, MChD, FCFMOS(CMSA), PhD
Director, Centre for Orthognathic Surgery,
Cape Town Mediclinic, Cape Town, South Africa
Honorary Professor, Department of Maxillofacial and Oral Surgery
University of the Western Cape, Cape Town, South Africa
Associate Professor, Division of Oral and Maxillofacial Surgery
Universidad Autonoma de Nuevo Leon, Monterrey, Mexico
Clinical Professor, Department of Oral and Maxillofacial Surgery
University of Oklahoma College of Dentistry, Oklahoma City, Oklahoma, USA
and University of Florida College of Dentistry, Gainesville, Florida, USA

## Cameron R. Smith, MD, PhD
Assistant Professor, Department of Anesthesiology
Division of Acute and Perioperative Pain Medicine
University of Florida College of Medicine, Gainesville, Florida, USA

## Yury Zasimovich, MD
Assistant Professor of Anesthesiology, Department of Anesthesiology
Division of Acute and Perioperative Pain Medicine
University of Florida College of Medicine, Gainesville, Florida, USA

# Dedication

To all the Fellows in Acute and Perioperative Pain Medicine,
who over so many years honored me by allowing me
to participate in their education.

# Chapter 1

## The Proximal Brachial Plexus

*Macroanatomy*
*Microanatomy*
*Sonoanatomy*
*Functional Anatomy*

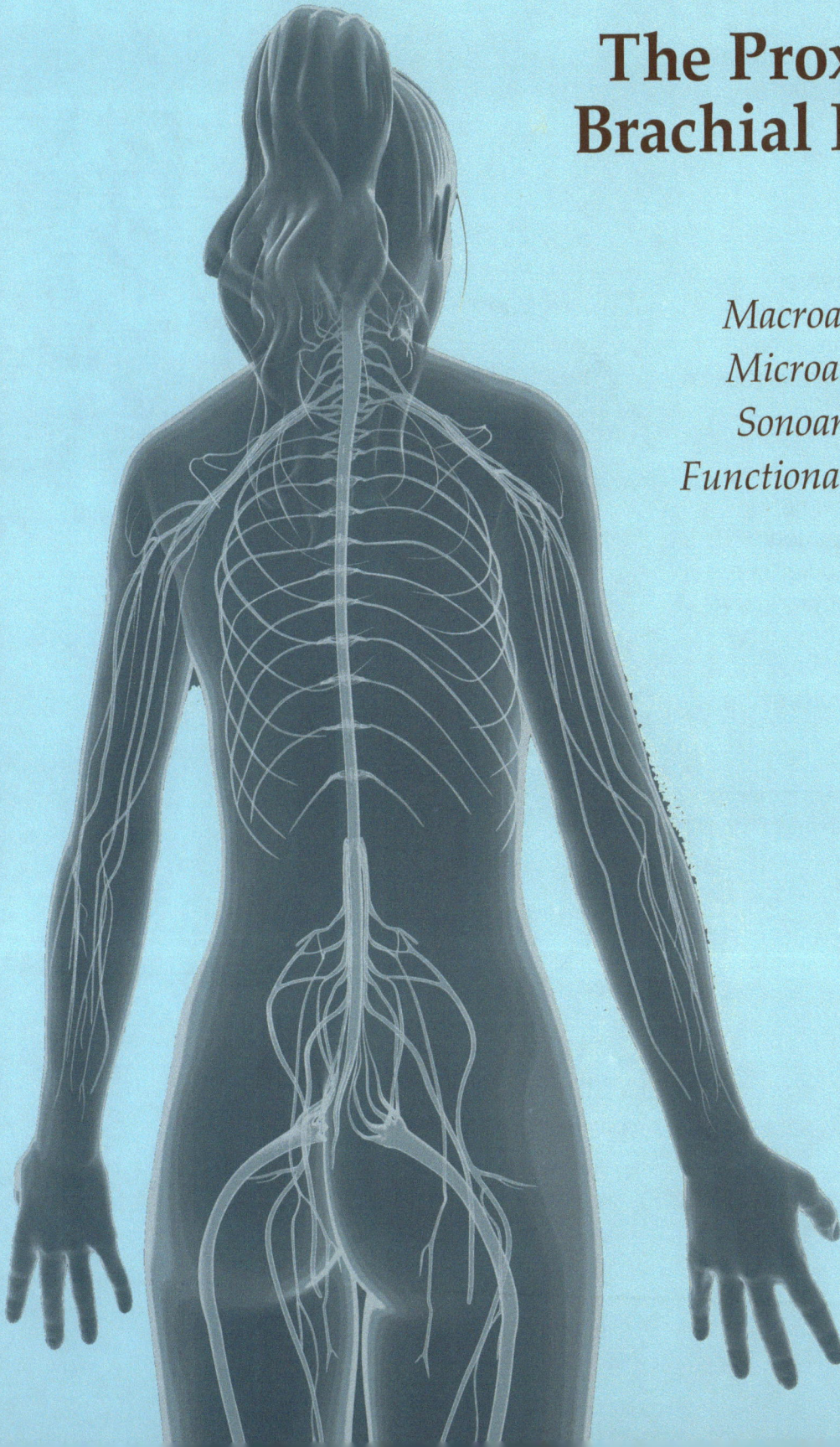

# Macroanatomy

1 Phrenic nerve
2 Nerve to Levator Scapulae
3 Spinal accessory nerve
4 Dorsal scapular nerve
5 Suprascapular nerve
6 Superior trunk
7 Middle trunk
8 Inferior trunk
9 Long thoracic nerve
10 Nerves to longus colli
   and scalene muscles
11 Nerve to subclavius muscle
12 Lateral cord
13 Posterior cord
14 Medial cord
15 Lateral pectoral nerve
16 Medial pectoral nerve
17 Upper subscapular nerve
18 Lower subscapular nerve
19 Medial cutaneous nerve
   of arm
20 Medial cutaneous nerve
   of upper arm
21 Axillary nerve
22 Musculocutaneous nerve
23 Radial nerve
24 Median nerve
25 Ulnar nerve

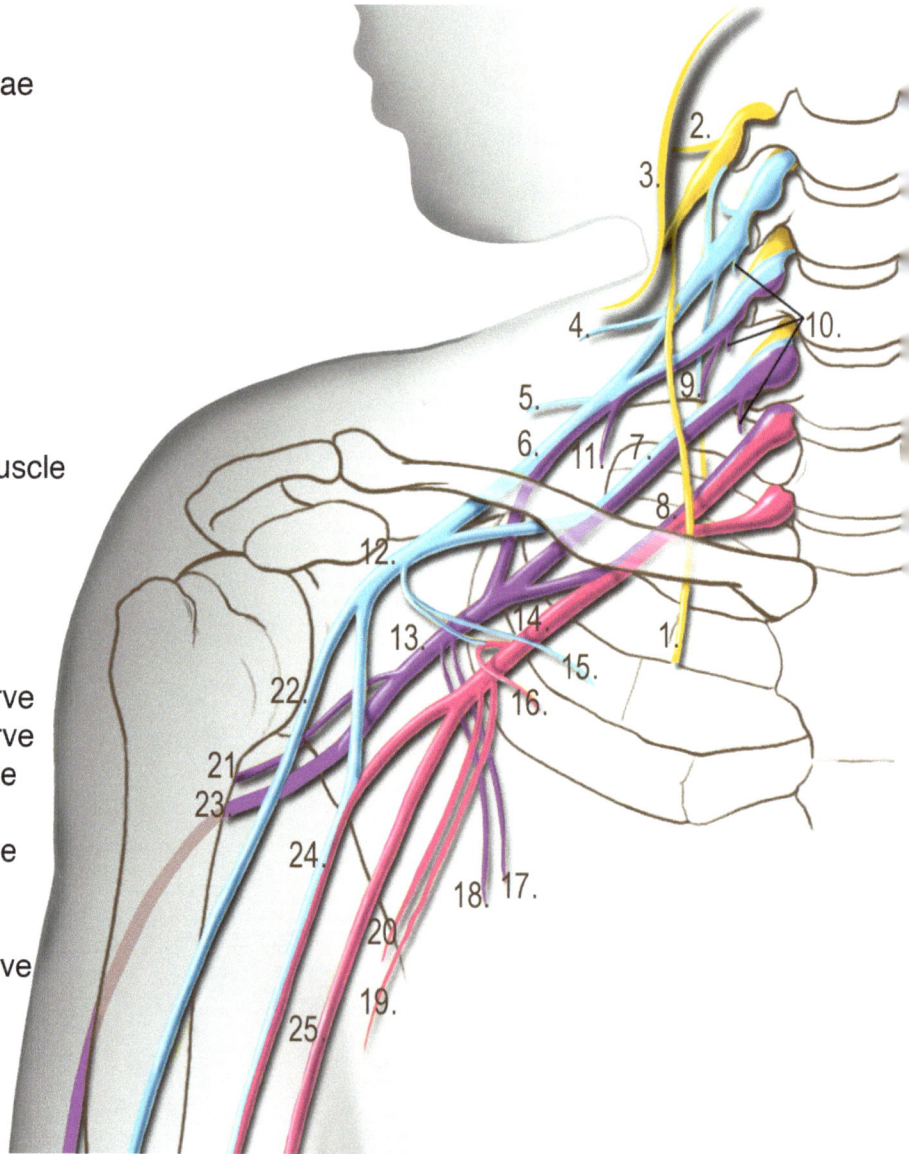

*Figure 1-1*

The phrenic nerve (1) originates mainly from 4th cervical spinal root (C4), receives a small branch from the 5th cervical spinal root (C5) of the brachial plexus, and runs caudad on the belly of the anterior scalene muscle. It supplies motor innervation to the diaphragm. The nerve to the levator scapulae muscle (2), the dorsal scapular nerve (4), and the supra-scapular nerve (5) also originate from the C4 and C5 roots. The long thoracic nerve (9) also stems from the C4, C5, and C6 roots. The accessory nerve (3) is a cranial nerve. The superior trunk (6) forms as the C5 and C6 spinal roots join, whereas the middle trunk is a continuation from the C7 spinal root. The inferior trunk forms as the 8th cervical (C8) and first thoracic spinal (T1) roots join. The C5 and C6 roots come together to form the upper (superior) trunk, which gives off a small branch to the subclavius muscle (11). In the cervical region, the spinal roots exit the neuroforamens of the vertebra above it. Thus, C5, for example, exits the neuroforamen between the 4th and 5th cervical vertebra. The first thoracic spinal root is the transition and exits below the 7th cervical vertebra and above the corresponding T1 vertebra. From there downward, all of the spinal roots of the thoracic and lumbar areas exit below the corresponding vertebra. From the three trunks that usually extend to the supraclavicular area, three divisions split away to form the three cords of the brachial plexus: the lateral cord (12), the medial cord (14), and the posterior cord (13).

# Dissection of the Posterior Triangle of the Neck

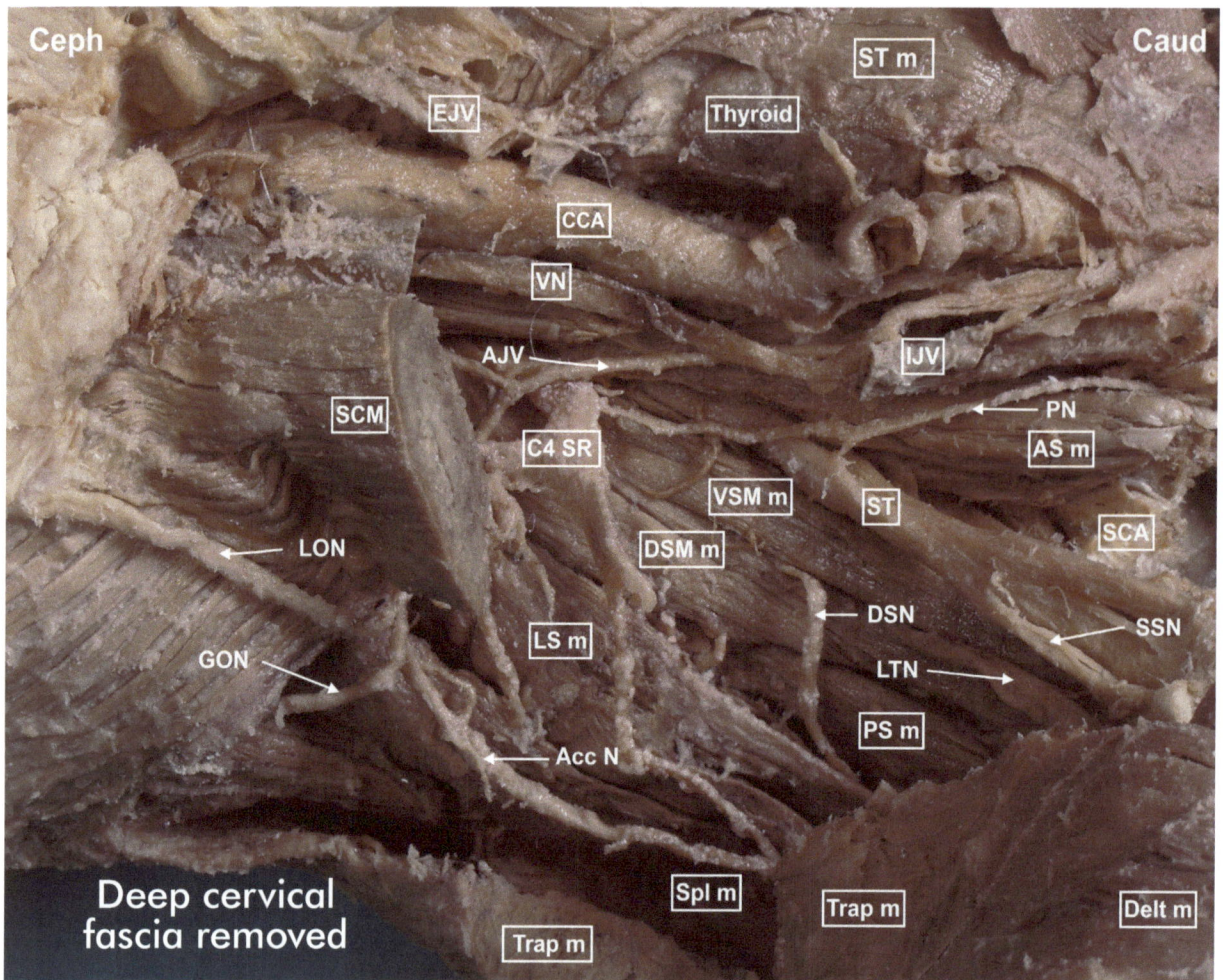

*Figure 1-2: Anatomical dissection of the posterior triangle of the neck: lateral vi*

| | | | |
|---|---|---|---|
| Acc N | Accessory nerve (CN XI) | LS m | Levator scapulae muscle |
| AJV | Anterior jugular vein | LTN | Long thoracic nerve |
| AS m | Anterior scalene muscle | PN | Phrenic nerve |
| C4 SR | 4th cervical spinal root | SCA | Subclavian artery |
| Caud | Caudad | SCM | Sternocleidomastoid muscle (cut) |
| CCA | Common carotid artery | Spl m | Splenius muscle |
| Ceph | Cephalad | SSN | Suprascapular nerve |
| Delt m | Deltoid muscle | ST | Superior trunk of the brachial plexus |
| DSM m | Dorsal part of middle scalene muscle | ST m | Sternothyroid muscle |
| DSN | Dorsal scapular nerve | Thyroid | Thyroid gland |
| EJV | External jugular vein (cut) | Trap m | Trapezius muscle (cut) |
| GON | Greater occipital nerve | VN | Vagus nerve (CN X) |
| IJV | Internal jugular vein (cut) | VSM m | Ventral part of middle scalene muscle |
| LON | Lesser occipital nerve | | |

# Posterior Triangle of the Neck

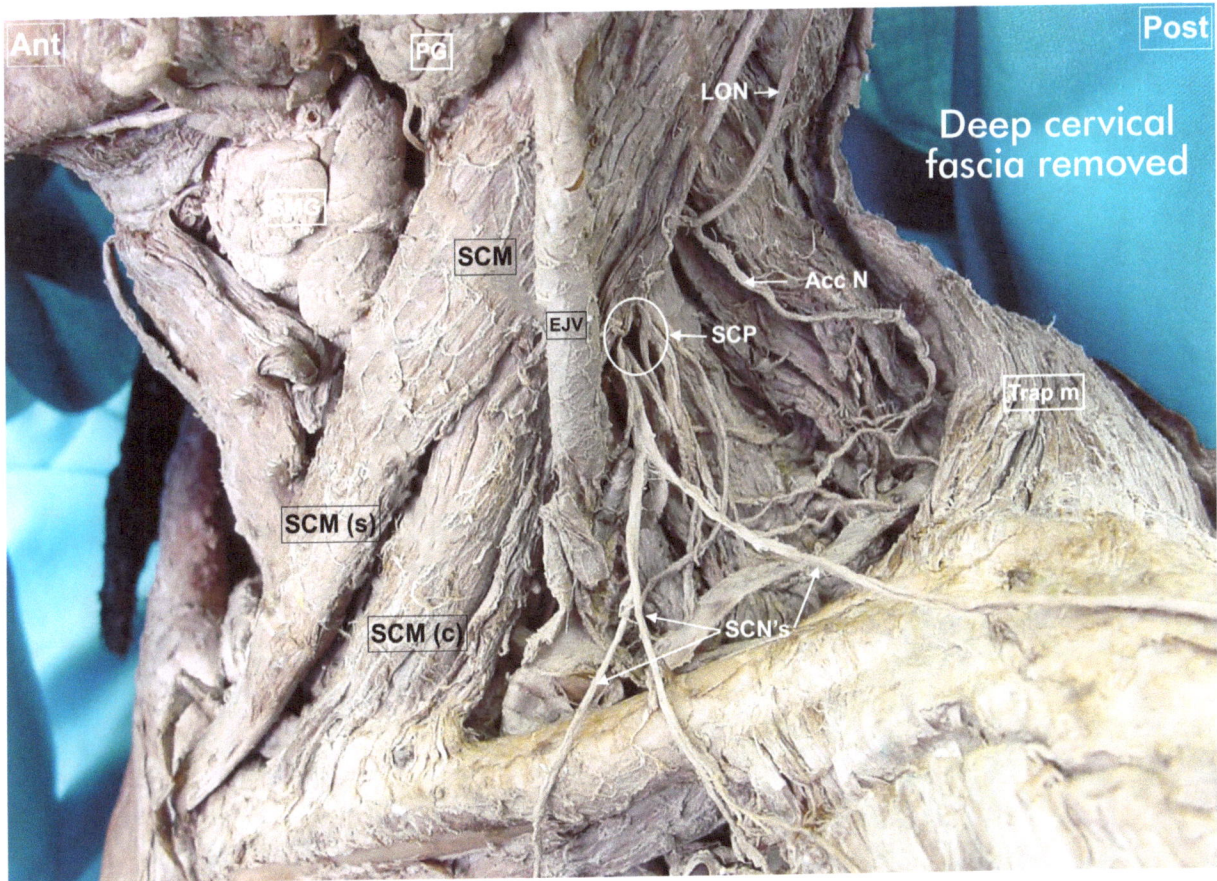

*Figure 1-3: Anatomical dissection of the posterior triangle of the neck depicting outer structures: antero-lateral view.*

Acc N    Accessory nerve
Ant      Anterior
EJV      External jugular vein
LON      Lesser occipital nerve
PG       Parotid gland
Post     Posterior
SCM(c)   Clavicular head of sternocleidomastoid muscle
SCM(s)   Sternal head of sternocleidomastoid muscle
SCM      Sternocleidomastoid muscle
SCN's    Supraclavicular veins
SCP      Superficial cervical plexus
SMG      Submandibular gland
Trap m   Trapezius muscle

# Posterior Triangle of the Neck

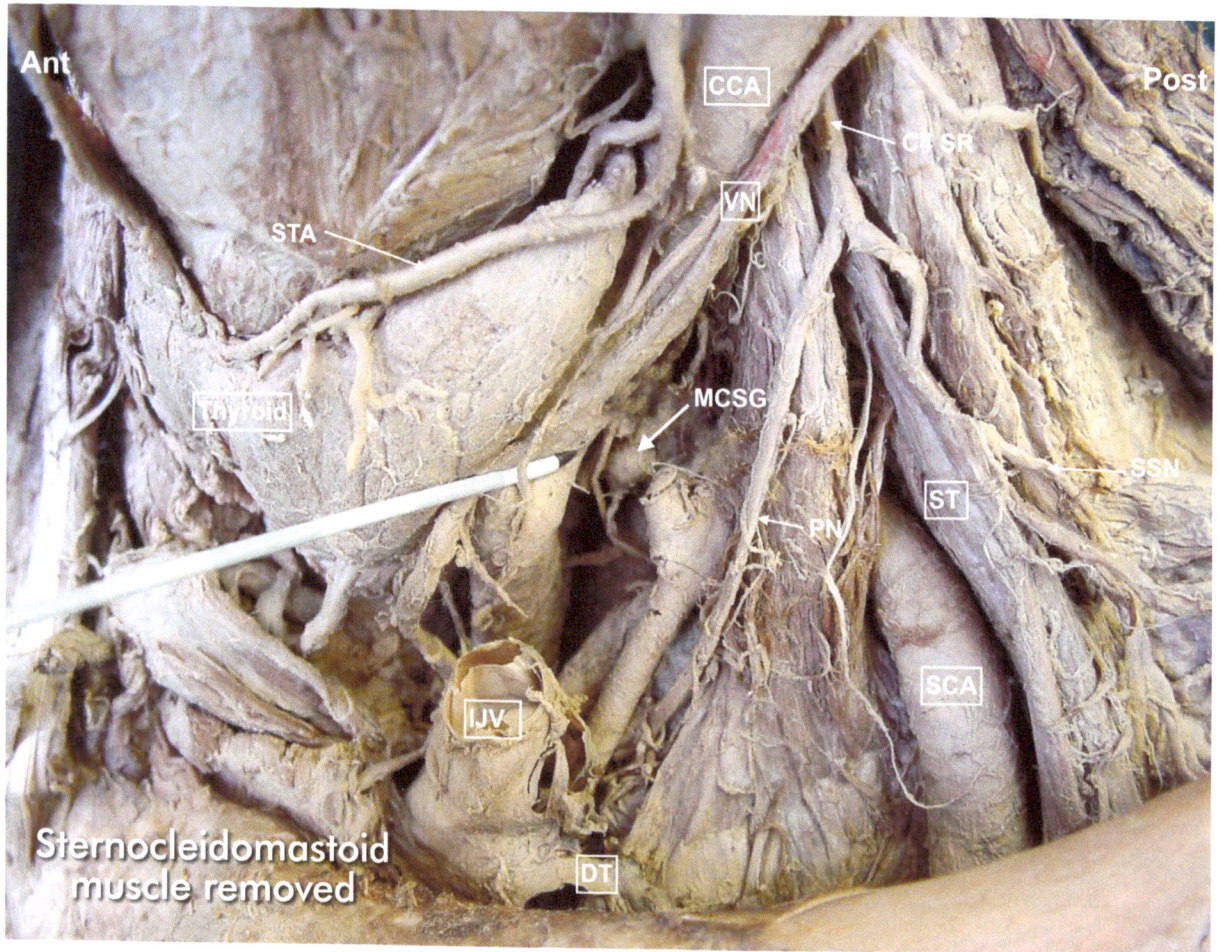

*Figure 1-4: Anatomical dissection of the posterior triangle of the neck depicting deeper structures: anterolateral view with sternocleidomastoid muscle removed.*

| | |
|---|---|
| Ant | Anterior |
| C4 SR | 4th cervical spinal root |
| CCA | Common carotid artery |
| DT | Ductus thoracicus |
| IJV | Internal jugular vein |
| MCSG | Middle cervical sympathetic ganglion |
| PN | Phrenic nerve |
| Post | Posterior |
| SCA | Subclavian artery |
| SSN | Suprascapular nerve |
| ST | Superior trunk of the brachial plexus |
| STA | Superior thoracic arter; |
| Thyroid | Thyroid gland |
| VN | Vagus nerve |

# Dissection of the Lateral Aspect of the Neck

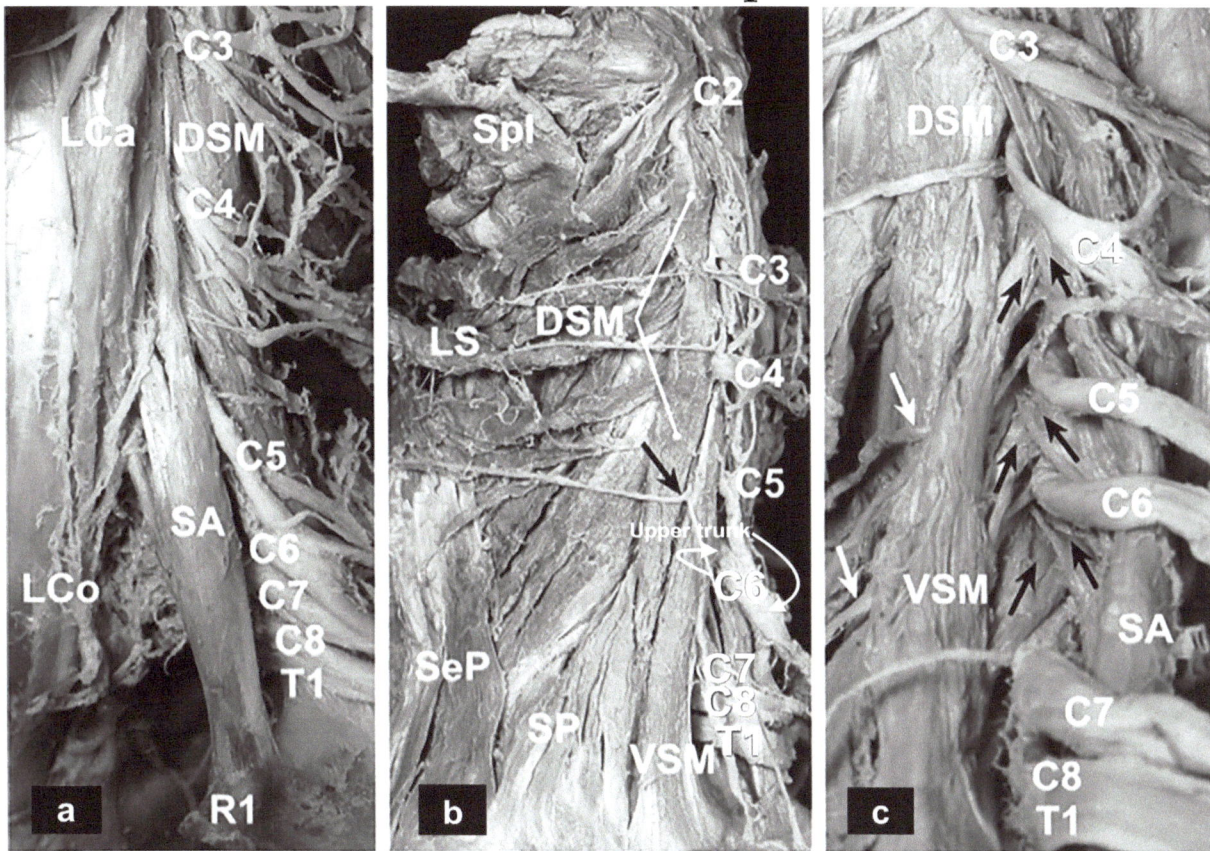

*Figure 1-5: Dissection of 2nd to 8th ventral rami of the cervical nerve roots (C2–C8).*

**(a)** Ventral aspect of the left anterior scalene muscle (SA). **(b)** Dorsal aspect of the right Ventral middle scalene muscle (VSM), dorsal middle scalene muscle (DSM), and posterior scalene muscle (SP). The black arrow in 8b indicates the common root of the dorsal scapular and long thoracic nerves. **(c)** Lateral aspect of the origins of the right ventral middle scalene muscle (VSM), dorsal middle scalene muscle (DSM), and anterior scalene muscle (SA). SA and VSM attach to the anterior and posterior tubercles respectively, and their fibers cross each other (black arrows in c). The upper and lower white arrows indicate the dorsal scapular and long thoracic nerves, respectively. It is important to note, as seen in this illustration by Sakamoto, that muscle fibers of the anterior and middle scalene muscles cross over between the spinal roots to form an enclosed paravertebral trough medial to the cross-over (Fig. 1-5b). This may explain the vertical spread of local anesthetic

agents along the vertebral column sometimes seen during cervical paravertebral block. Sakamoto also clarified the anatomical variations in the relationships of the five scalene muscles to the brachial plexus.

| | |
|---|---|
| DSM | Dorsal part of scalenus medius |
| LCa | Longus capitis |
| LCo | Longus colli |
| LS | Levator scapulae |
| R1 | First rib |
| SA | Scalenus anterior |
| SeP | Serratus posterior superior |
| SP | Scalenus posterior |
| Spl | Splenius capitis |
| T1 | First thoracic ventral ramus |
| VSM | Ventral part of scalenus medius |

*Reprinted from Sakamoto Y. Spatial relationship between the morphologies & innervations of the scalene, anterior & vertebral muscles. Ann Anat 2012;194: 381-88. Ref: Boezaart AP, Ihnatsenka BV. Cervical paravertebral block for elbow & wrist surgery: Reg Anesth Pain Med 2014;39:361-62.*

# Oblique Fluoroscopic View of the Neck

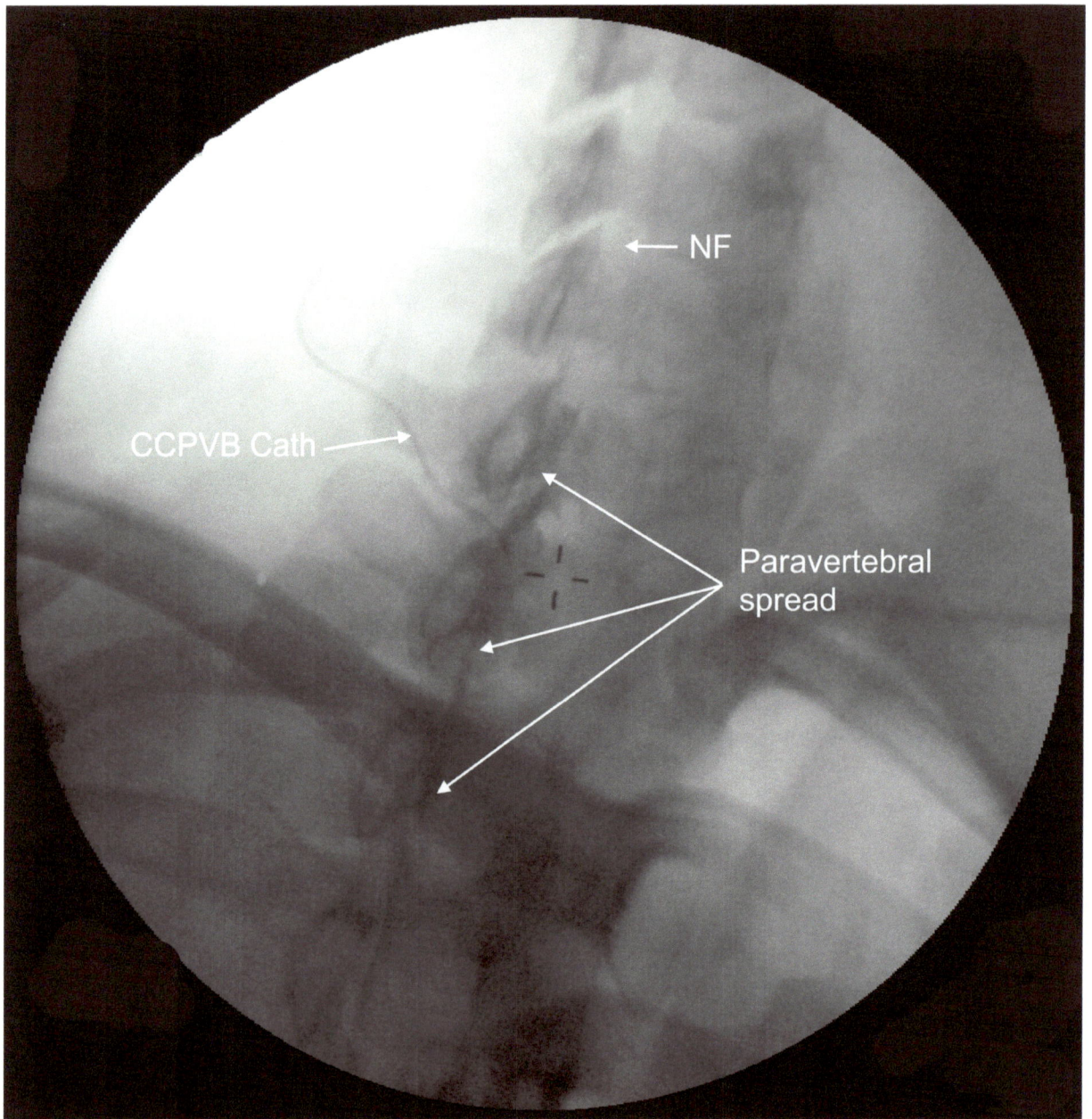

*Figure 1-6: Oblique X-ray of cervical spine with contrast showing longitudinal paravertebral spread in the paravertebral "trough."*

| | |
|---|---|
| CCPVB Cath | Catheter for continuous cervical paravertebral block placed at the level of the 7th cervical vertebra through the dorsal scalene muscle |
| NF | Neuroforamen |
| ⟶ | Longitudinal paravertebral spread of contrast medium |

# Posterior Triangle of the Neck

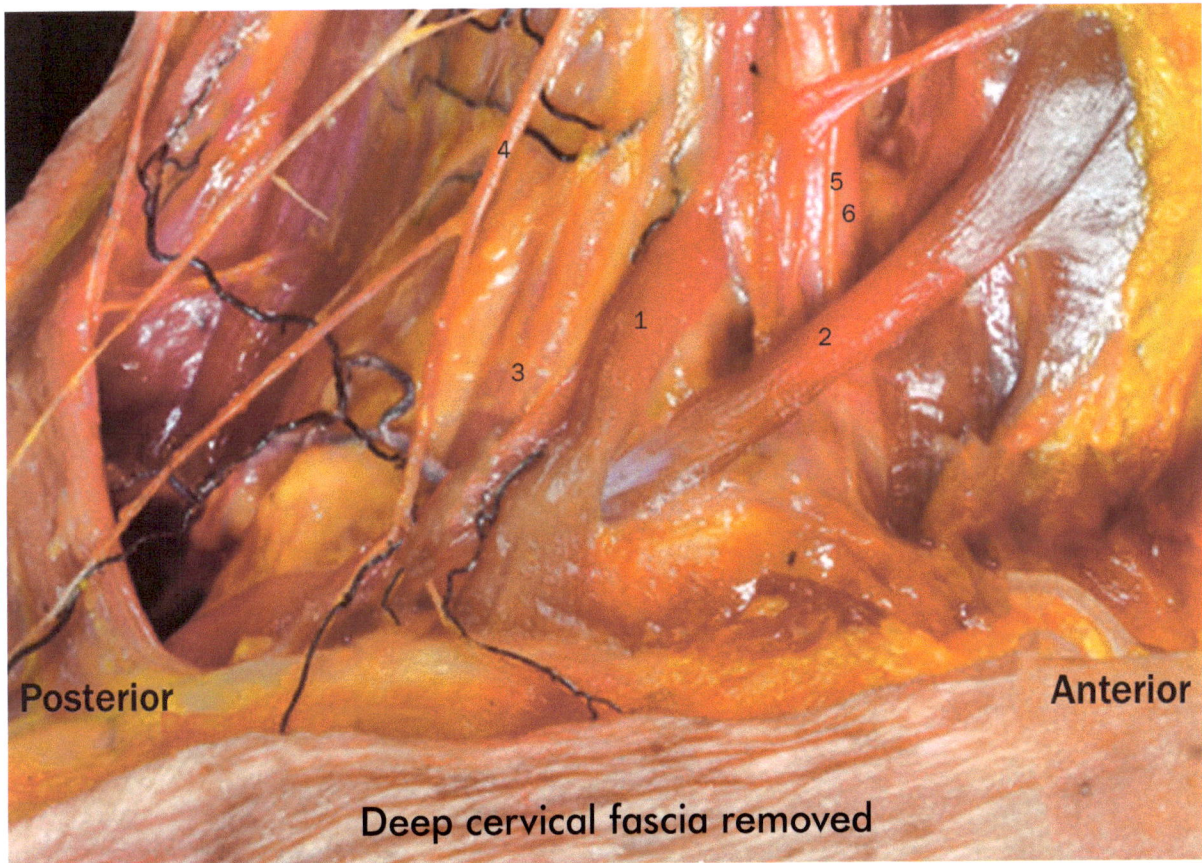

*Figure 1-7: Lateral dissection of the neck showing three of the five scalene muscles including scalene minimi.*

There are five scalene muscles: the anterior (6), the ventral (3), and dorsal (not shown on this dissection) middle, the posterior (not shown on this dissection), and the minimus scalene (1) muscles. The phrenic nerve (5) is shown on the belly of the anterior scalene muscle (6). The number (4) depicts the anterior ramus of C4 and number 2 depicts the omohyoid muscle.

# Transection of the Neck at the Level of C6

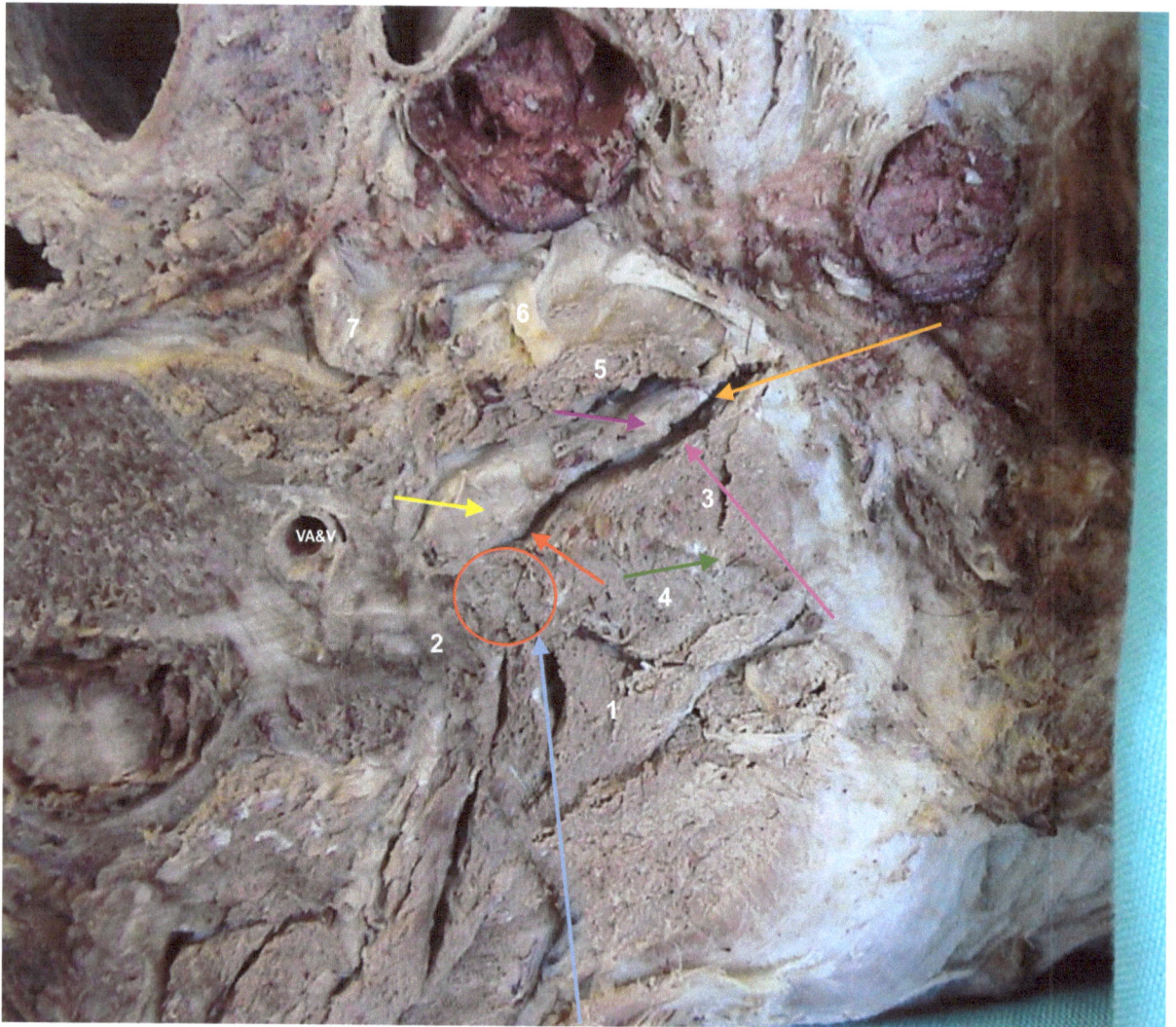

*Figure 1-8: Anatomical axial section through the neck at the level of the 6th cervical vertebra.*

| | | | |
|---|---|---|---|
| 1 | Posterior scalene muscle | → | needle path for cervical paravertebral block |
| 2 | Posterior tubercle of transverse process of C6 | → | epimyseal space around C6 spinal root |
| 3 | Ventral middle scalene muscle | → | C6 spinal root |
| 4 | Dorsal middle scalene muscle | → | C5 spinal root that joins C6 to form upper trunk |
| 5 | Anterior scalene muscle | | |
| 6 | Phrenic nerve | → | needle path of posterior approach interscalene block |
| 7 | Stellate ganglion | | |
| VA&V | Vertebral artery and vein | | |
| ○ | Slips of origin of posterior scalene muscle attached to posterior tubercle of transverse process of C5, 6 & 7 | ▶ | needle path of lateral approach interscalene block |

Please note:

The posterior scalene muscle (1) attaches to posterior spinous process of C5, C6, C7 (2).

Slips of origin of posterior scalene muscle (red oval) is tendinous (aponeurotic).

The blue arrow indicates path of the needle during cervical paravertebral block placement.

Loss of resistance is felt when the space (red arrow) between the slips of origin (red oval) and brachial plexus roots of C6 (yellow arrow) is entered. This is the sub-epimyseal space, which extends around the anterior scalene muscle.

The C5 root is indicated by the purple arrow. Further caudad, at the C7 level, these two roots merge to form the upper trunk. The fibers of the anterior (5) and middle (3 & 4) scalene muscles cross medial to the upper trunk (see Figures 1-5, 1-6).

The dorsal scapular and long thoracic nerves (green arrow) are between the ventral (3) and dorsal (4) middle scalene muscles.

The pink arrow indicates the posterior approach to the interscalene block.

The orange arrow indicates the longitudinal or lateral approach to the interscalene block.

The phrenic nerve (6) and superior cervical sympathetic ganglion (7), (stellate ganglion) are in the subepimyseal space (red arrow).

VA&V depict the vertebral artery and vein.

**Please refer to standard textbooks for indications for and techniques of performing any of the blocks referred to in this book.**

# Transection of the Neck at the Level of C6

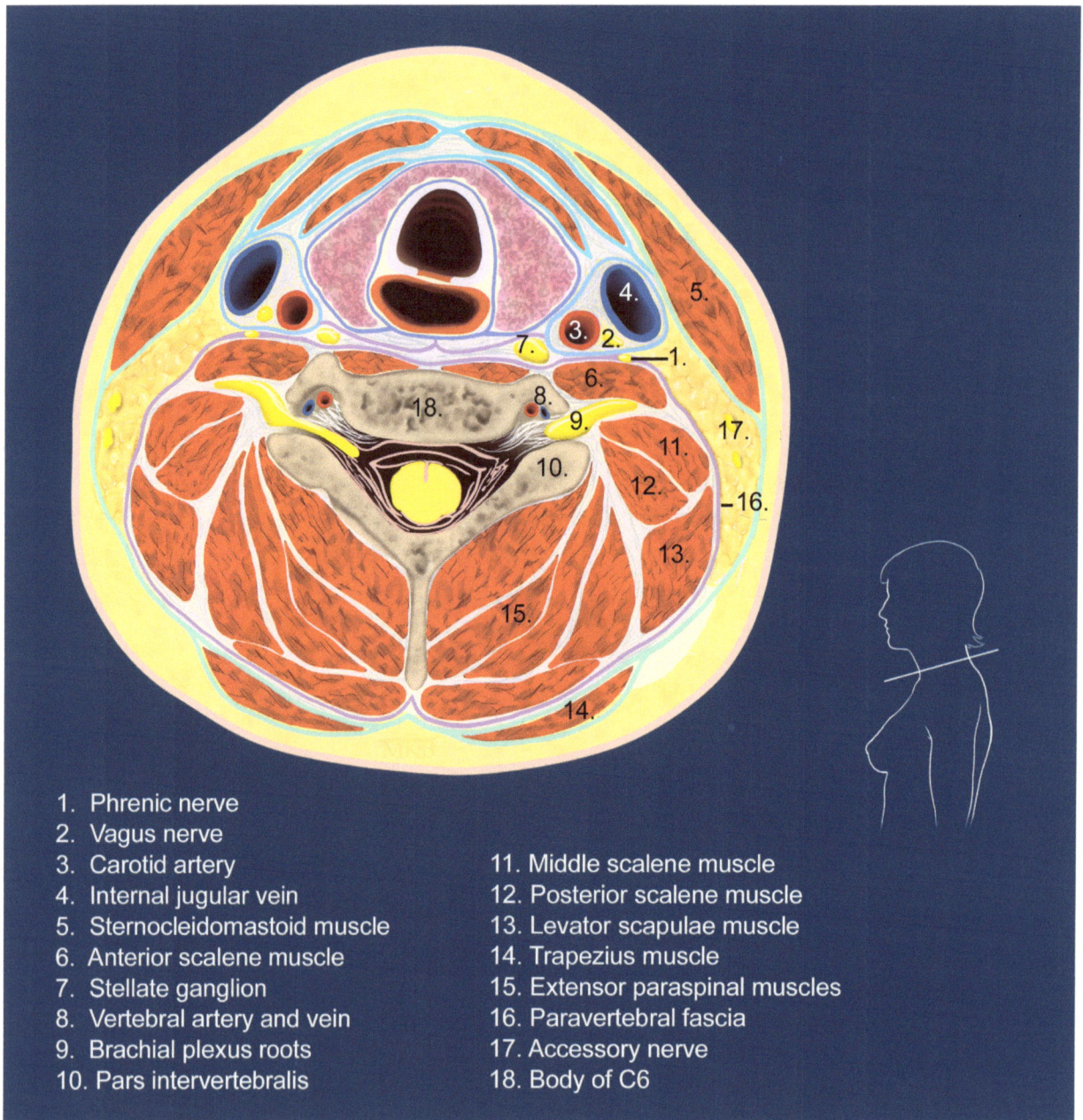

1. Phrenic nerve
2. Vagus nerve
3. Carotid artery
4. Internal jugular vein
5. Sternocleidomastoid muscle
6. Anterior scalene muscle
7. Stellate ganglion
8. Vertebral artery and vein
9. Brachial plexus roots
10. Pars intervertebralis
11. Middle scalene muscle
12. Posterior scalene muscle
13. Levator scapulae muscle
14. Trapezius muscle
15. Extensor paraspinal muscles
16. Paravertebral fascia
17. Accessory nerve
18. Body of C6

*Figure 1-9: Trans-section of the neck through the 6th cervical vertebra area.*

Please note: The extensor paraspinal muscles (15) are usually tender; penetrating these with a needle or catheter may cause pain. There is a "natural pathway" between the levator scapulae muscle (13) and trapezius muscle (14). The posterior scalene muscle (12) attaches to the posterior tubercle of the C5, C6, and C7 transverse processes. At the C7 level (where the cervical paravertebral block is performed), the muscle is tendinous (aponeurotic) and when a needle exits the anterior border of the posterior scalene muscle (between 12 and 9), there is a distinct loss of resistance to air or D5W.

*Ref: Boezaart AP, Lucas SD, Elliott CE. Paravertebral block: cervical, thoracic, lumbar & sacral. Curr Opin Anaesthesiol 2009;22:637-43.*

# Mid-Clavicular Sagittal Section

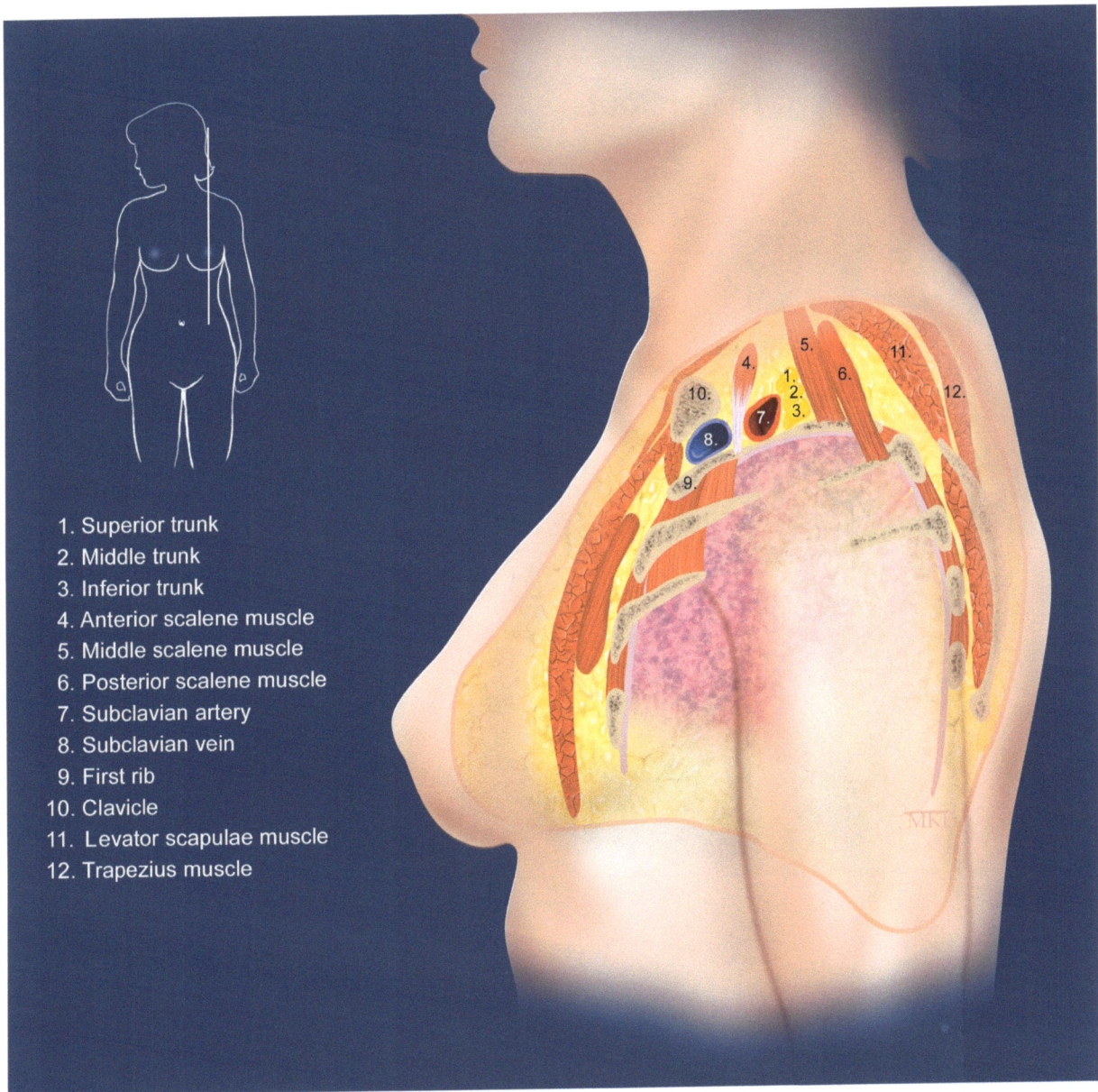

1. Superior trunk
2. Middle trunk
3. Inferior trunk
4. Anterior scalene muscle
5. Middle scalene muscle
6. Posterior scalene muscle
7. Subclavian artery
8. Subclavian vein
9. First rib
10. Clavicle
11. Levator scapulae muscle
12. Trapezius muscle

*Figure 1-10: Sagittal view of the area where the brachial plexus crosses the first rib in mid-clavicular plane.*

The anterior (4) and middle (5) scalene muscles implant onto the first rib (9) and the subclavian artery (7) and brachial plexus trunks or divisions (1, 2, and 3) run between them. The posterior scalene muscle (6) implants on the second rib. The subclavian vein (8) passes anterior to the anterior scalene muscle (4), where it implants onto the first rib. The artery, vein, and inferior trunk course over the pleura of the dome of the lung before they reach the first rib. In the subclavian area, therefore, the three trunks of the brachial plexus (1, 2, 3) can be seen posterior and lateral to the artery (7), and all four of these structures are between the anterior (4) and middle (5) scalene muscles. This is where the supraclavicular block is typically performed.

# Midline Sagittal Section

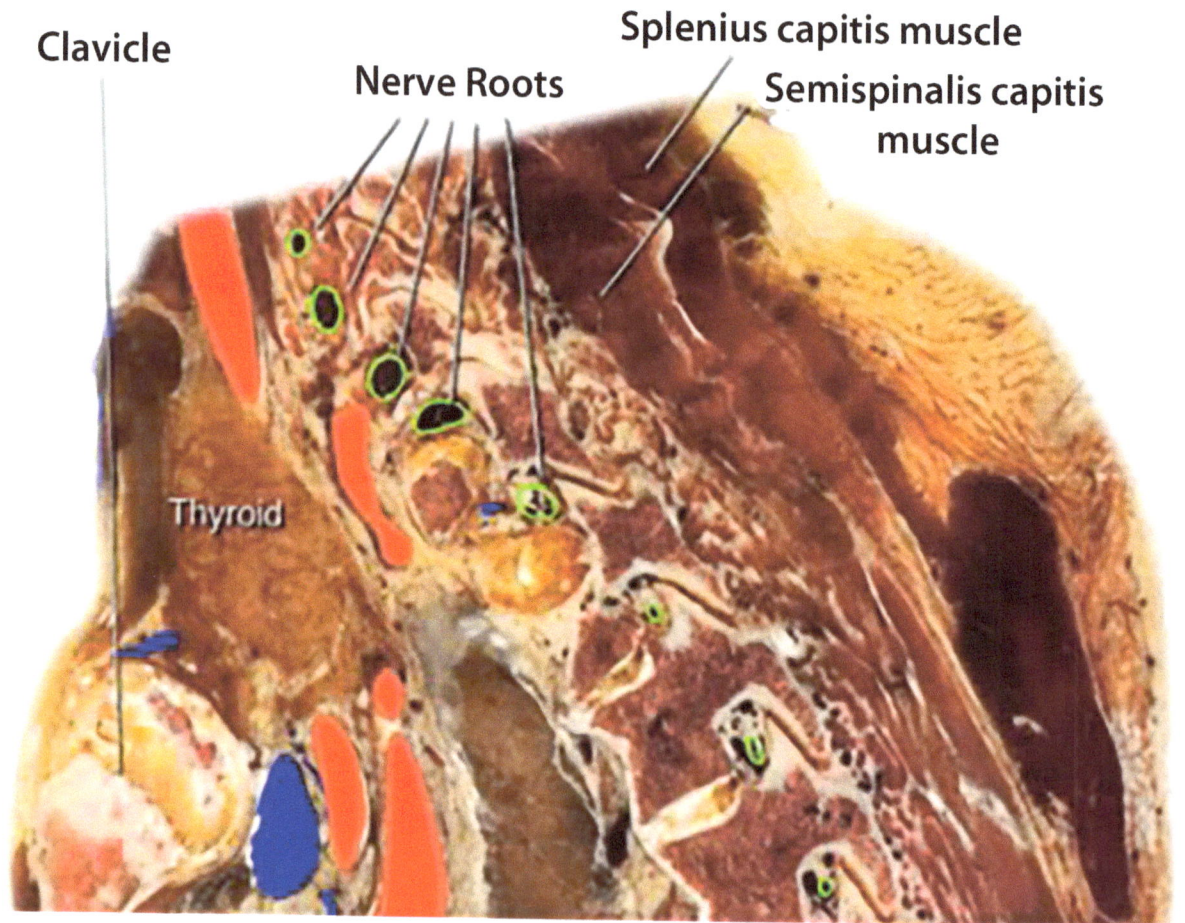

Figure 1-11: Anatomic sagittal section through the paramedian section showing the five roots of the brachial plexus.

The dural sheaths are colored in green.

See RAEducation.com - Acute Pain Medicine - Anatomy - Sagittal Anatomy: Brachial plexus above the clavicle

Video and photograph courtesy of Paul Bigeleisen, Nizar Moayeri, Gerbrand Groen. UMC Utrecht, The Netherlands

# Just Lateral of Midline Sagittal Section

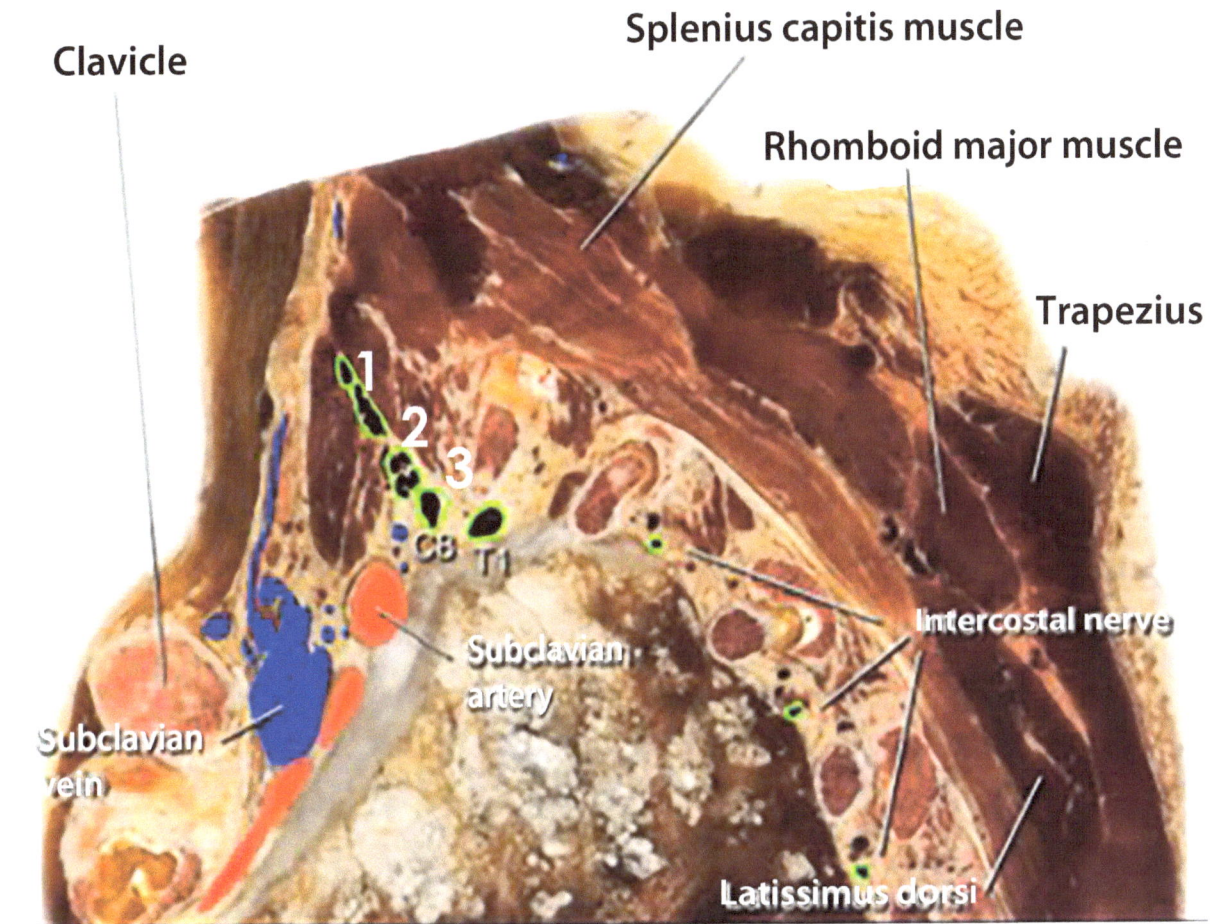

*Figure 1-12: Anatomical sagittal section lateral to the transverse processes of the cervical vertebrae.*

This sections shows the 5th and 6th cervical spinal root joining to form the upper or superior trunk, the middle trunk (1), the 8th cervical spinal root (2), and the 1st thoracic spinal root not yet together to form the inferior trunk (3).

The intercostal nerves are also shown. Also, note the position of the subclavian artery and vein.

The dural sheaths are colored in green.

*Photograph courtesy of Paul Bigeleisen, Nizar Moayeri, Gerbrand Groen. UMC Utrecht, The Netherlands*

# More Lateral of Midline Sagittal Section

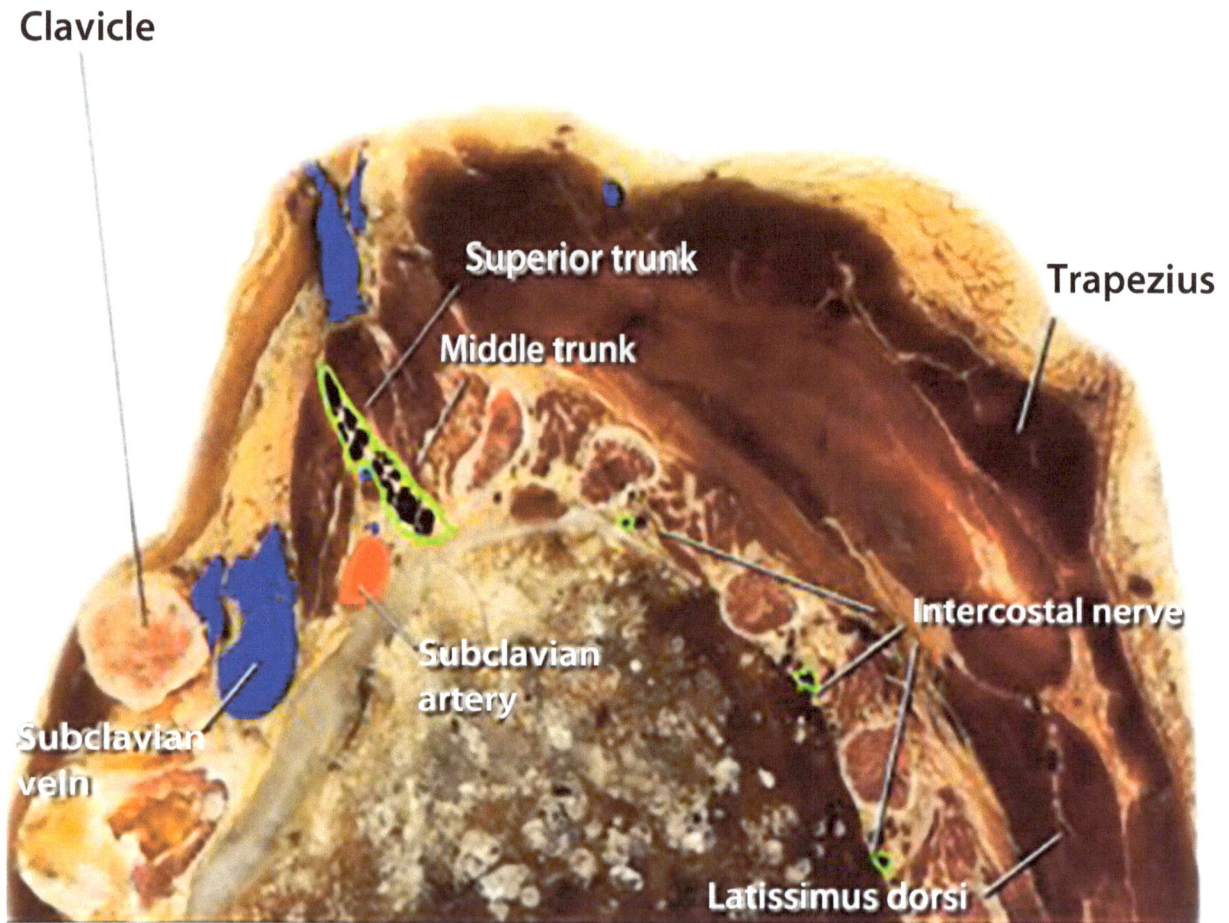

**Clavicle**

**Superior trunk**

**Trapezius**

**Middle trunk**

**Intercostal nerve**

**Subclavian artery**

**Subclavian vein**

**Latissimus dorsi**

*Figure 1-13: Anatomical sagittal section in the semi-mid-clavicular region.*

This section depicts the formation of all three trunks of the brachial plexus. (Inferior trunk is not marked).

The dural sheaths are colored in green.

*Photograph courtesy of Paul Bigeleisen, Nizar Moayeri, Gerbrand Groen. UMC Utrecht, The Netherlands*

Please note:

1. In this figure (basically a redraw of the photograph in Figure 1-17, the parasagittal view is of a longitudinal "cut," as illustrated in the figure on the right.

2. The phrenic nerve (22) is in the prevertebral layer of the deep fascia (1) and lies anterior on the belly of the anterior scalene muscle (2). This is an extension of the epimysium (12) between the muscles, blood vessels and the nerve roots and is the potential space between the layers is the sub-epimyseal space (13), which forms the "doughnut" around the roots if "hydro-dissected" with fluid.

3. The middle scalene muscle has a ventral part (3) and dorsal part (4), and the dorsal scapular nerve (23), which innervates the rhomboid muscles, and long thoracic nerve (24), which innervates the serratus anterior muscle lie between them.

4. The posterior scalene muscle slips of origin (6) are aponeurotic here, thus more of a tendon.

5. The fibers of the anterior and middle scalene muscles cross over between the spinal roots (5). This also happens between the C5 and C6 roots, but more medial to where this "cut" has been made. Where this cut is made is more lateral and caudad where the two roots have already penetrated the cross-over fibers and are in the process of joining to form the upper or superior trunk.

6. The scalene minimi muscle (7) often separates the middle trunk (10) from the C8 root (11).

7. At the level of this "cut", the T1 spinal root has not yet joined the C8 spinal root to form the inferior trunk. The T1 root is caudad of the Subclavian artery (25) at the level of this "cut", and thus not visible here.

8. The nerve roots are covered by dura (16) and arachnoid (17) mater and the endoneurium contains cerebrospinal fluid (18).

9. The spinal roots have a posterior (dorsal) sensory root (20) and an anterior (ventral) motor root (21).

10. The middle trunk (10) has epineurium (10) around it. At the current state of our understanding this is thought to originate from the paravertebral fascia. The dura here moves inward and form septae, which later close to form nerve fascicles (see Figure 1-24).

11. At the current state of our knowledge, and based on the strong arguments forwarded by the Reina group, and their convincing microscopic photographs, after staining the tissue with Masson's trichrome stain, specifically to show this layer (See Figure 1-17), it appears that all the spinal roots and trunks have a circumneural (also known as paraneural) sheath (14) that surrounds the roots and all peripheral nerves. There is, therefore also a sub-circumneural space (15) between the dura (16) and the circumneural sheath (14) also called the paraneural sheath in older texts. For a continuous nerve block, catheter placement within this space would appear to be ideal, but much more research has to be done to finally clarify this.

12. Outside the circumneural sheath is a sub-epimyseal space (13), which is surrounded by the epimysium (12). Please note that the phrenic nerve is also in this space.

13. The subclavian artery (25) is in close relationship to the lower spinal roots and trunks.

# Microanatomy

## Upper & Middle Trunks in the Interscalene Region

Masson's trichrome stained to show circumneurium (AKA paraneurium) This histological section and that of Figure 1-17 inspired the drawing of Figure 1-15.

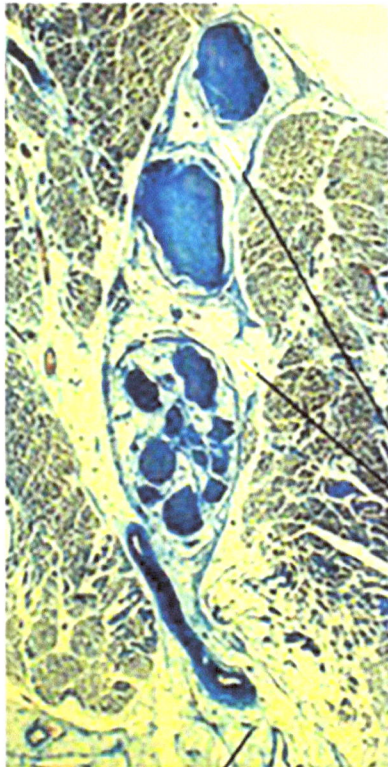

**Paraneurium (Circumneurium)**

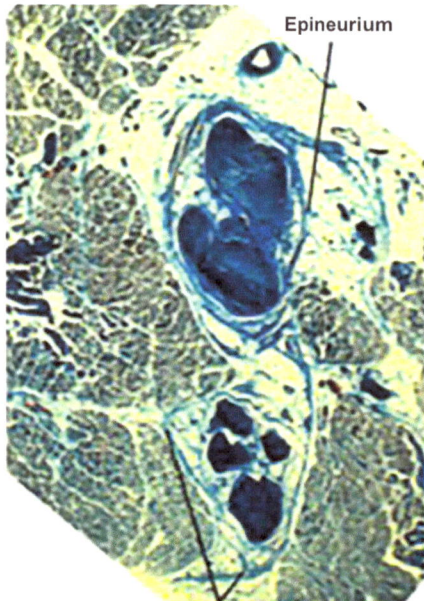

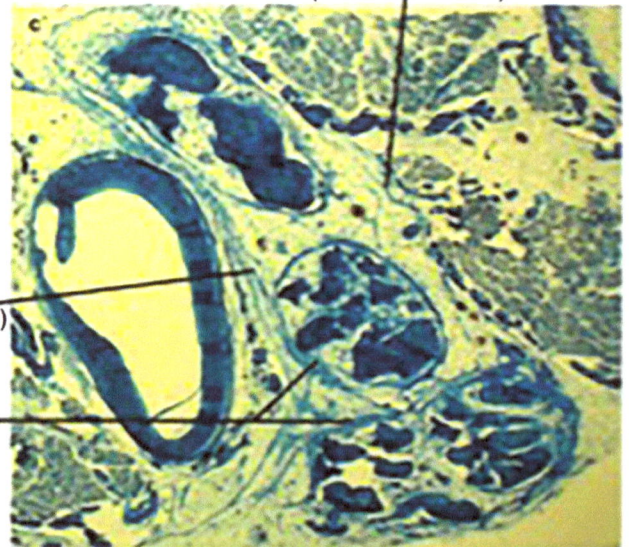

**Paraneurium (Circumneurium)**

**Paraneurium (Circumneurium)**

**Epineurium**

**Paraneurium (Circumneurium)**

**Epineurium**

**Paraneurium (Circumneurium)**

Please note:
Paraneurium should more correctly be named circumneurium, since "para" refers to next to, while "circum" refers to around or surrounding. This was previously known as the "gliding apparatus" of the nerve.

*Figure 1-16: Internal structure of a nerve root in the interscalene region.*

Reprinted with permission from. Reina MA, Dominquez MF, Tardieu I. Origin of the fascicles & intraneural plexus. In: Reina MA, Ed. Atlas of Functional Anatomy for Regional Anesthesia & Pain Medicine. New York: Springer, 2015, 185. Ref: Boezaart AP. The Sweet Spot of the Nerve: Is the "Paraneural Sheath" Named Correctly, & Does It Matter? Reg Anesth Pain Med 2014;39:557-8. Ref: Millesi H, Zoch G, Rath T. The gliding apparatus of peripheral nerve & its clinical significance. Ann Chir Main Memb Super. 1990; 9:87-97.

# Upper & Middle Trunks in the Interscalene Region

Masson's trichrome stained to specifically show the circumneurium (paraneurium).

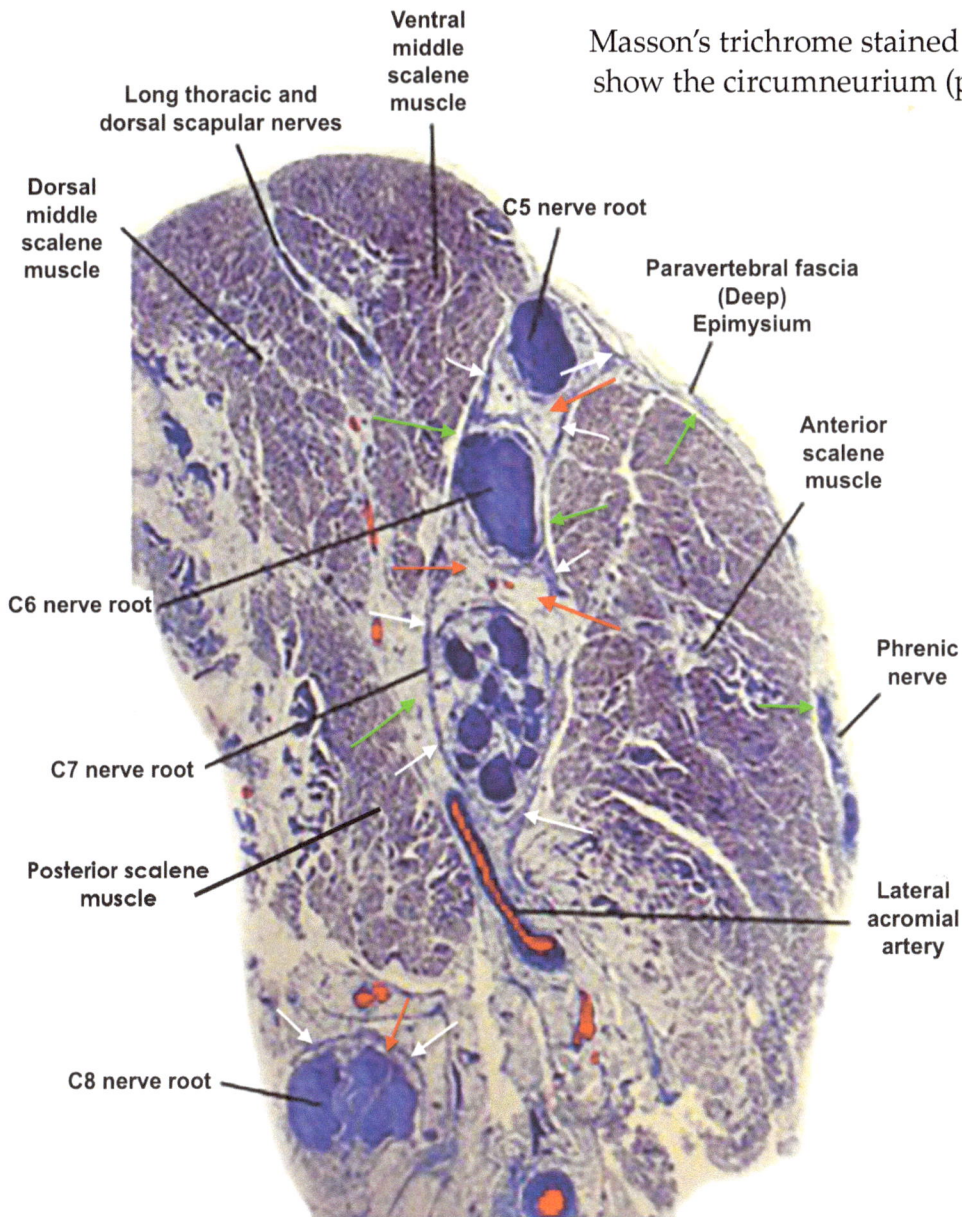

*Fig 1-17: Cross-sectional microanatomy of the brachial plexus at the interscalene region.*

Please note: White arrows point to circumneurium (paraneurium), green arrows to sub-epimyseal space, and red arrows to sub-circumneural (sub-paraneural) space Phrenic nerve is in sub-epimyseal space (green arrows).

The long thoracic and dorsal scapular nerves lie between the ventral and dorsal parts of the middle scalene muscles. The drawing of Figure 1-15 is an illustration of this microscopic photograph.

*Reprinted with permission from: Reina MA, Dominquez MF, Tardieu I. Origin of the fascicles & intraneural plexus. In: Reina MA, Ed. Atlas of Functional Anatomy for Regional Anesthesia & Pain Medicine. New York: Springer, 2015, 162.Ref: Boezaart AP. The Sweet Spot of the Nerve: Is the "Paraneural Sheath" Named Correctly, & Does It Matter? Reg Anesth Pain Med 2014; 39:557-8.*

# Membranes Surrounding Spinal Roots

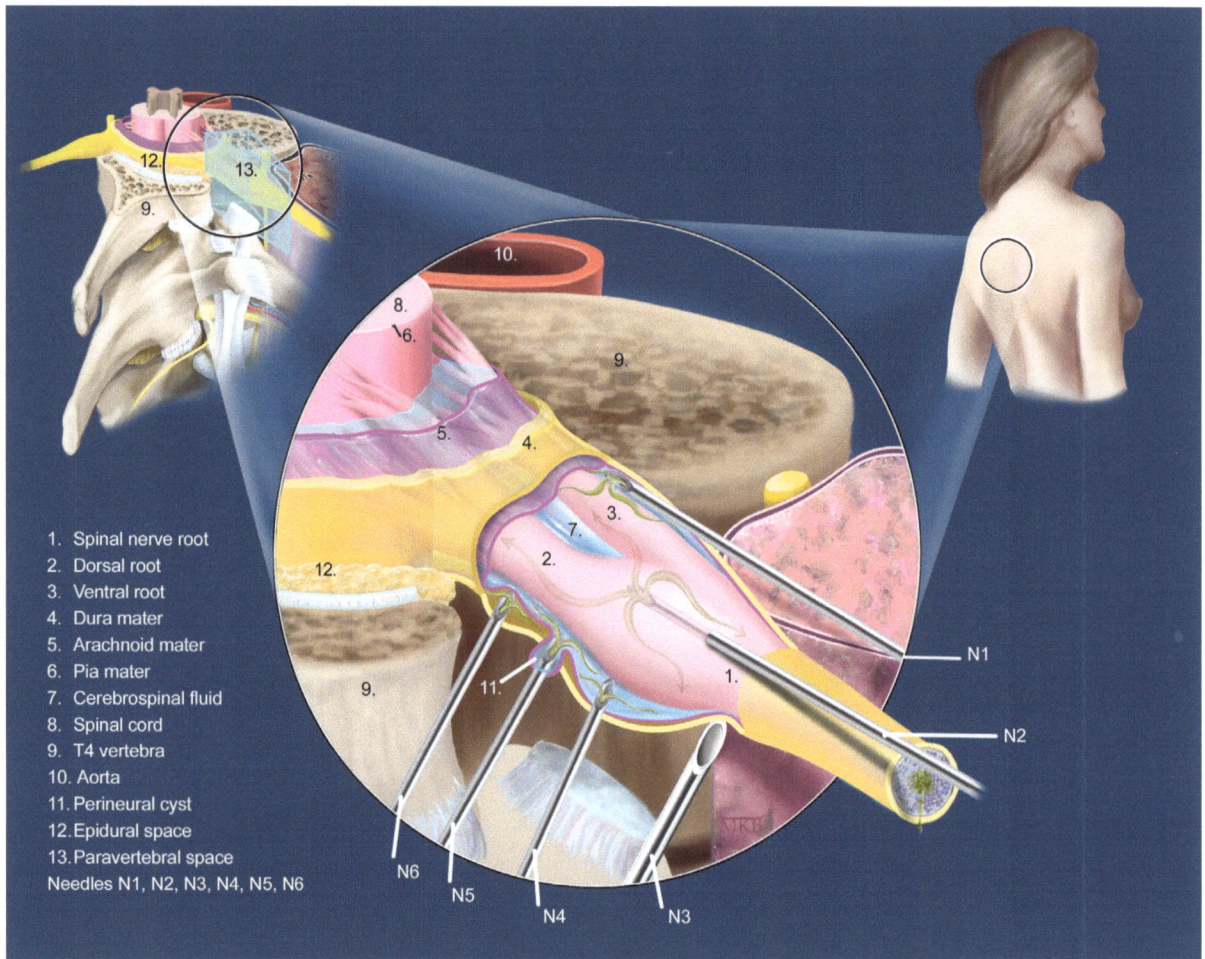

1. Spinal nerve root
2. Dorsal root
3. Ventral root
4. Dura mater
5. Arachnoid mater
6. Pia mater
7. Cerebrospinal fluid
8. Spinal cord
9. T4 vertebra
10. Aorta
11. Perineural cyst
12. Epidural space
13. Paravertebral space
Needles N1, N2, N3, N4, N5, N6

*Figure 1-18: Schematic representation of the thoracic paravertebral space and the meninges surrounding the spinal root.*

**Please Note: This is similar for all levels of paravertebral blocks: Cervical, Thoracic, Lumbar or Sacral**

Six possible needle placements are illustrated:

Needle 1 (N1): Subarachnoid placement of a relatively thin needle during a transforaminal injection (usually steroids).

Needle 2 (N2): Intra-parenchymal placement of relatively thin needle during a nerve root block (e.g., interscalene block at cervical level) or an intercostal nerve block.

Needle 3 (N3): Extradural Tuohy needle placement during a paravertebral block.

Needle 4 (N4): Subarachnoid placement of relatively thin needle during a paravertebral block.

Needle 5 (N5): Needle placement into a perineural cyst during a paravertebral block.

Needle 6 (N6): Subdural (extra-arachnoid) needle placement during a paravertebral block.

# Endoneurium

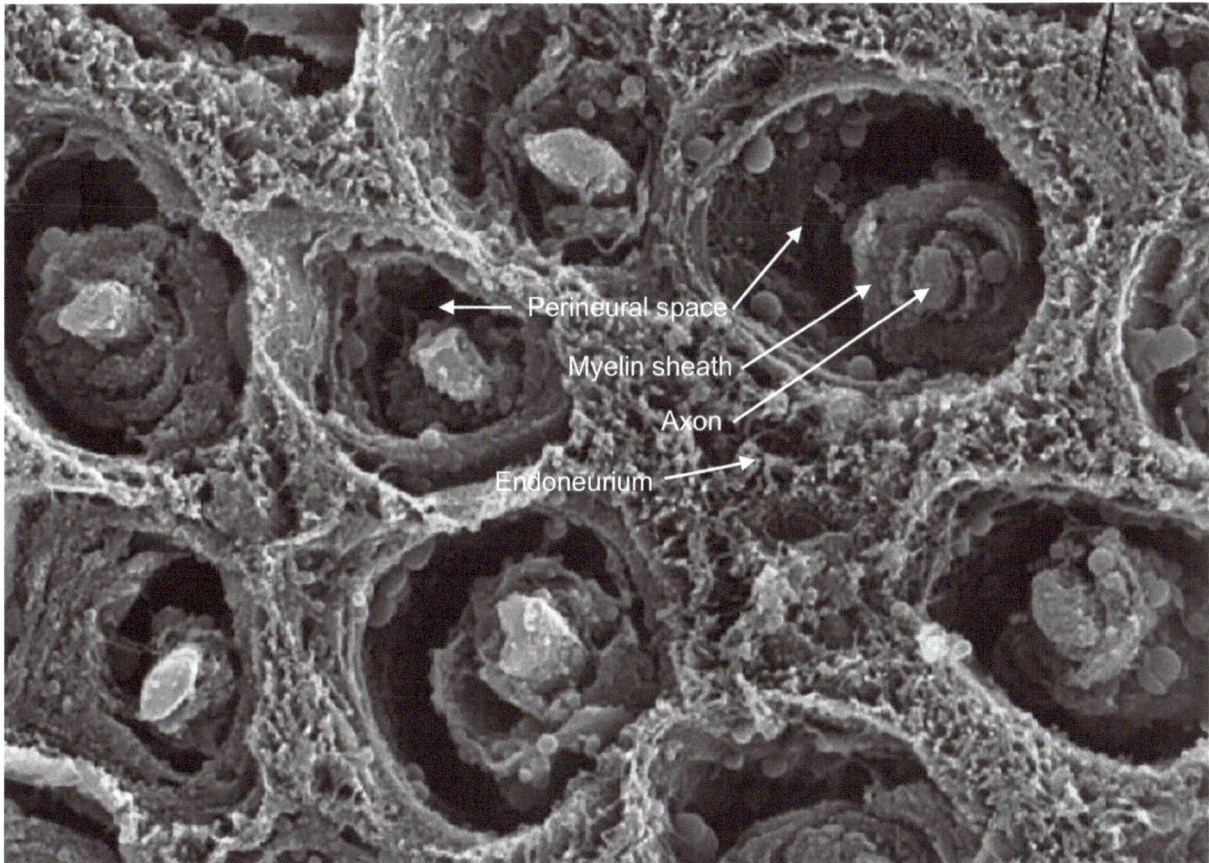

*Figure 1-19: Perineural spaces. Scanning electron microscopy, magnification × 2000.*

Please note: Up until 2017, it was thought that drugs injected into a fascicle of a peripheral nerve or into the parenchyma of a spinal root or trunk would spread centrally via these spaces. In the spinal cord, the drug can (depending on the type, volume, and pressure used for the injection) cause ischemic or toxic damage to the spinal cord, which may or may not result in syrinx formation and neurological damage such as mono-, para-, or quadriplegia – depending on the extent and location of the injury. Newer work by the Reina and Boezaart group has convincingly shown that what was thought to be perineural spaces on this photograph are in fact artifacts. The endoneurium is in fact a solid structure. There are no paraneural spaces and the proximal spread seems to be via the interfascicular spaces that are filled with adipocytes and also within the cells that form the perineurium. (Please visit the 2018 papers of the Reina group for more clarity on this.)

*Reprinted with permission from Reina MA, Navarro RA, Mateos EMD. Ultrastructure of myelinated & unmyelinated axons. In: Reina MA, Ed. Atlas of Functional Anatomy For Regional Anesthesia & Pain Medicine. New York: Springer, 2015; 3-18. (Annotations by author) Ref: Moore DC, Hain RF Ward A, Bridenbaugh LD. Importance of the perineural spaces in nerve blocking. JAMA 1954;156:1050-5.*

# Microanatomy of the Brachial Plexus Roots

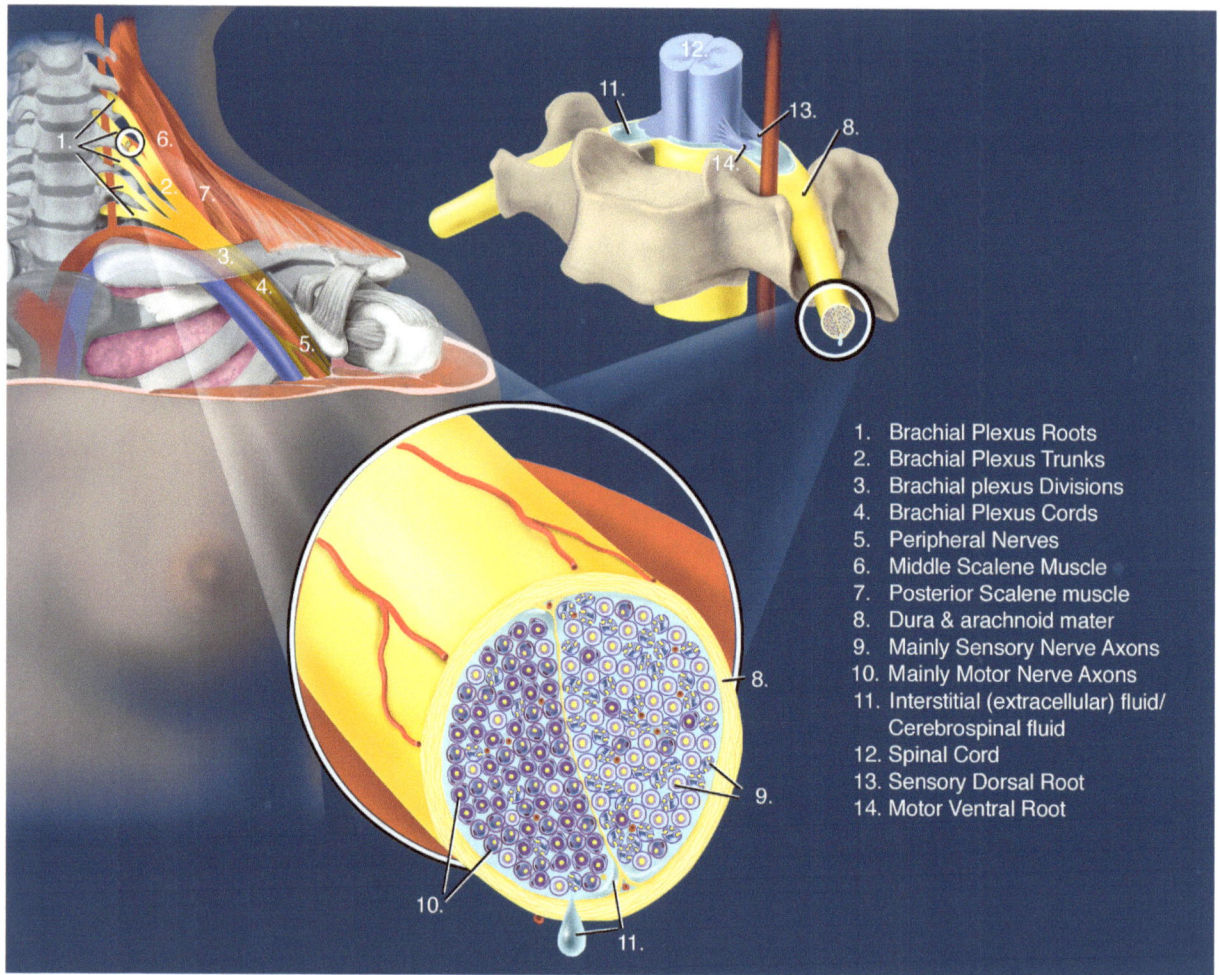

1. Brachial Plexus Roots
2. Brachial Plexus Trunks
3. Brachial plexus Divisions
4. Brachial Plexus Cords
5. Peripheral Nerves
6. Middle Scalene Muscle
7. Posterior Scalene muscle
8. Dura & arachnoid mater
9. Mainly Sensory Nerve Axons
10. Mainly Motor Nerve Axons
11. Interstitial (extracellular) fluid/
    Cerebrospinal fluid
12. Spinal Cord
13. Sensory Dorsal Root
14. Motor Ventral Root

*Figure 1-20: Micro-structure of a spinal root.*

Please note: The root is surrounded by dura, arachnoid and pia mater (8). The interstitial fluid inside the root (11) is cerebrospinal fluid. The posterior part of the root (9) contains mainly sensory fibers. The anterior part of the root (10) contains mainly motor fibers. The circumneurium (paraneurium) has been omitted in this drawing (see Figs. 1-15, 1-16, 1-17). Central spread of drugs injected inside the parenchyma of the root will be via the perineural spaces (Fig. 1-19).

*Ref: Boezaart AP. That which we call a rose by any other name would smell as sweet - and its thorns would hurt as much. Reg Anesth Pain Med 2009;34:3-7.*

# Microanatomy of the Brachial Plexus Trunks

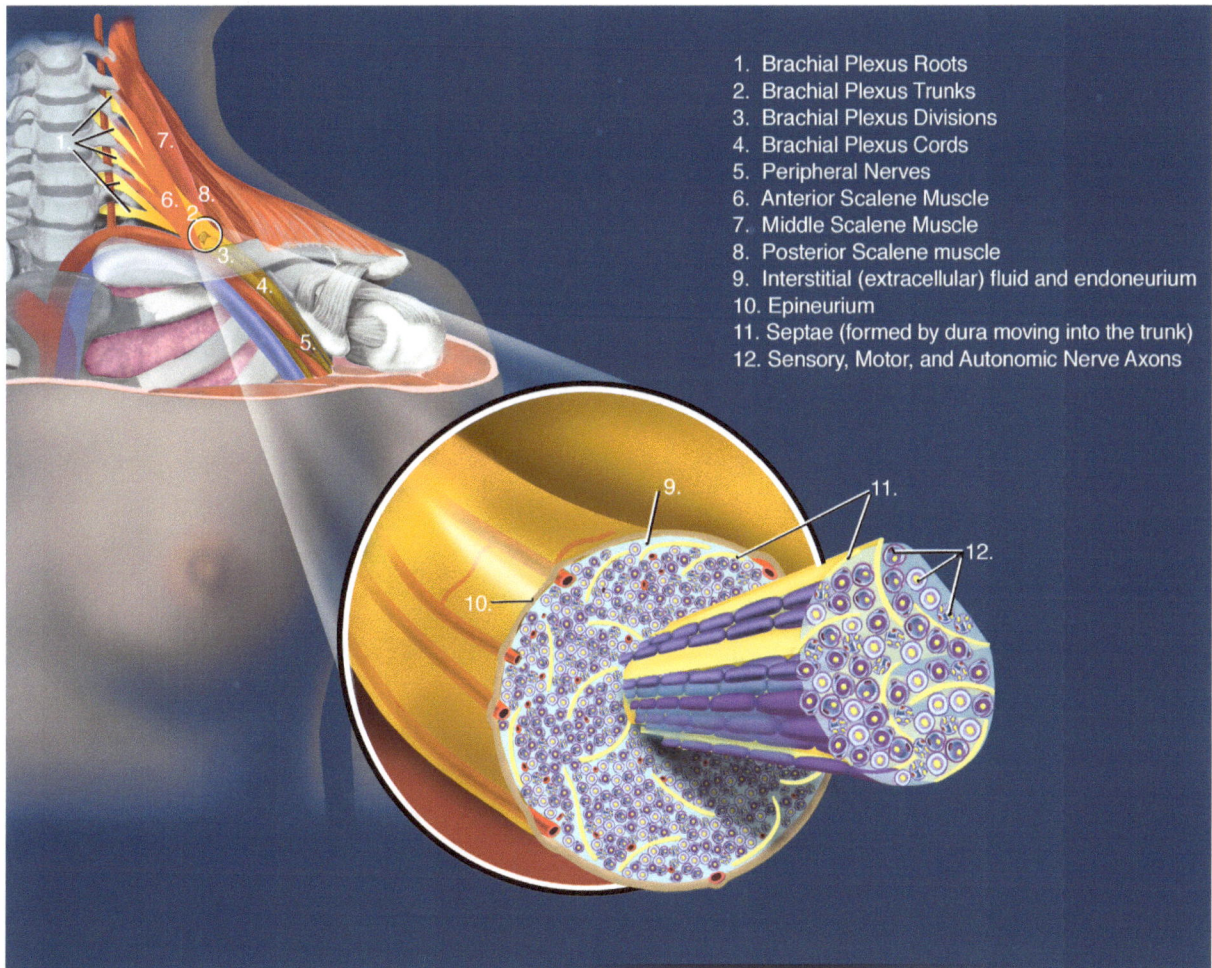

1. Brachial Plexus Roots
2. Brachial Plexus Trunks
3. Brachial Plexus Divisions
4. Brachial Plexus Cords
5. Peripheral Nerves
6. Anterior Scalene Muscle
7. Middle Scalene Muscle
8. Posterior Scalene muscle
9. Interstitial (extracellular) fluid and endoneurium
10. Epineurium
11. Septae (formed by dura moving into the trunk)
12. Sensory, Motor, and Autonomic Nerve Axons

*Figure 1-21: Micro-structure of a brachial plexus trunk.*

Please note: The yellow septae (11) that now form on the level of the trunk originate from the dura mater that surrounded the roots (see Figure 1-20), which now "break up" to form the septae. Later, these septae close to form fascicles in peripheral nerves.

Ref: Boezaart AP. That which we call a rose by any other name would smell as sweet - and its thorns would hurt as much. Reg Anesth Pain Med 2009;34:3-7.

# Microanatomy of the Spinal Root

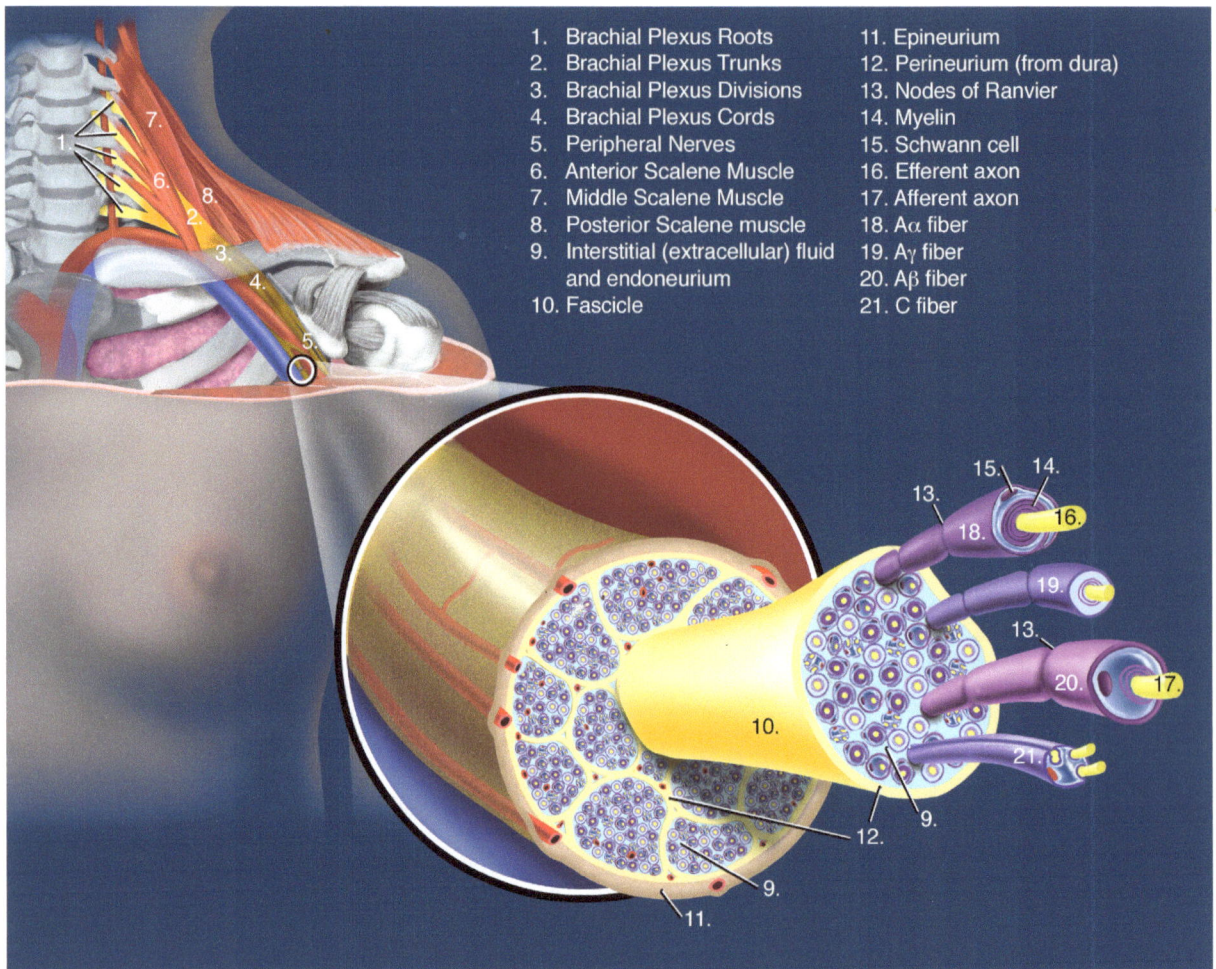

1. Brachial Plexus Roots
2. Brachial Plexus Trunks
3. Brachial Plexus Divisions
4. Brachial Plexus Cords
5. Peripheral Nerves
6. Anterior Scalene Muscle
7. Middle Scalene Muscle
8. Posterior Scalene muscle
9. Interstitial (extracellular) fluid and endoneurium
10. Fascicle
11. Epineurium
12. Perineurium (from dura)
13. Nodes of Ranvier
14. Myelin
15. Schwann cell
16. Efferent axon
17. Afferent axon
18. Aα fiber
19. Aγ fiber
20. Aβ fiber
21. C fiber

*Figure 1-22: Micro-structure of a peripheral nerve. [Circumneural (paraneural) sheath not depicted].*

Please note: That the perineurium (12) that surrounds the fascicle (10) originates from the dura. That the interstitial fluid inside the fascicle (9) is cerebrospinal fluid, whereas the interstitial fluid inside the nerve itself, which is surrounded by the epineurium (11), is lymph that is removed by the lymphatic flow to the lymph nodes, and blood flow. The epineurium most probably originates from the paravertebral fascia.

*Ref: Boezaart AP. That which we call a rose by any other name would smell as sweet - and its thorns would hurt as much. Reg Anesth Pain Med 2009;34:3-7.*

# Sonoanatomy

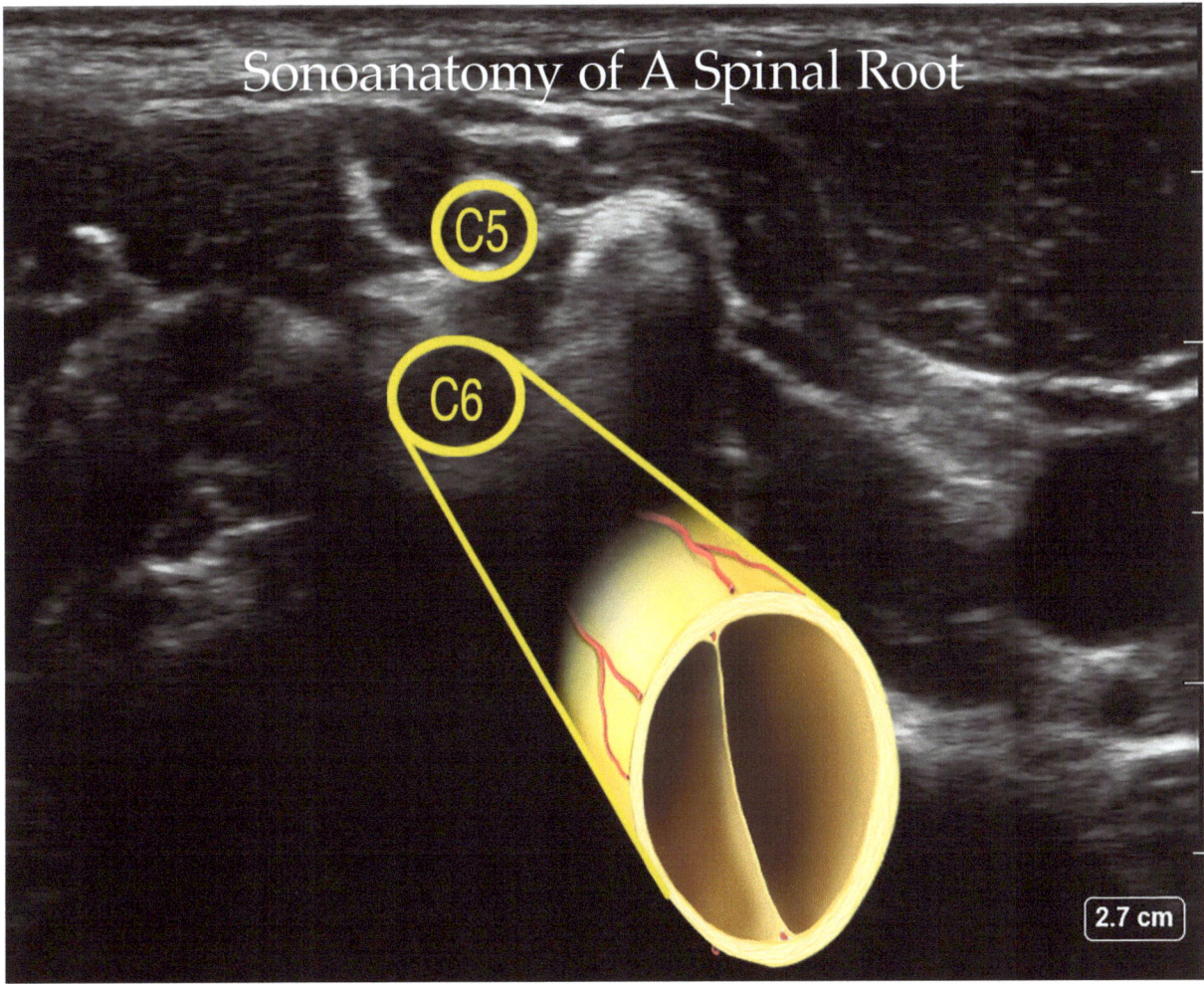

Figure 1-23: Hypoechoic appearance of spinal root nerve.

C5        5th cervical nerve root
C6        6th cervical nerve root

Please note:
The root is basically a fluid-filled (hypoechoic) space structure.

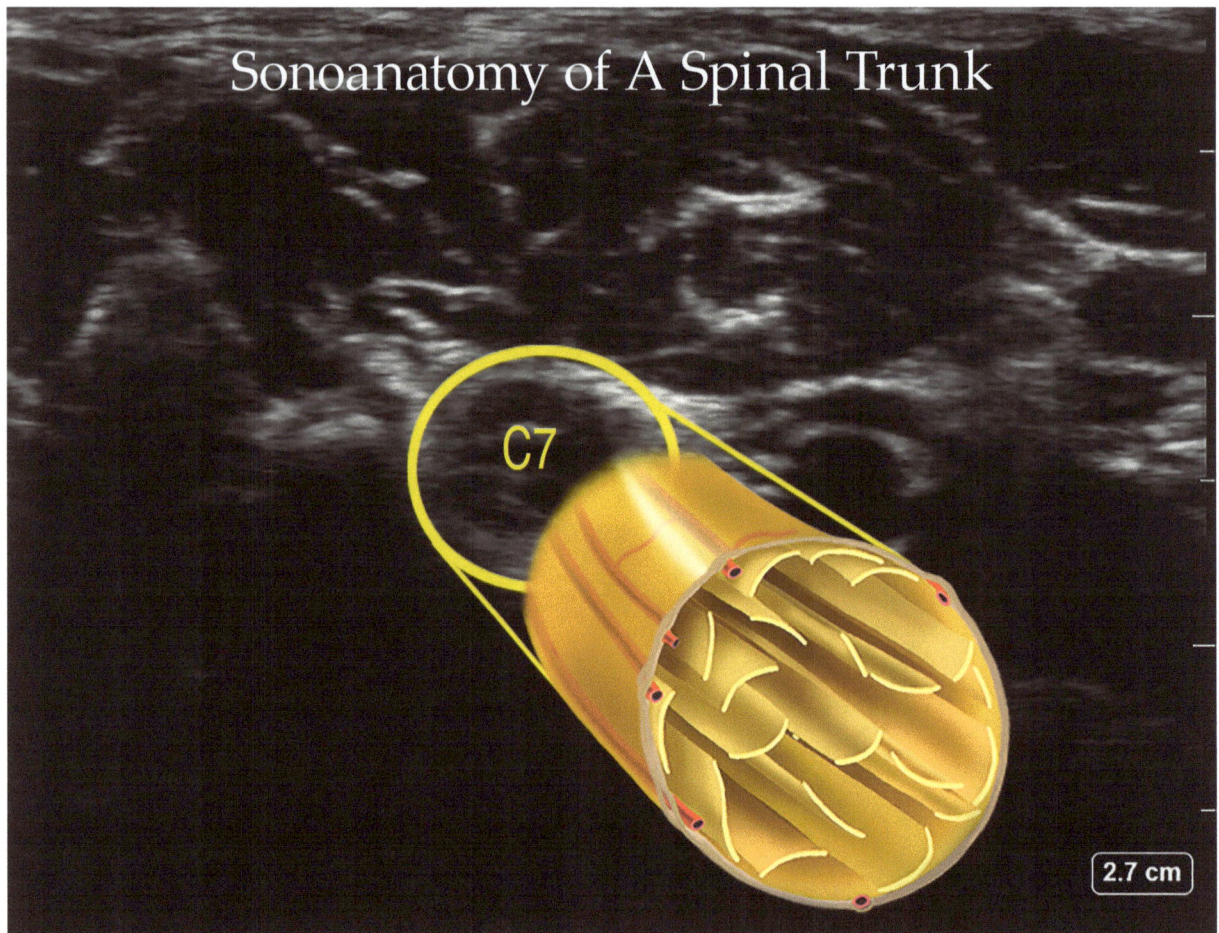

Figure 1-24: More hyperechoic appearance of a brachial plexus trunk nerve.

Please note: At the trunk level, the septae have formed from dura and the trunk has a more hyperechoic appearance.

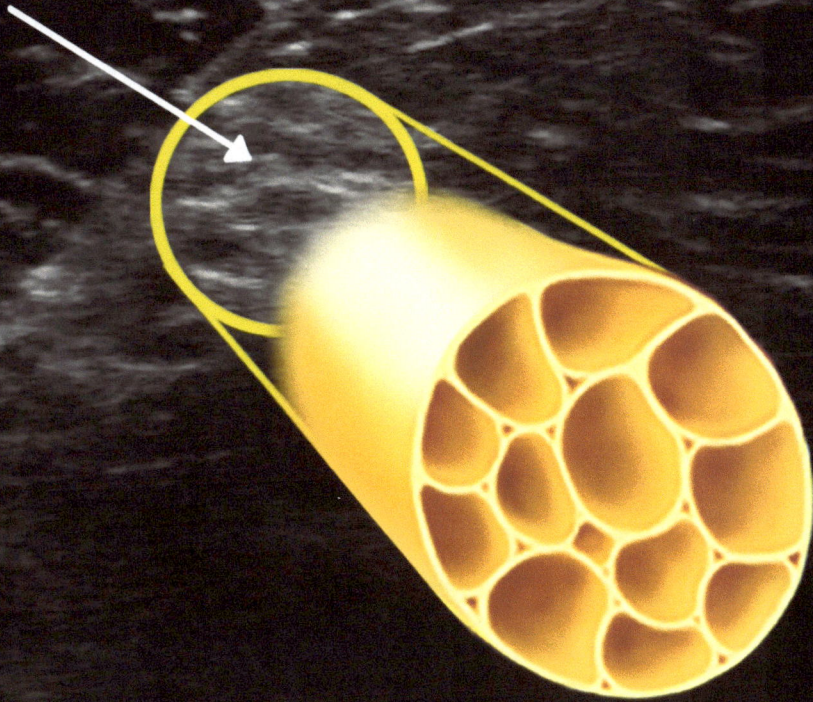

Figure 1-25: "Honeycomb" appearance of a peripheral nerve.

# 3D Illustration of Sonoanatomy of the Brachial Plexus

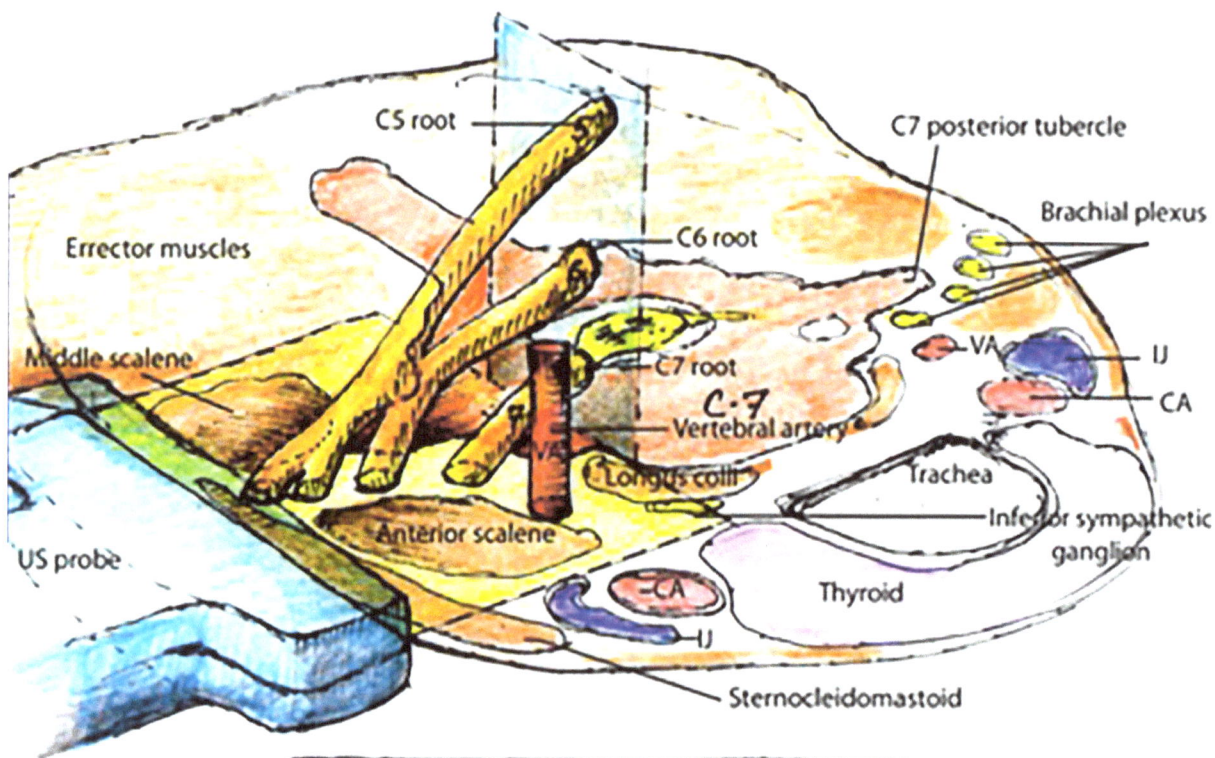

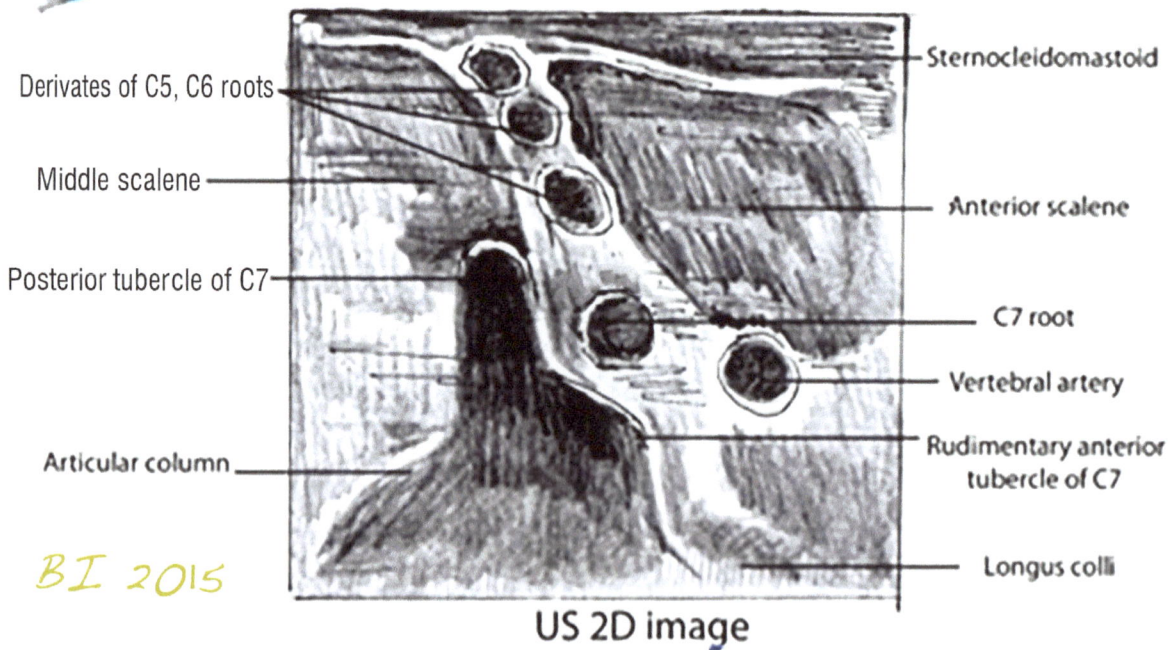

**Top illustration labels:**
- C5 root
- C7 posterior tubercle
- Brachial plexus
- Errector muscles
- C6 root
- VA
- IJ
- Middle scalene
- CA
- C7 root
- C·7
- Vertebral artery
- Inferior sympathetic ganglion
- Longus colli
- Trachea
- Anterior scalene
- CA
- Thyroid
- US probe
- IJ
- Sternocleidomastoid

**Bottom ultrasound image labels:**
- Derivates of C5, C6 roots
- Sternocleidomastoid
- Middle scalene
- Anterior scalene
- Posterior tubercle of C7
- C7 root
- Vertebral artery
- Rudimentary anterior tubercle of C7
- Articular column
- Longus colli

BI 2015

**US 2D image**

*Figure 1-26: Schematic three-dimensional view of the posterior triangle of the neck through the transverse process of the 7th cervical vertebra.*

| | |
|---|---|
| CA | Carotid artery |
| IJ | Internal jugular vein |
| US probe | Ultrasound transducer probe |
| VA | Vertebral artery |

*Drawing: Barys V. Ihnatsenka, MD*

# Supraclavicular Ultrasound

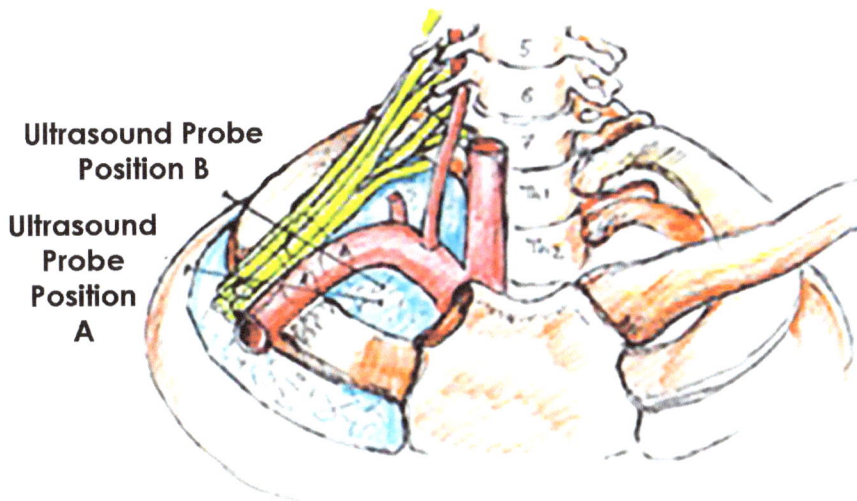

**Ultrasound Probe Position B**

**Ultrasound Probe Position A**

1.  Subclavian artery
2.  Brachial plexus
3.  First rib
4.  Pleura and lung

**Ultrasound Probe Position A**

US picture

Drawing

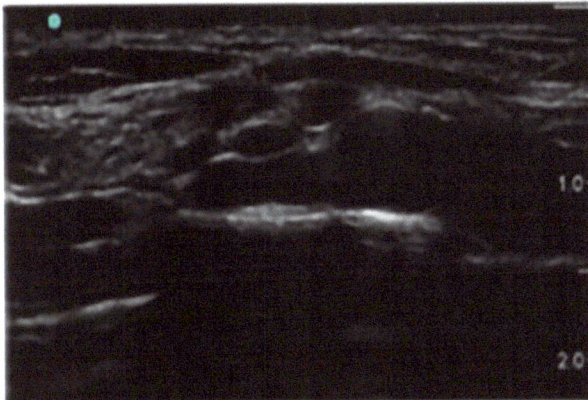
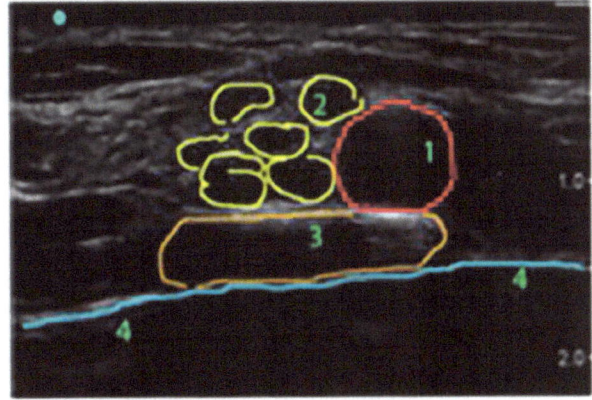

**Position B**

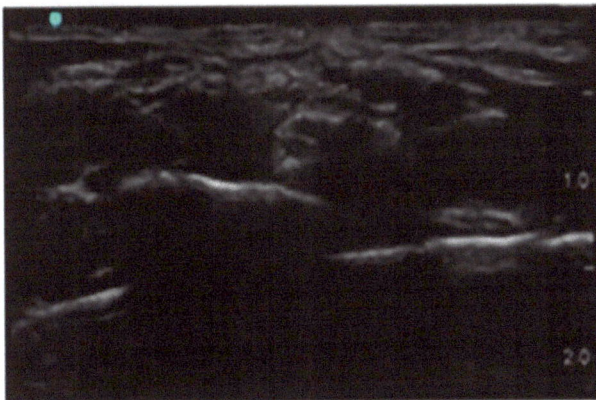
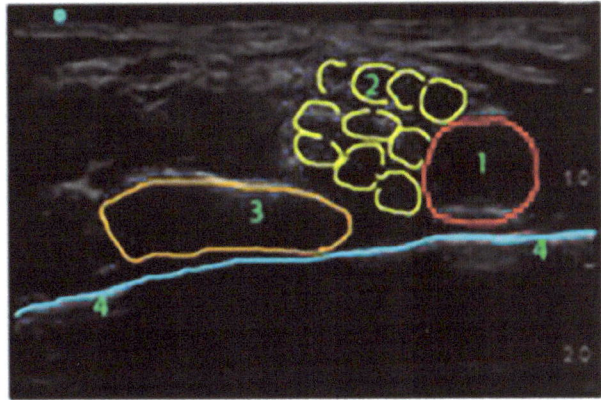

*Figure 1-27: Sonoanatomy of the supraclavicular area.*

View video at RAEducation.com
Acute Pain Medicine - Anatomy
Sonoanatomy - Dynamic -
Supraclavicular Brachial Plexus

*Drawing: Barys V. Ihnatsenka, MD*

# Supraclavicular Ultrasound

## Trunks & Artery are on first rib (Position A, Figure 1-27)

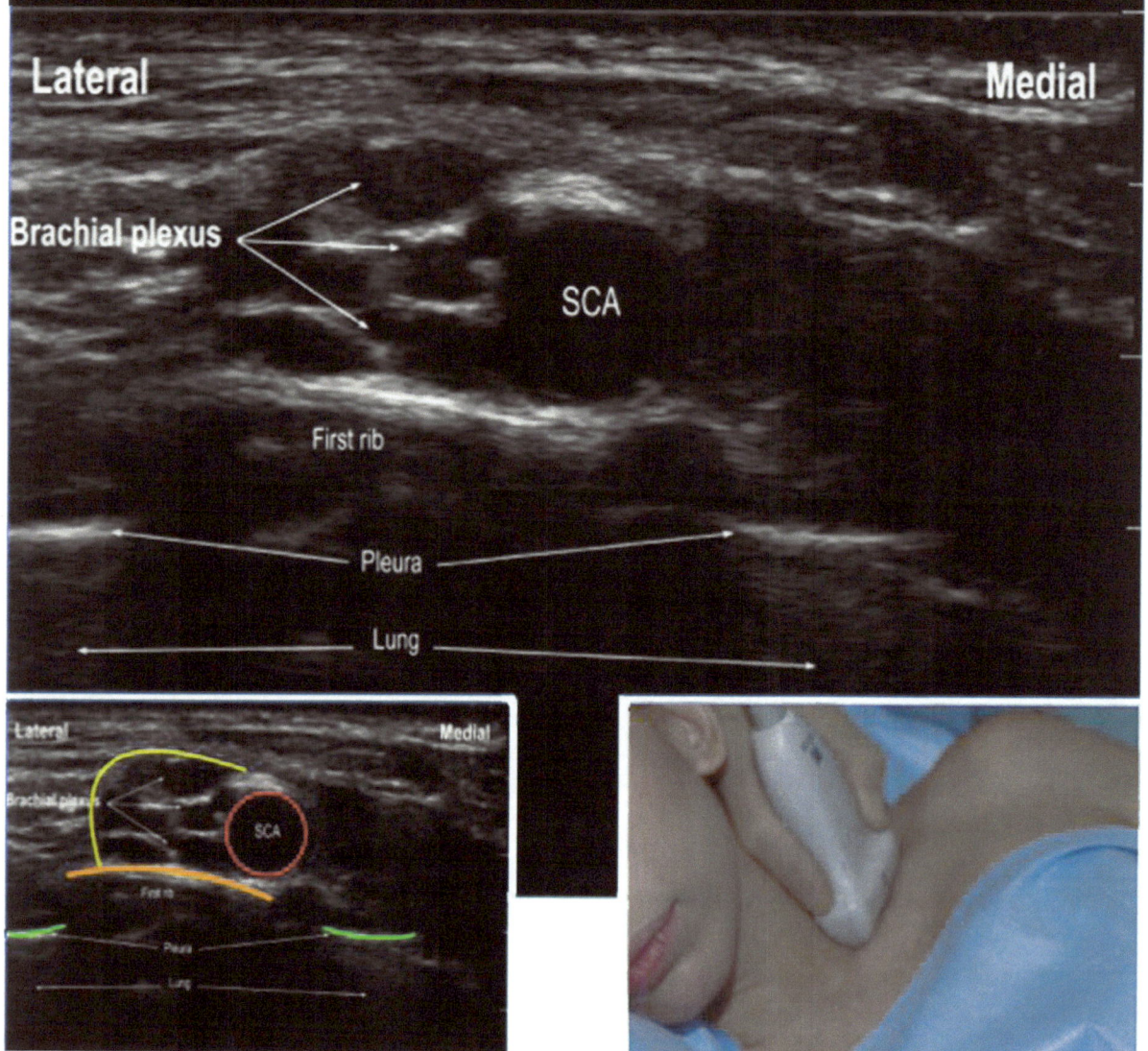

Figure 1-28: Sonoanatomy of the supraclavicular brachial plexus. Subclavian artery viewed on the first rib.

SCA    Subclavian artery

# Supraclavicular Ultrasound

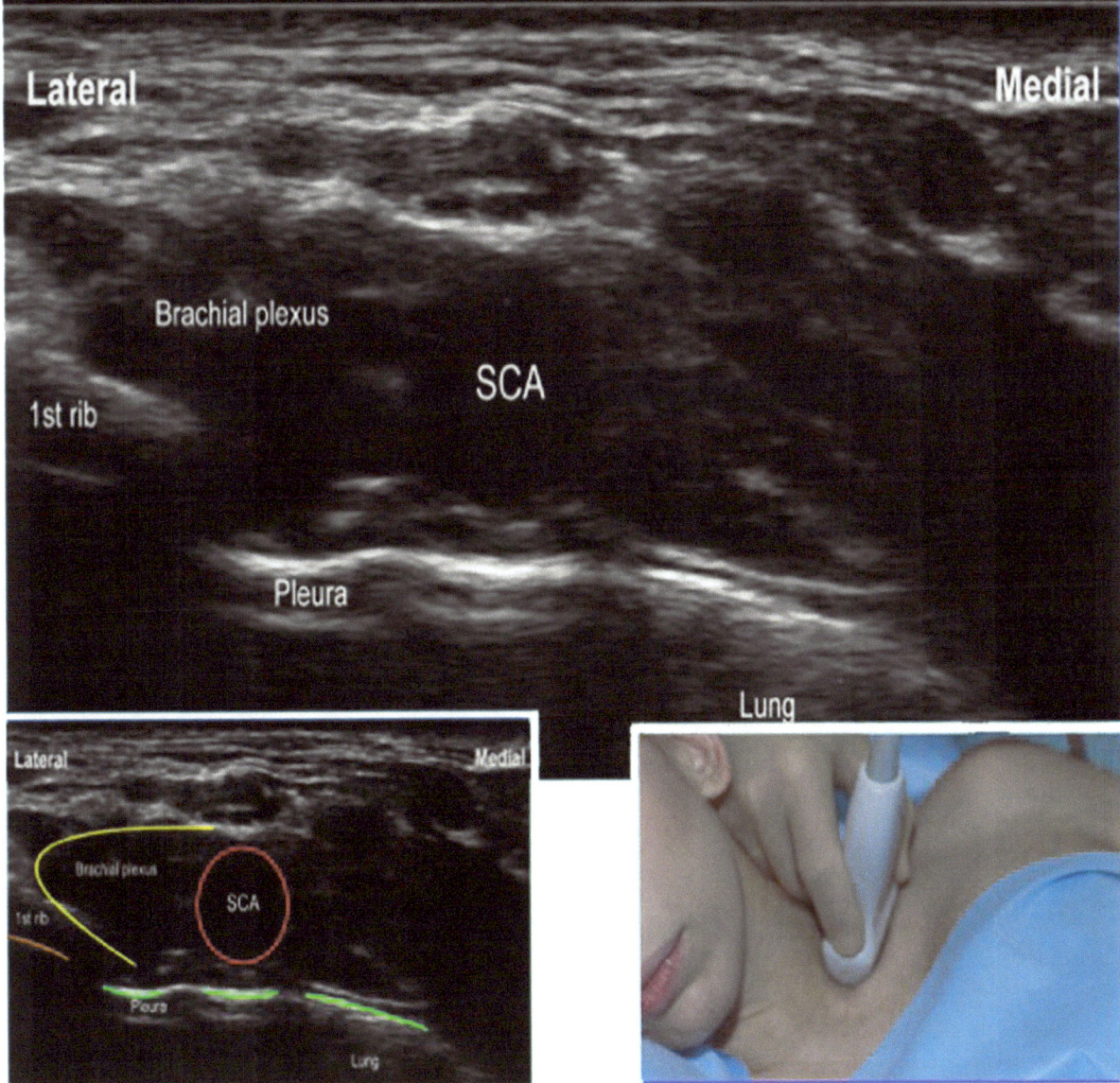

Figure 1-29: Sonoanatomy of supraclavicular brachial plexus. Subclavian artery viewed on the pleura.

SCA     Subclavian artery

# Supraclavicular Ultrasound

Position B - Figure 1-27            Position A - Figure 1-27

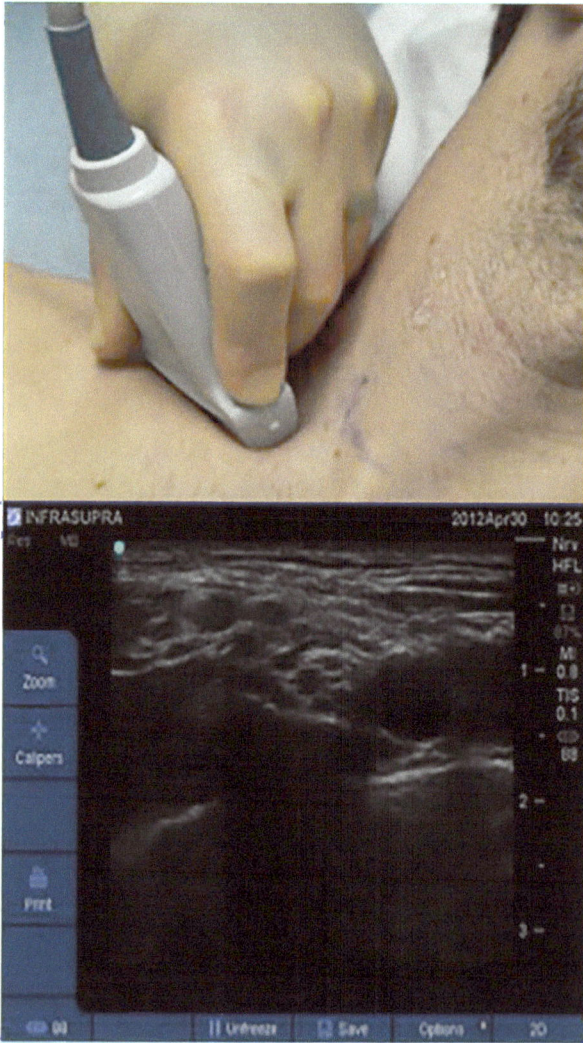

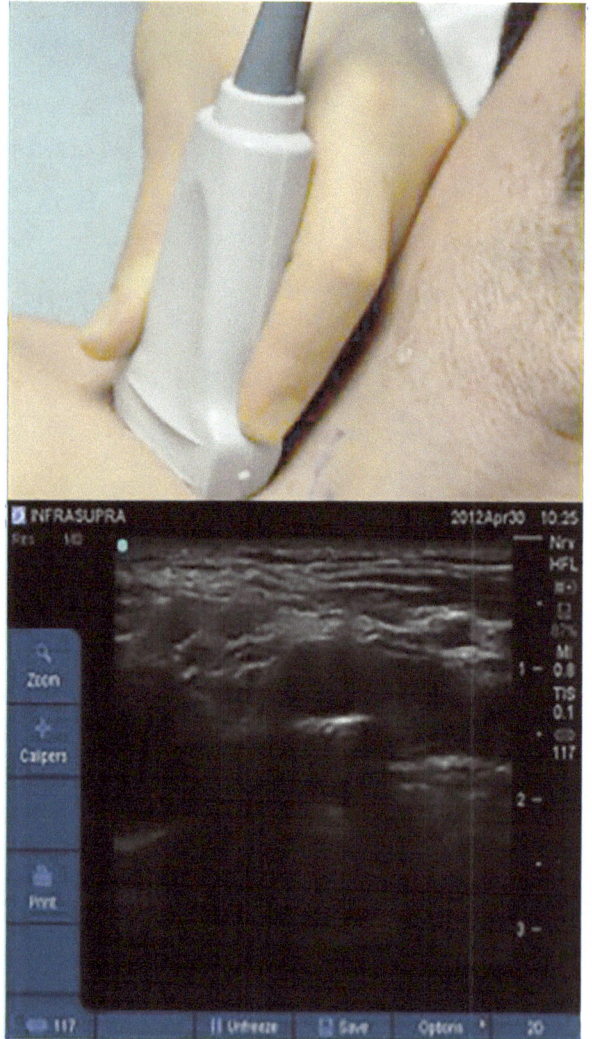

*Figure 1-30: Ultrasound transducer positioning for supraclavicular block.*

On the left hand top photograph, the ultrasound beam is pointed dorsally or posterior, and the ultrasound image below it illustrates the subclavian artery where it is situated on the pleura of the lung.

In the right hand photograph, the probe is tilted such that the ultrasound beam is directed ventrally or anterior, and the image below it (right) is now of the subclavian artery situated on the first rib.

# The Dorsal Scapular Artery

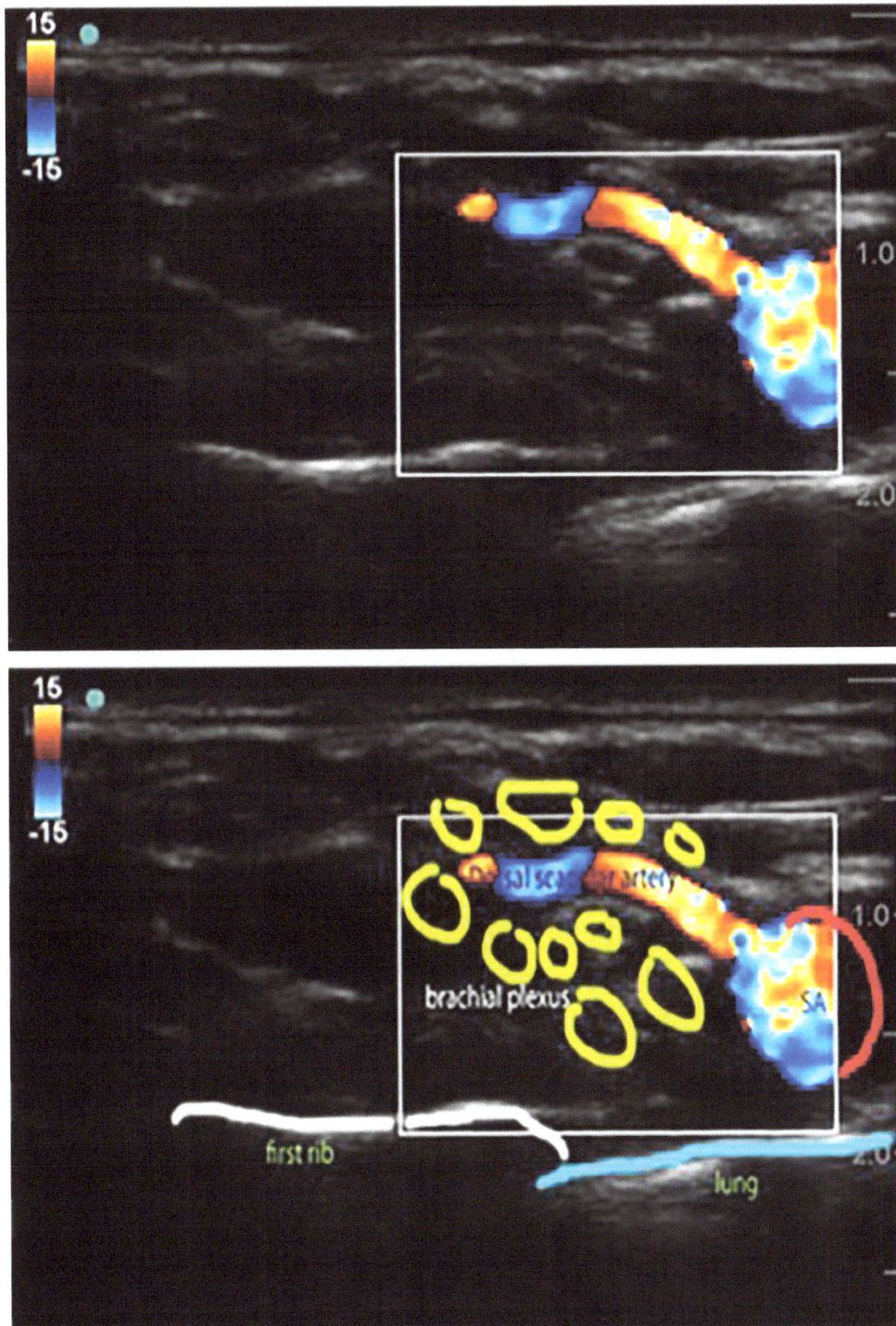

*Figure 1-31: Dorsal scapular artery.*

When the Doppler function of the ultrasound is applied, we can clearly see the dorsal scapular artery where it comes off of the subclavian artery. It frequently courses between the nerves of the brachial plexus, where it splits it into superficial and deeper parts – most commonly, the upper and medial trunks.

# Lateral Neck Ultrasound at level of First Rib

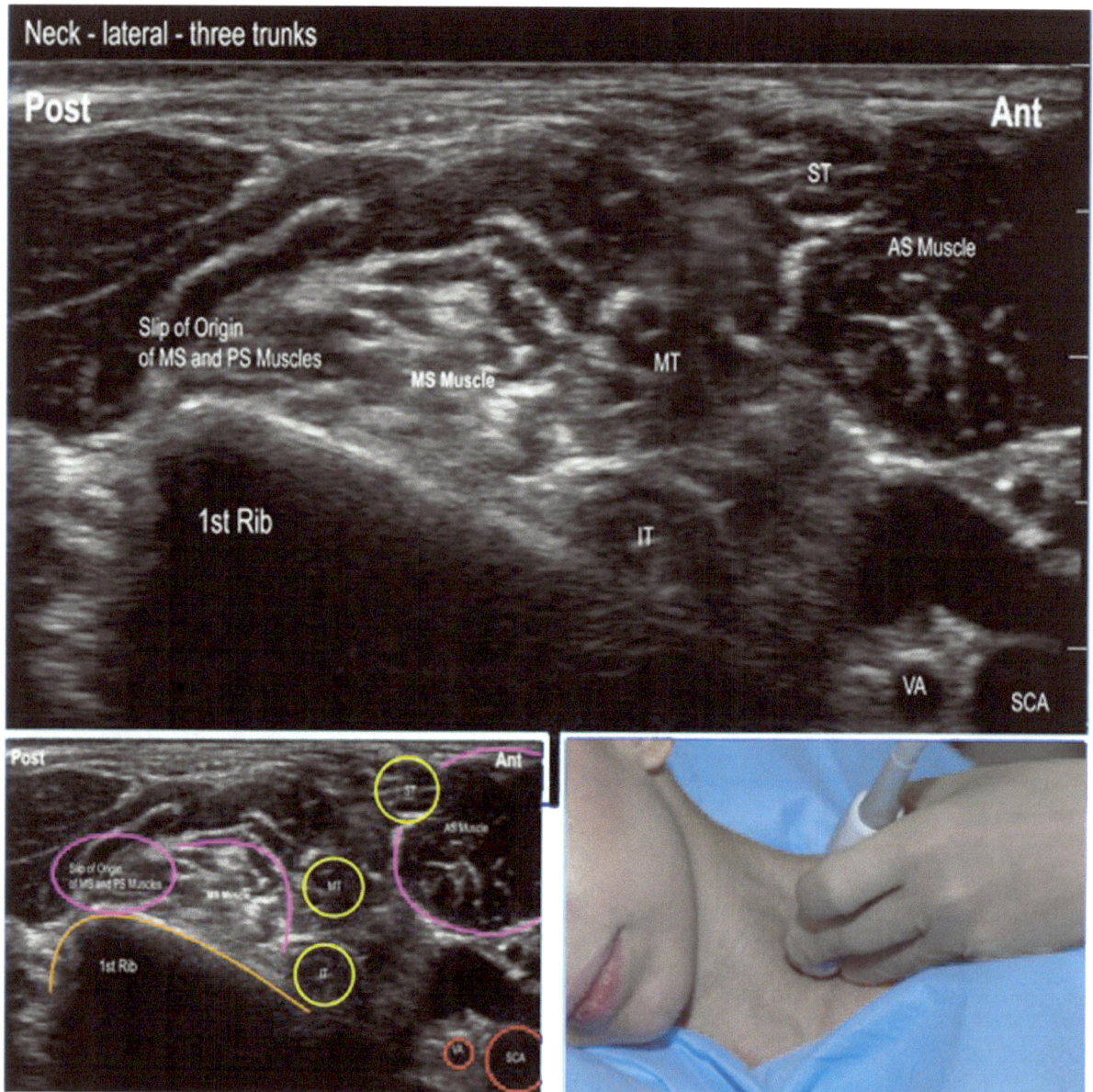

Figure 1-32: Sonoanatomy of the posterior triangle of the neck. Three trunks – lateral view.

| | | | |
|---|---|---|---|
| Ant | Anterior | ST | Superior trunk of the brachial plexus where C5-C6 have fused |
| AS Musc | Anterior scalene muscle | | |
| IT | Inferior or lower trunk, which is formed by the fusion of the 8th cervical and 1st thoracic spinal nerve roots | MT | Middle trunk, which is formed from the 7th spinal nerve root |
| | | VA | Vertebral artery |
| MS Mus | Middle scalene muscle | | |
| Post | Posterior | | |
| PS Mus | Posterior scalene muscle | | |
| SCA | Subclavian artery | | |

**View Video at RAEducation.com
- Acute Pain Medicine - Anatomy
Sonoanatomy - Dynamic
Brachial plexus above the clavicle**

# Lateral Neck Ultrasound on C7 Level

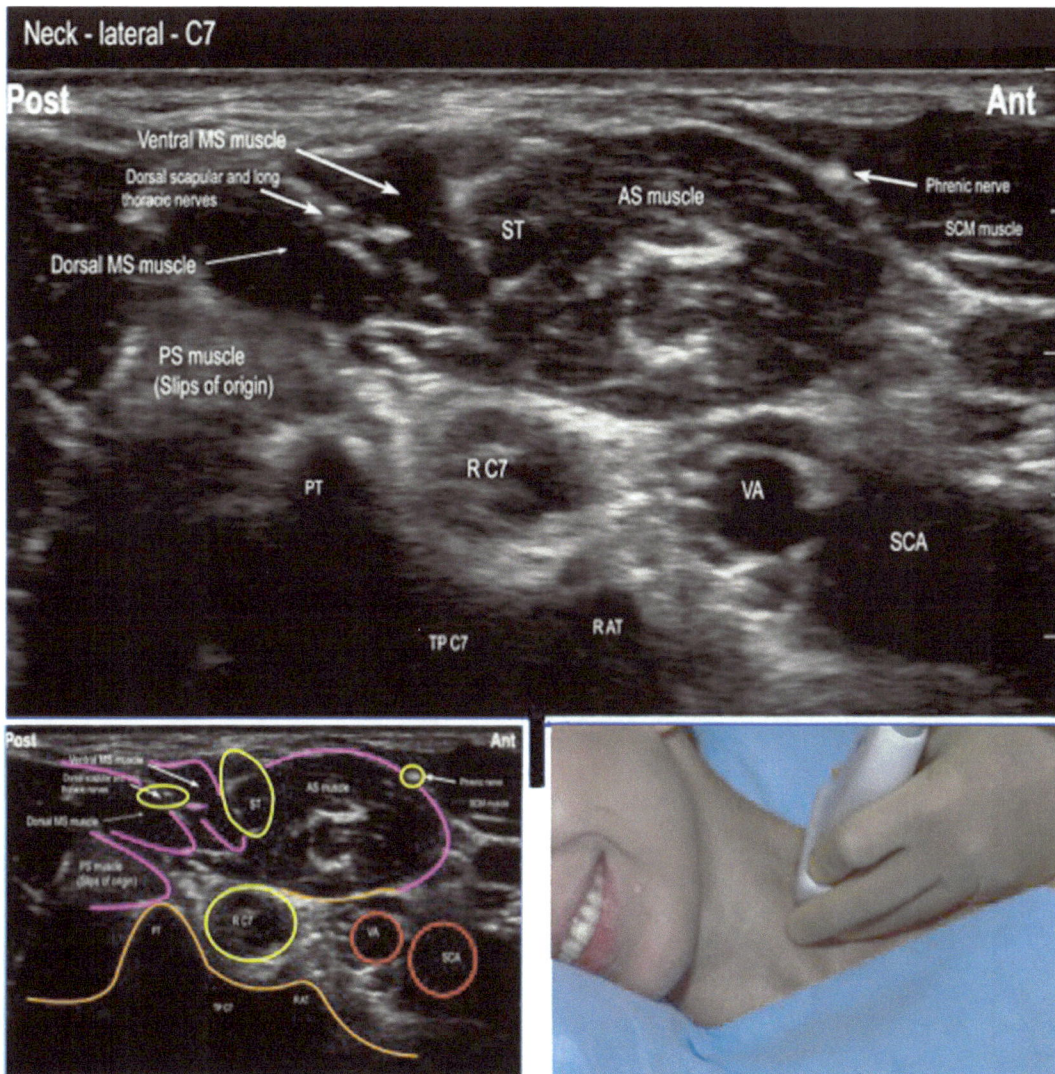

*Figure 1-33: Sonoanatomy of the posterior triangle of the neck. C7 – lateral view.*

| | |
|---|---|
| Ant | Anterior |
| AS Musc | Anterior scalene muscle |
| Dorsal MS | Dorsal middle scalene muscle |
| Post | Posterior |
| PS musc | Posterior scalene muscle (slips of origin) |
| PT | Posterior tubercle of the transverse process |
| R AT | Rudimentary anterior tubercle of the transverse process of C7 |
| R C7 | 7th cervical spinal nerve root (C7) |
| SCA | Subclavian artery |
| ST | Superior trunk of the brachial plexus where C5-C6 have fused. (Please note, in this |

image, these two roots are about to fuse together to form the upper or superior trunk)

| | |
|---|---|
| TP C7 | Transverse process of the 6th cervical vertebra |
| SCM Mus | Sternocleidomastoid muscle |
| VA | Vertebral artery |
| Vent MS | Ventral middle scalene muscle |

Please note: The phrenic nerve on anterior scalene muscle (AS muscle) and the dorsal scapular nerve between the ventral MS and dorsal MS muscles. The long thoracic nerve also exits here with the dorsal scapular nerve

# Lateral Neck Ultrasound on C6 Level

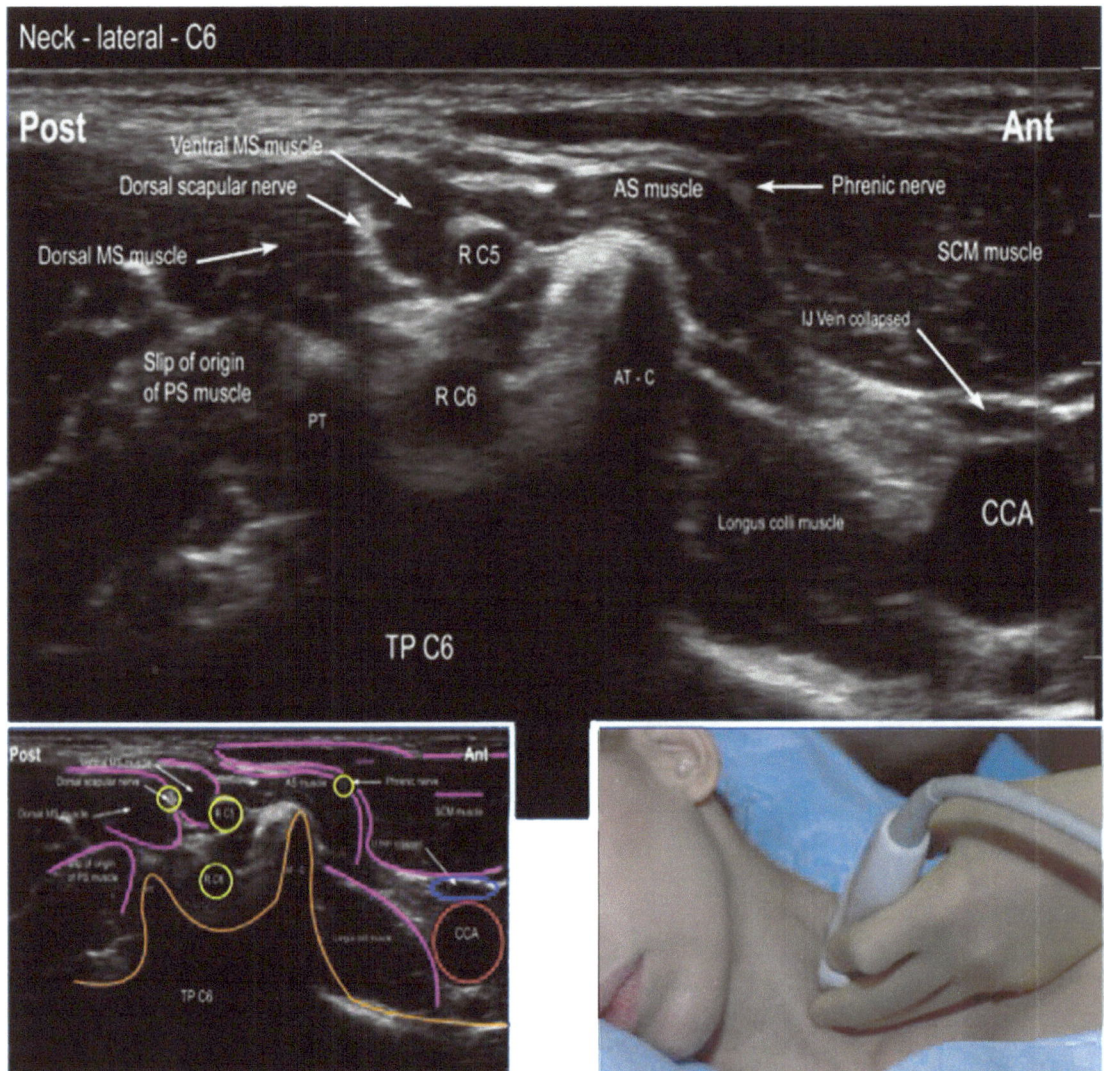

*Figure 1-34: Sonoanatomy of the posterior triangle of the neck. C6 – lateral view.*

| | | | |
|---|---|---|---|
| Ant | Anterior | PT | Posterior tubercle of the transverse process |
| AS | Slips of origin of the anterior scalene muscle | | |
| | | R C5 | 5th cervical spinal nerve root (C5) |
| AT C | Large anterior tubercle of the transverse process also called the Carotid or Chassaignac's tubercle | R C6 | 6th cervical spinal nerve root (C6) |
| | | SCM | Sternocleidomastoid muscle |
| | | TP C6 | Transverse process of the 6th cervical vertebra |
| CCA | Common carotid artery | | |
| Dorsal MS | Dorsal middle scalene muscle | VentMS | Ventral middle scalene muscle |
| IJ Vein | Internal jugular vein (collapsed) | | |
| Post | Posterior | | |
| PS | Slips of origin of the posterior scalene muscle | | |

(Please note the dorsal scapular nerve between the ventral and dorsal MS muscles. The long thoracic nerve also exits here with the dorsal scapular nerve)

# Lateral Neck Ultrasound on C5 Level

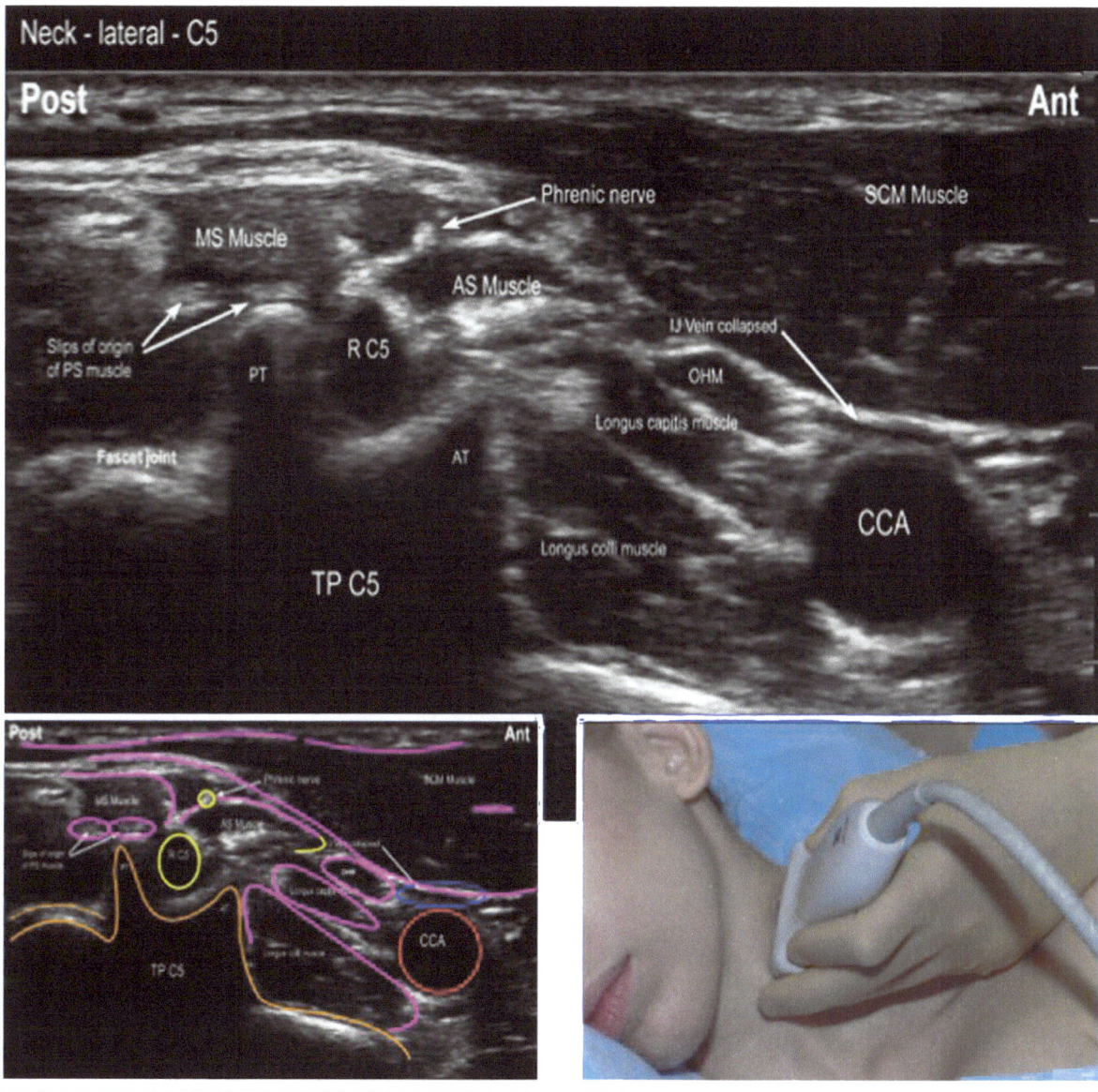

*Figure 1-35: Sonoanatomy of the posterior triangle of the neck. C5 – lateral view.*

| | | | |
|---|---|---|---|
| Ant | Anterior | Post | Posterior |
| AS Mus | Anterior scalene muscle (Please note: The phrenic nerve on its belly close to the C5 spinal nerve root at this level) | PS Mus | Slips of origin of the posterior scalene muscle |
| | | PT | Posterior tubercle of the transverse process of C5 |
| AT | Anterior tubercle of the transverse process of C5 | R C5 | 5th cervical spinal nerve root (C5) |
| CCA | Common carotid artery | SCM Mus | Sternocleidomastoid muscle |
| IJ Vein | Internal jugular vein (collapsed) | TP C5 | Transverse process of the 5th cervical vertebra |
| MS Mus | Middle scalene muscle | | |

# Lateral Neck Ultrasound on C5 Level

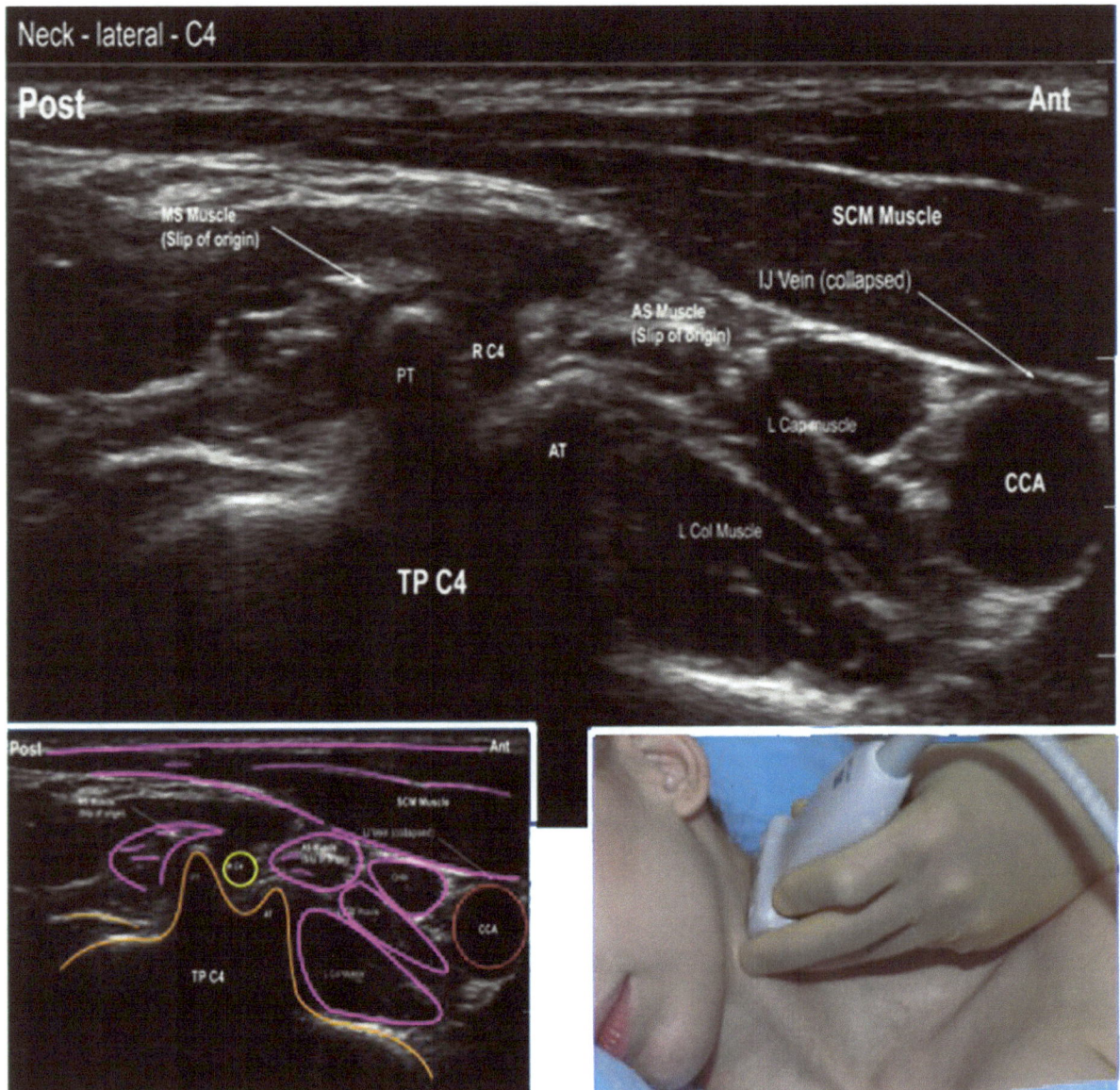

Neck - lateral - C4

Post     Ant

MS Muscle (Slip of origin)

SCM Muscle

IJ Vein (collapsed)

AS Muscle (Slip of origin)

R C4

PT

L Cap muscle

AT

CCA

L Col Muscle

TP C4

*Figure 1-36: Sonoanatomy of the posterior triangle of the neck. C4 – lateral view.*

| | | | |
|---|---|---|---|
| Ant | Anterior | MS Mus | Slips of origin of the middle scalene muscle |
| AS Mus | Slips of origin of the anterior scalene muscle | Post | Posterior |
| AT | Anterior tubercle of the transverse process | PT | Posterior tubercle of the transverse process |
| CCA | Common carotid artery | R C4 | 4th cervical spinal nerve root (C4) |
| IJ Vein | Internal jugular vein (collapsed) | SCM Mus | Sternocleidomastoid muscle |
| LCapMus | Longus capitis muscle | TP C4 | Transverse process of the 4th cervical vertebra |
| LColMus | Longus colli muscle | | |

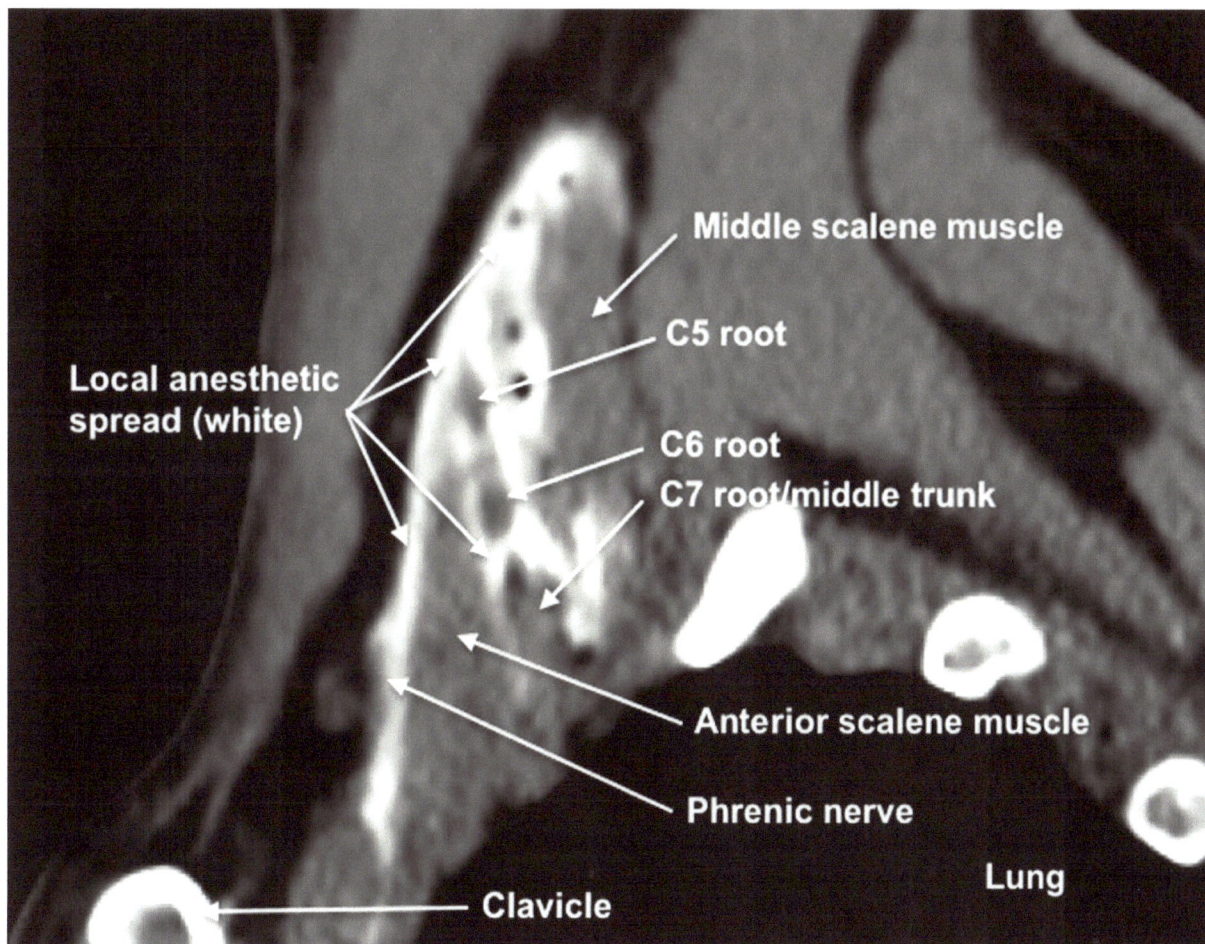

*Figure 1-37: Sagittal anatomy of neck lateral view.*

This is a sagittal CT scan of the neck after contrast has been injected into the interscalene sub-epimyseal space during an interscalene block (See Figs. 1-15 , 1-16, 1-17.)

Please note: The phrenic nerve also lies inside the sub-epimyseal space.

# Functional Anatomy

## Dermatomes of the Upper Extremity

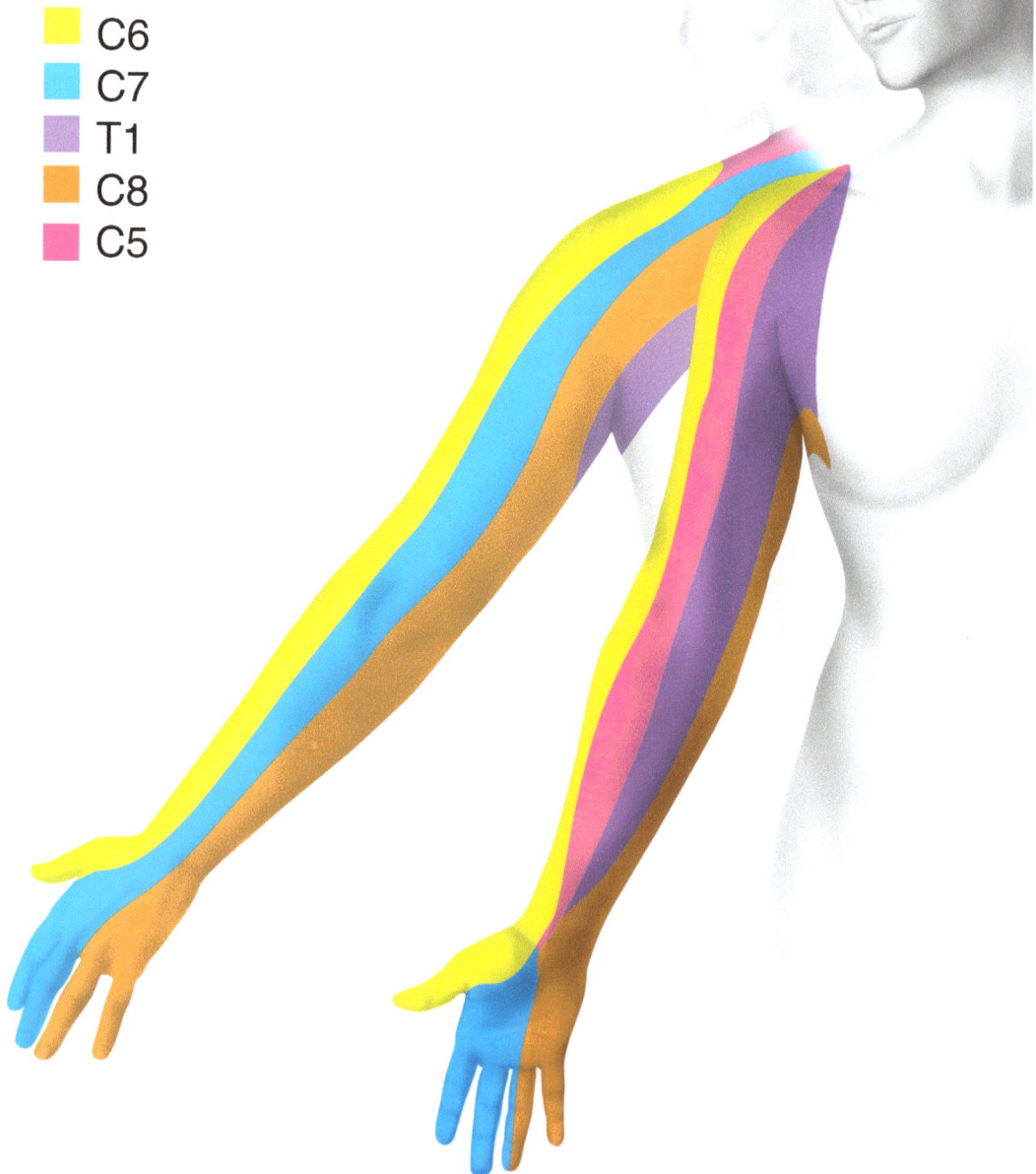

- **C6** (yellow)
- **C7** (blue)
- **T1** (purple)
- **C8** (orange)
- **C5** (pink)

*Figure 1-38: Schematic demarcation of the dermatomes of the upper limb.*

These demarcations are not distinct segments as depicted here because there is significant overlap between adjacent dermatomes. C5, C6, C7, C8, and T1 are cervical (C5-C8) and thoracic (T1) spinal roots.

# Osteotomes of the Upper Extremity

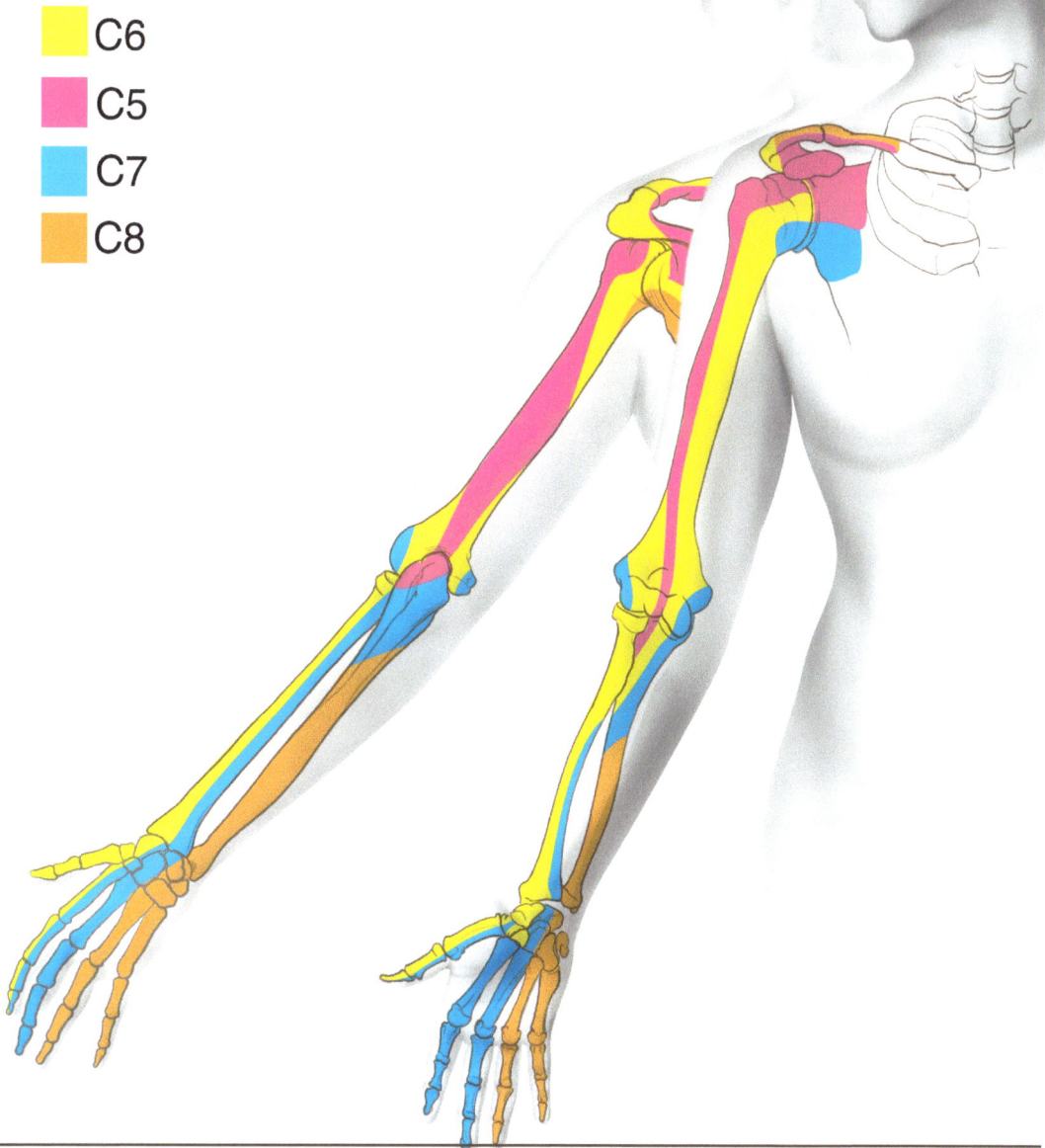

- ■ C6 (yellow)
- ■ C5 (pink)
- ■ C7 (blue)
- ■ C8 (orange)

*Figure 1-39: Schematic demarcation of the osteotomes of the upper limb.*

These demarcations are not distinct segments as depicted here because there is significant overlap between adjacent osteotomes. C5, C6, C7, C8, and T1 are cervical (C5-C8) spinal roots. Although the spinal roots represent corresponding sensory dermatomes and osteotomes, the individual peripheral nerves innervate different areas of the upper limb, represented by neurotomes.

# Neurotomes of the Upper Extremity

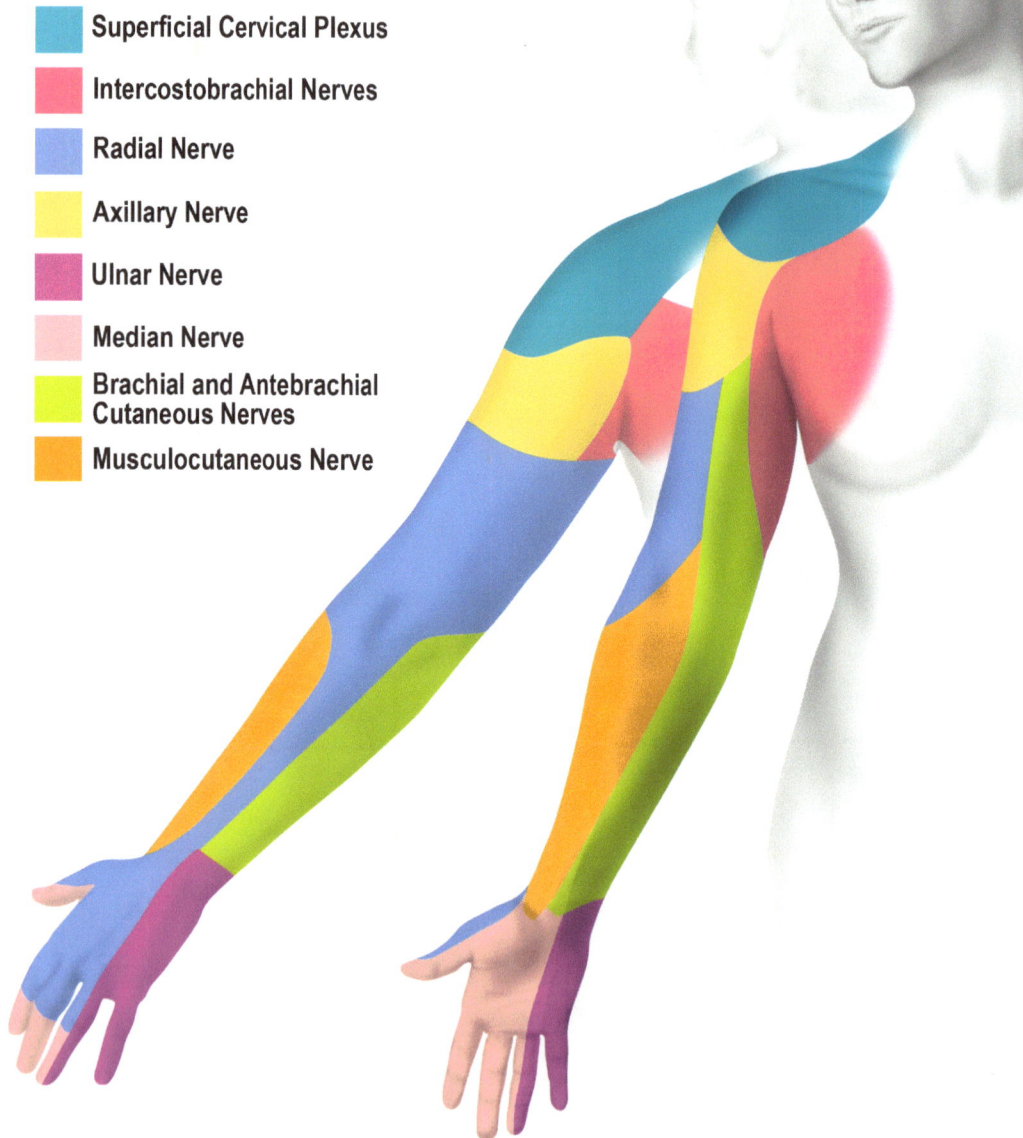

- Superficial Cervical Plexus
- Intercostobrachial Nerves
- Radial Nerve
- Axillary Nerve
- Ulnar Nerve
- Median Nerve
- Brachial and Antebrachial Cutaneous Nerves
- Musculocutaneous Nerve

Figure 1-40: Schematic demarcation of the neurotomes of the upper limb.

These demarcations are not distinct areas as depicted here because there is significant overlap between adjacent neurotomes.

# Chapter 2

## The Distal Brachial Plexus

*Macroanatomy*
*Microanatomy*
*Sonoanatomy*
*Functional Anatomy*

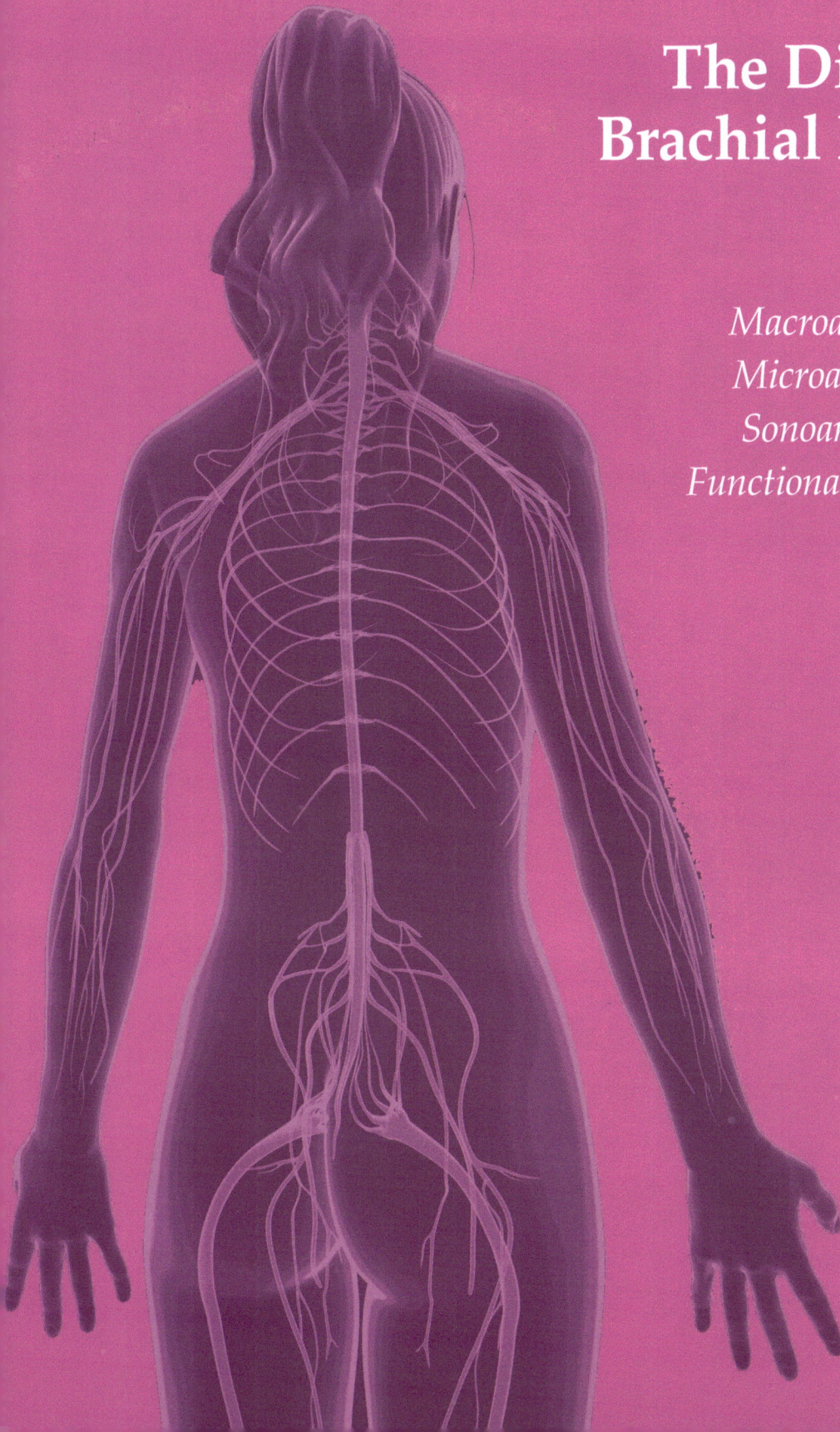

# Macroanatomy
## Sagittal Section through Lateral Clavicular Line

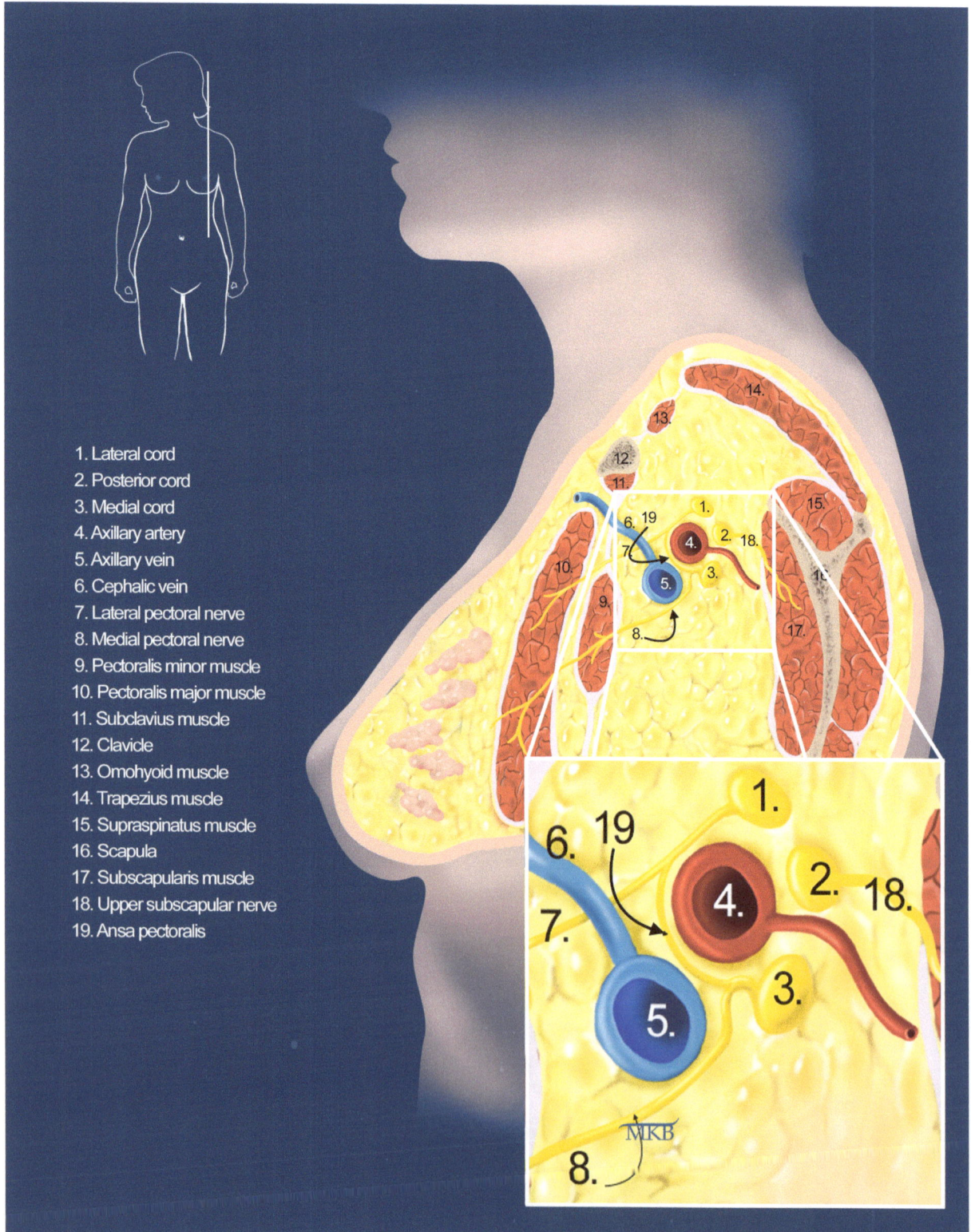

1. Lateral cord
2. Posterior cord
3. Medial cord
4. Axillary artery
5. Axillary vein
6. Cephalic vein
7. Lateral pectoral nerve
8. Medial pectoral nerve
9. Pectoralis minor muscle
10. Pectoralis major muscle
11. Subclavius muscle
12. Clavicle
13. Omohyoid muscle
14. Trapezius muscle
15. Supraspinatus muscle
16. Scapula
17. Subscapularis muscle
18. Upper subscapular nerve
19. Ansa pectoralis

*Figure 2-1: Sagittal macroanatomy through the medial deltopectoral groove.*

Please note the ansa pectoralis communicating branch (19) (arrow), which is also sometimes referred to as the Martin-Gruber nerve, between lateral pectoral nerve (7) and medial pectoral nerve (8). The lateral pectoral nerve gives off an articular branch; a pure sensory nerve, that runs over the coracoid process and supplies sensory innervation to the acromioclavicular and subacromial joints. These two joints thus receive sensory innervation from both the medial and lateral pectoral nerves – therefore from the 5th, 6th, 7th and 8th cervical spinal roots and the 1st thoracic spinal root (See Figure 1-1).  The middle part of the clavicle and sternoclavicular joint receives sensory innervation from the superficial cervical plexus (C2 to C4). The sternoclavicular joint can also receive sensory innervation from the T2 root.

# The Proximal Infraclavicular Area

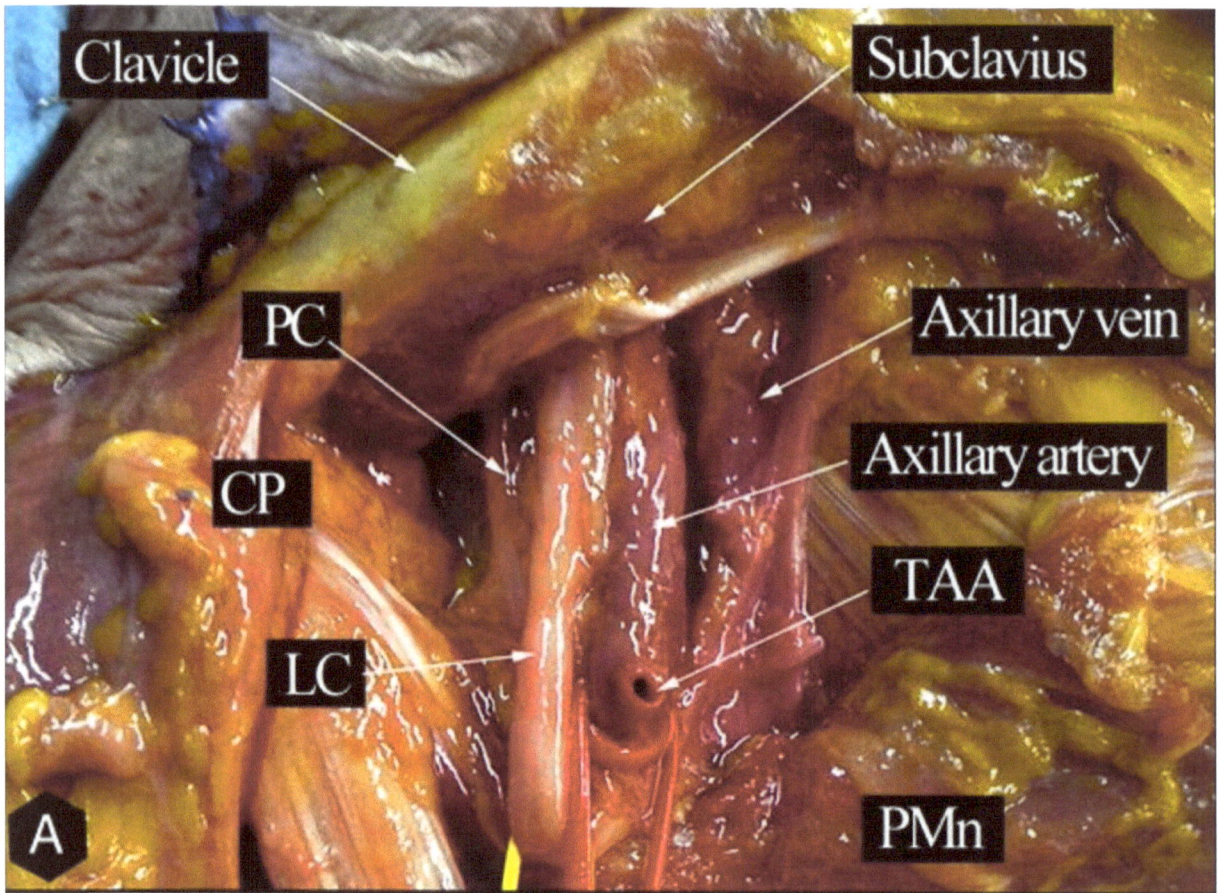

*Figure 2-2: Cadaver anatomic dissection of the right medial infraclavicular fossa (MICF).*

This dissection is below the middle-third of the clavicle and above the medial border of the pectoralis minor muscle, showing the anterior view of the relations of the cords of the brachial plexus to the first part of the axillary artery. The pectoralis minor muscle (PMn) has been cut at its origin from the coracoid process (CP) and reflected medially.

This figure shows the lateral (LC) and posterior (PC) cords lying lateral and parallel to the axillary artery and the PC lying posterolateral to the LC. The medial cord (MC) is not visible in this image. Also note the origin of the thoraco-acromial artery (TAA) from the axillary artery. Subclavius denotes the subclavius muscle.

*Reprinted with permission from: Sala-Blanch X, Reina MA, Pangthipampai P, Karmakar MK. Anatomic basis for brachial plexus block at the costoclavicular space: a cadaver anatomic study. Reg Anesth Pain Med 2016;41:387-91.*

# Macroanatomy of the Proximal Subclavicular Area

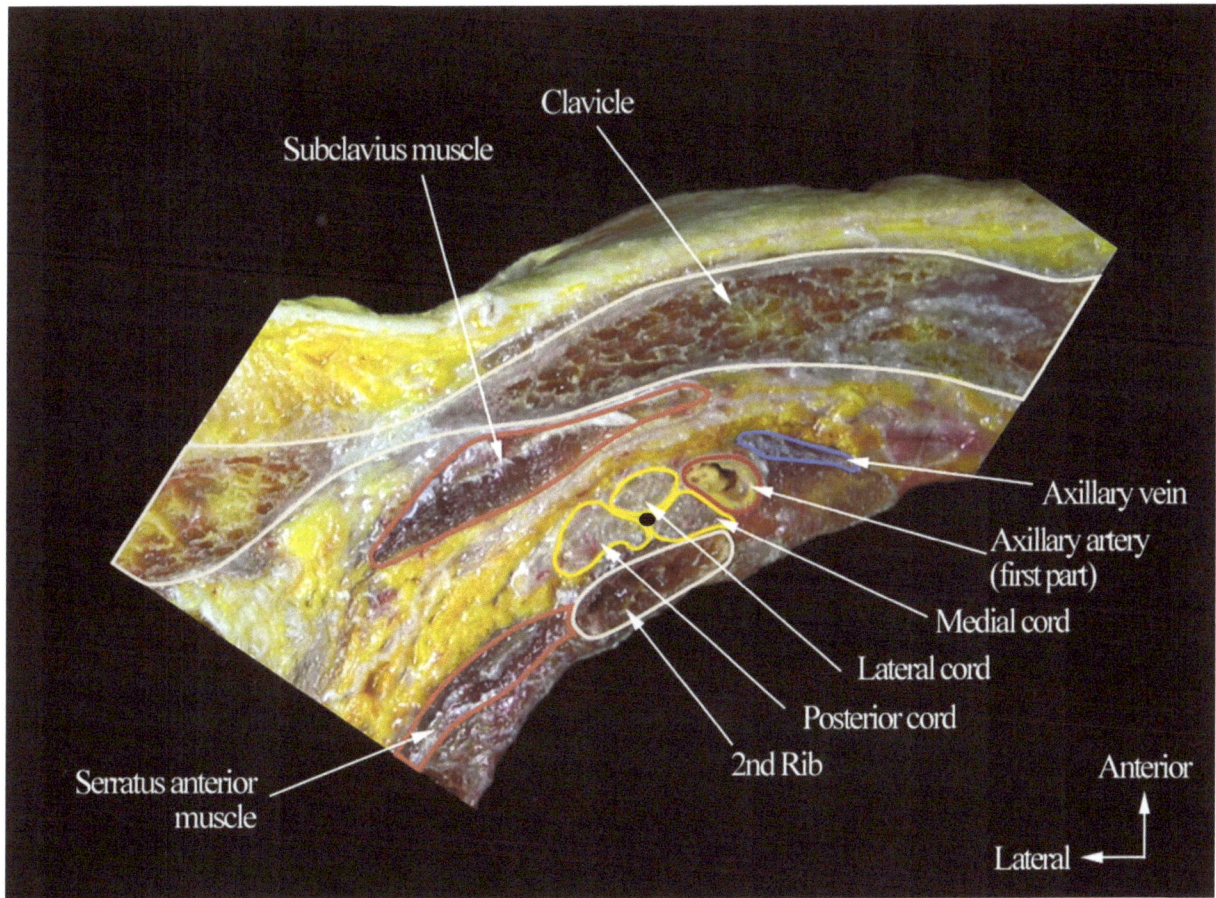

*Figure 2-3: Transverse anatomic section through the right costo-clavicular space (CCS) showing the anatomic arrangement and relations of the cords of the brachial plexus.*

The anatomy is presented as though one were looking at it from caudal to cranial (caudo-cranial view). This (black dot), where the three cords are bundled together, and more important, where they are in the same communal circumneural sheath would represent the ideal position to place a catheter for a continuous nerve block for the management of acute pain associated with elbow, wrist and other distal upper extremity surgery (black dot placed by author).

*Reprinted with permission from: Sala-Blanch X, Reina MA, Pangthipampai P, Karmakar MK. Anatomic basis for brachial plexus block at the costoclavicular space: a cadaver anatomic study. Reg Anesth Pain Med 2016; 41: 387 - 391.*

# Macroanatomy of the Subclavian Area

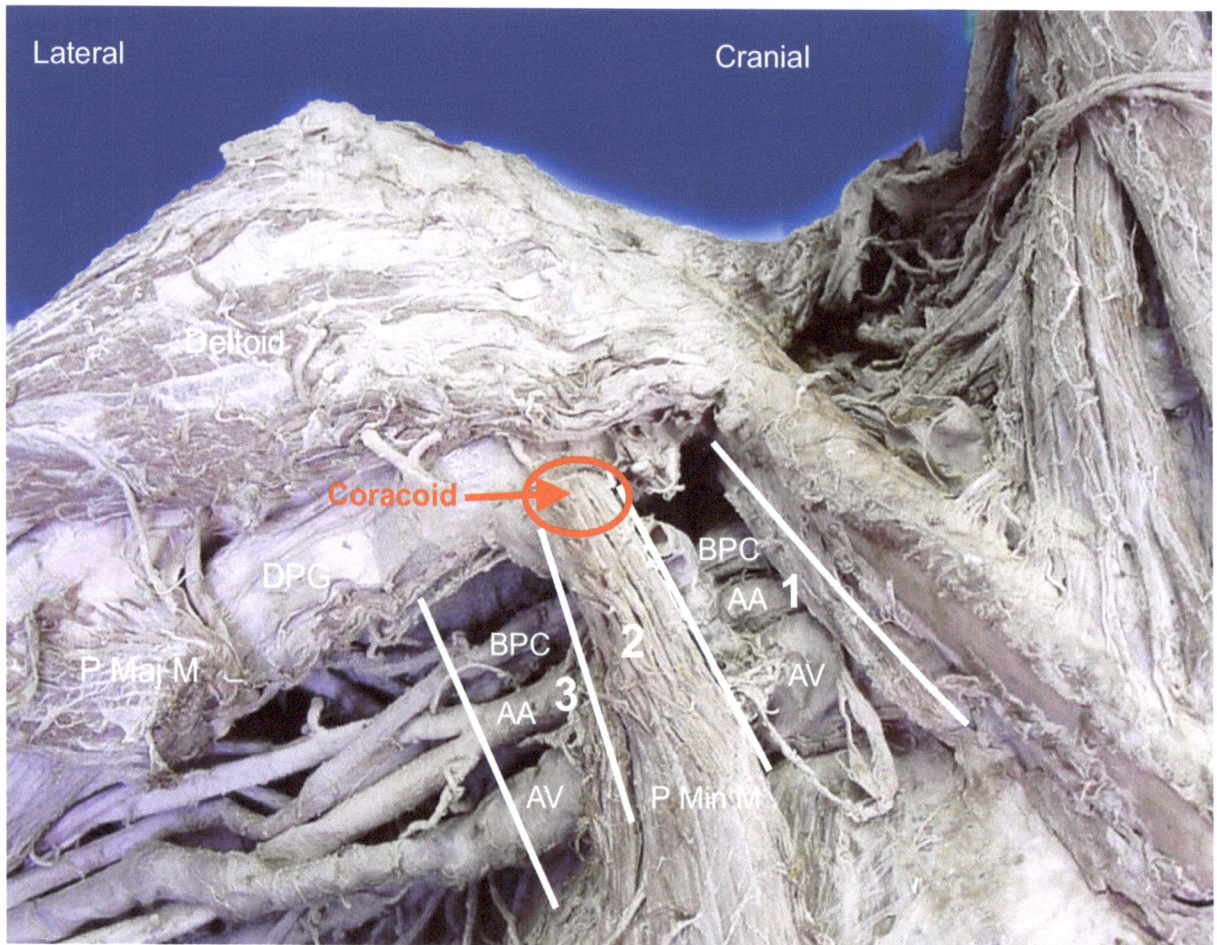

*Figure 2-4: Macroanatomy of the three parts of the infraclavicular axillary artery.*

| | |
|---|---|
| 1 | 1st part of axillary artery |
| 2 | 2nd part of axillary artery |
| 3 | 3rd part of axillary artery |
| AA | Axillary artery |
| AV | Axillary vein |
| BPC | Brachial plexus cords |
| Coracoid | Coracoid process |
| DPG | Deltopectoral groove |
| P Min M | Minor pectoral muscle |
| P Maj M | Major pectoral muscle (removed) |

# Sagittal Section through Midclavicular Area

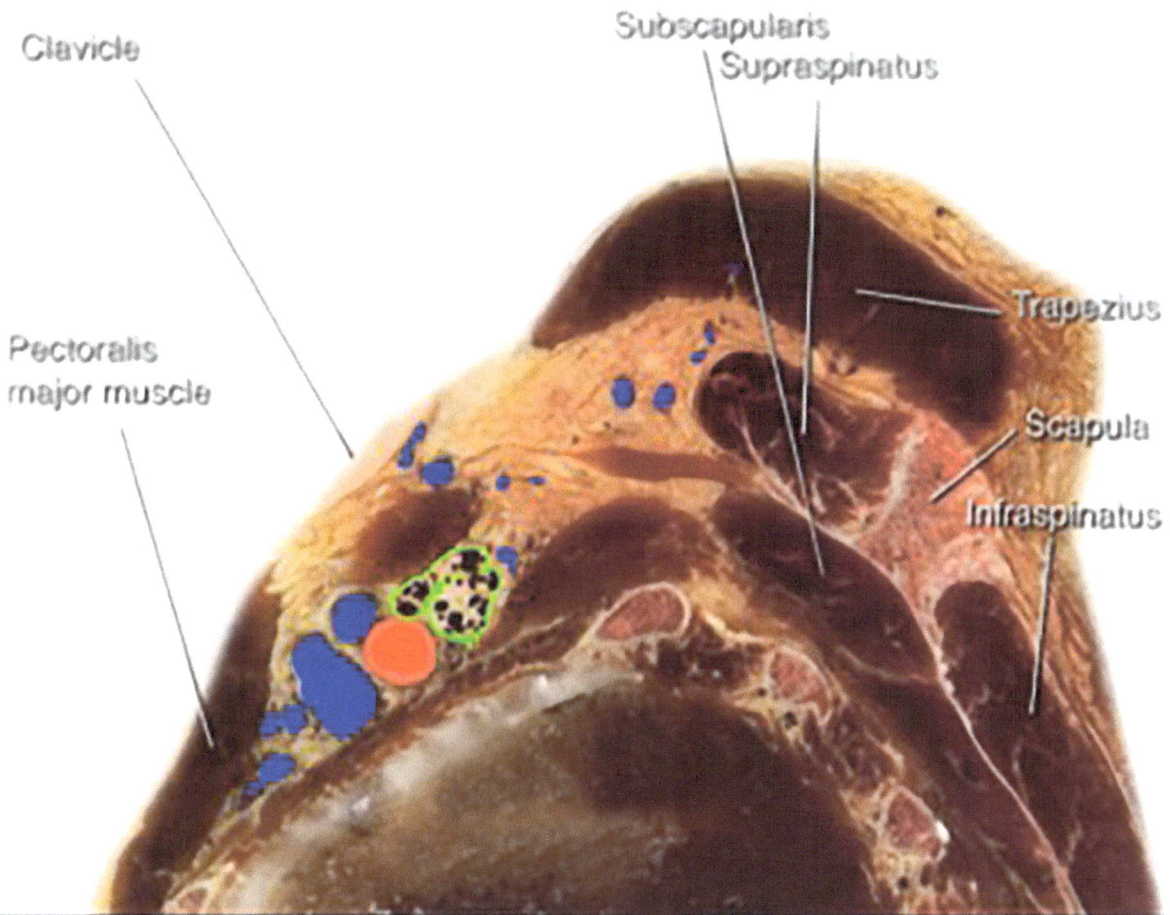

*Figure 2-5: Sagittal anatomy of the brachial plexus cords through the 1st part of the axillary artery: proximal mid-clavicular infraclavicular area.*

Please note:
At this level, the three cords are bundled together.

**View video at RAEducation.com**
**- Acute Pain Medicine - Anatomy -**
**Sagittal Anatomy**
**Brachial plexus below the clavicle**

*Photograph & video courtesy of Paul Bigeleisen, Nizar Moayeri, Gerbrand Groen. UMC Utrecht, The Netherlands*

# Sagittal Section through Lateral Clavicular Area

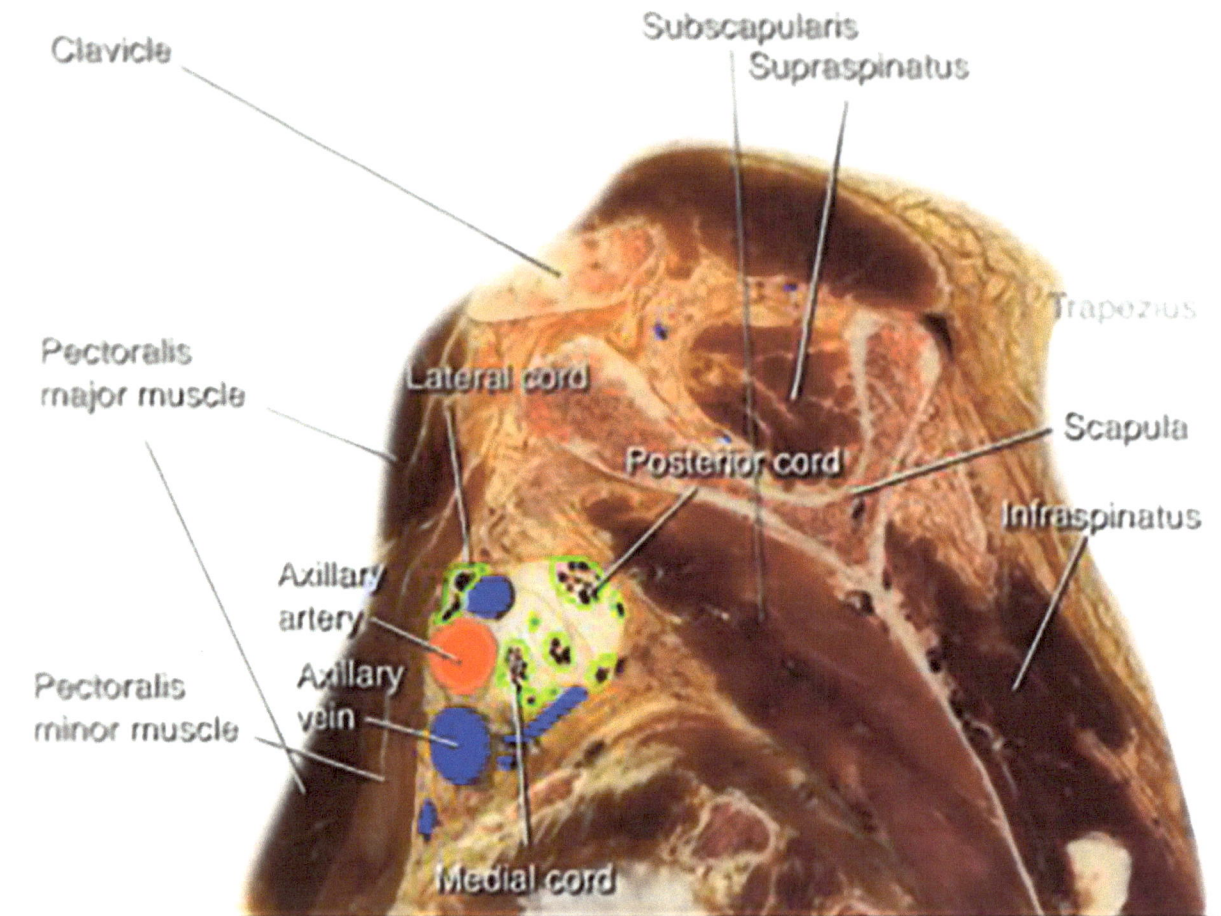

Figure 2-6: Sagittal anatomy of the brachial plexus cords through the second part of the axillary artery: more distal mid-clavicular infraclavicular area.

Please note: At this more distal level, the cords are starting to move into an arrangement around the axillary artery.

The brachial plexus of this particular cadaver was infiltrated by lung carcinoma tissue – the so-called Pancoast Tumor.

Photograph: Paul Bigeleisen, Nizar Moayeri, Gerbrand Groen. UMC Utrecht, The Netherlands

# Sagittal Section through Apex of the Axilla

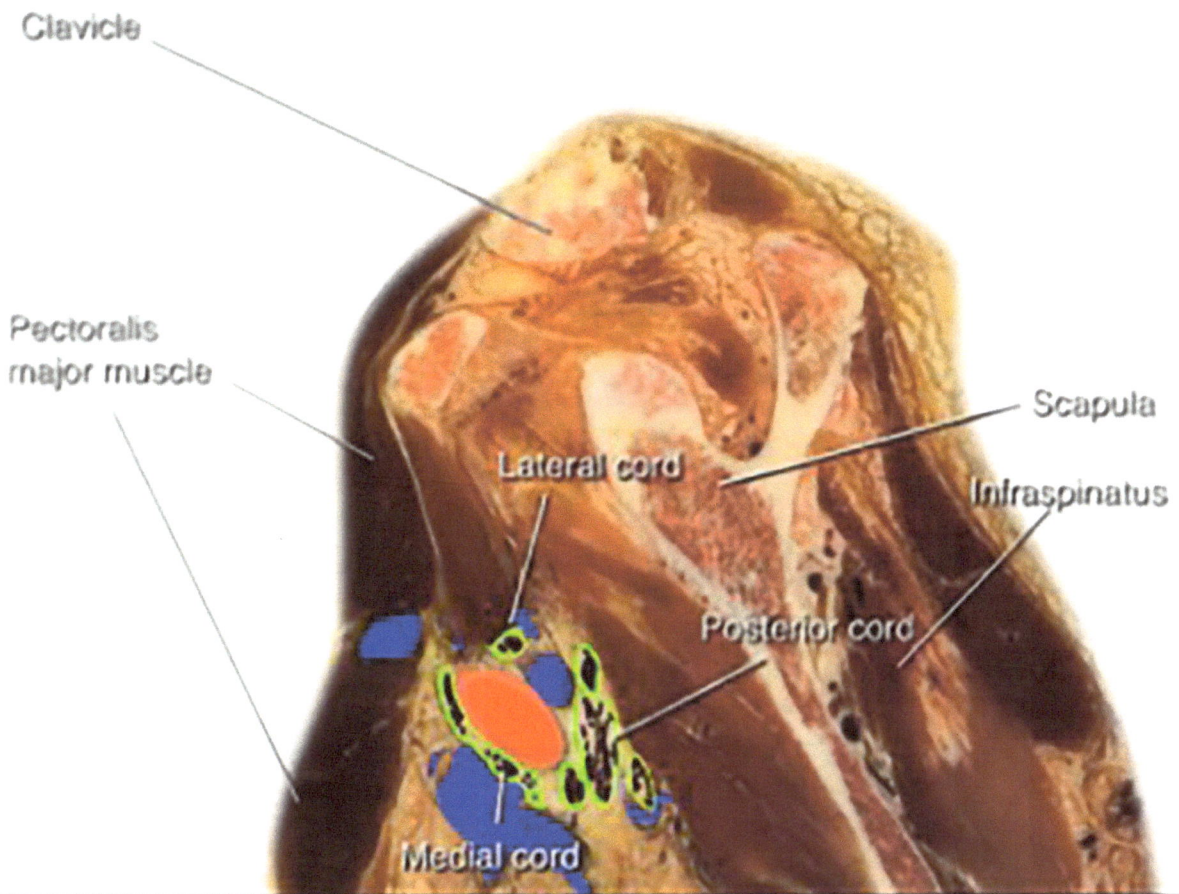

Clavicle

Pectoralis major muscle

Lateral cord

Scapula

Infraspinatus

Posterior cord

Medial cord

*Figure 2-7: Sagittal anatomy of the brachial plexus cords through the third part of the axillary artery: distal deltopectoral groove infraclavicular area.*

Please note: In the distal clavico-costal space (CCS), the brachial plexus is arranged around the axillary artery.

*Photograph: Paul Bigeleisen, Nizar Moayeri, Gerbrand Groen. UMC Utrecht, The Netherlands*

# Cross Section of Area near the Axilla

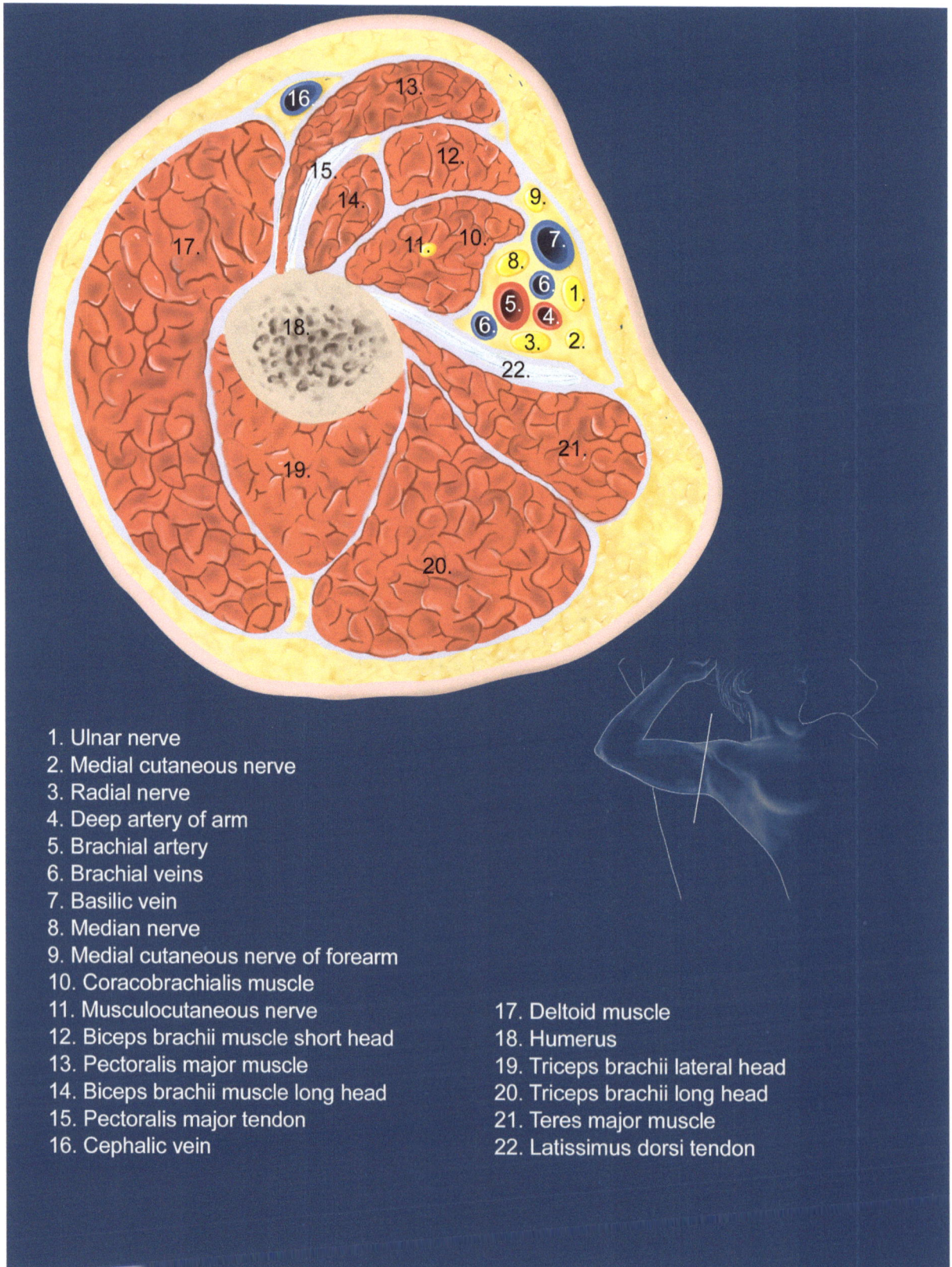

1. Ulnar nerve
2. Medial cutaneous nerve
3. Radial nerve
4. Deep artery of arm
5. Brachial artery
6. Brachial veins
7. Basilic vein
8. Median nerve
9. Medial cutaneous nerve of forearm
10. Coracobrachialis muscle
11. Musculocutaneous nerve
12. Biceps brachii muscle short head
13. Pectoralis major muscle
14. Biceps brachii muscle long head
15. Pectoralis major tendon
16. Cephalic vein

17. Deltoid muscle
18. Humerus
19. Triceps brachii lateral head
20. Triceps brachii long head
21. Teres major muscle
22. Latissimus dorsi tendon

*Figure 2-8: Cross-section through the upper arm close to the axilla.*

In the axilla, the musculocutaneous nerve (11) lies between the biceps (12, 14) and coracobrachialis (13) muscles, but more proximal, it lies inside the coracobrachialis muscle. The medial cutaneous nerve of the forearm (9) lies anterior and superficially in the neurovascular bundle, usually anterolateral to the basilica vein, while the ulnar nerve (1) lies anterior to the brachial artery (5) and vein (6) and inferomedial to the basilic vein (7). The median nerve (8) is situated anterolateral to the brachial artery (5), while the radial nerve (3) and median cutaneous nerve of the arm (2) are posteromedial.

# Microanatomy
## The Proximal Infraclavicular Area

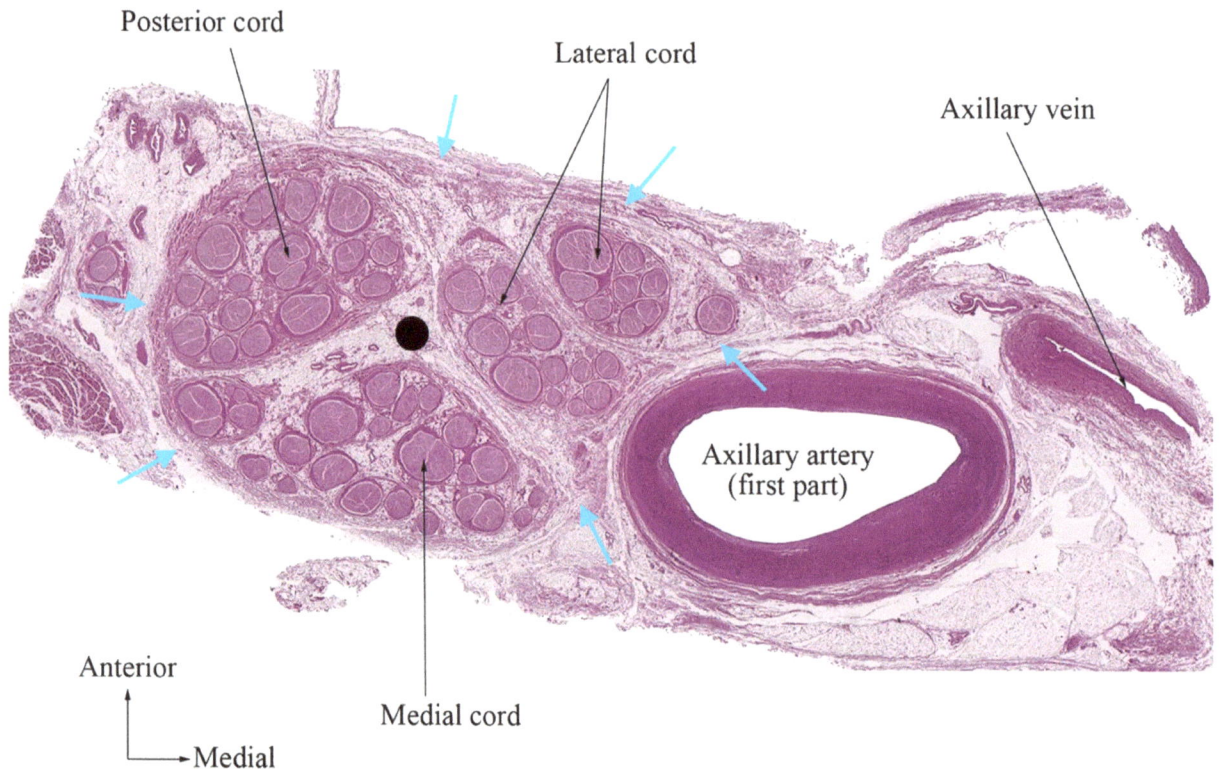

*Figure 2-9: Histological section from the right costo-clavicular space (CCS).*

The tissue in this section has been stained with hematoxylin and eosin, showing the anatomic arrangement and relations of the cords of the brachial plexus (caudo-cranial view).

Note: The red arrows represent the circum-neurium (also known as the paraneurium), although the section has not specifically stained for it.

The black dot (•) represents the ideal position to place a catheter for a continuous nerve block for the management of acute pain associated with elbow, wrist and other distal upper extremity surgery (black dot and arrows placed by author).

*Reprinted with permission from: Sala-Blanch X, Reina MA, Pangthipampai P, Karmakar MK. Anatomic basis for brachial plexus block at the costoclavicular space: a cadaver anatomic study. Reg Anesth Pain Med 2016; 41: 387 - 391.*

# The Proximal Infraclavicular Area

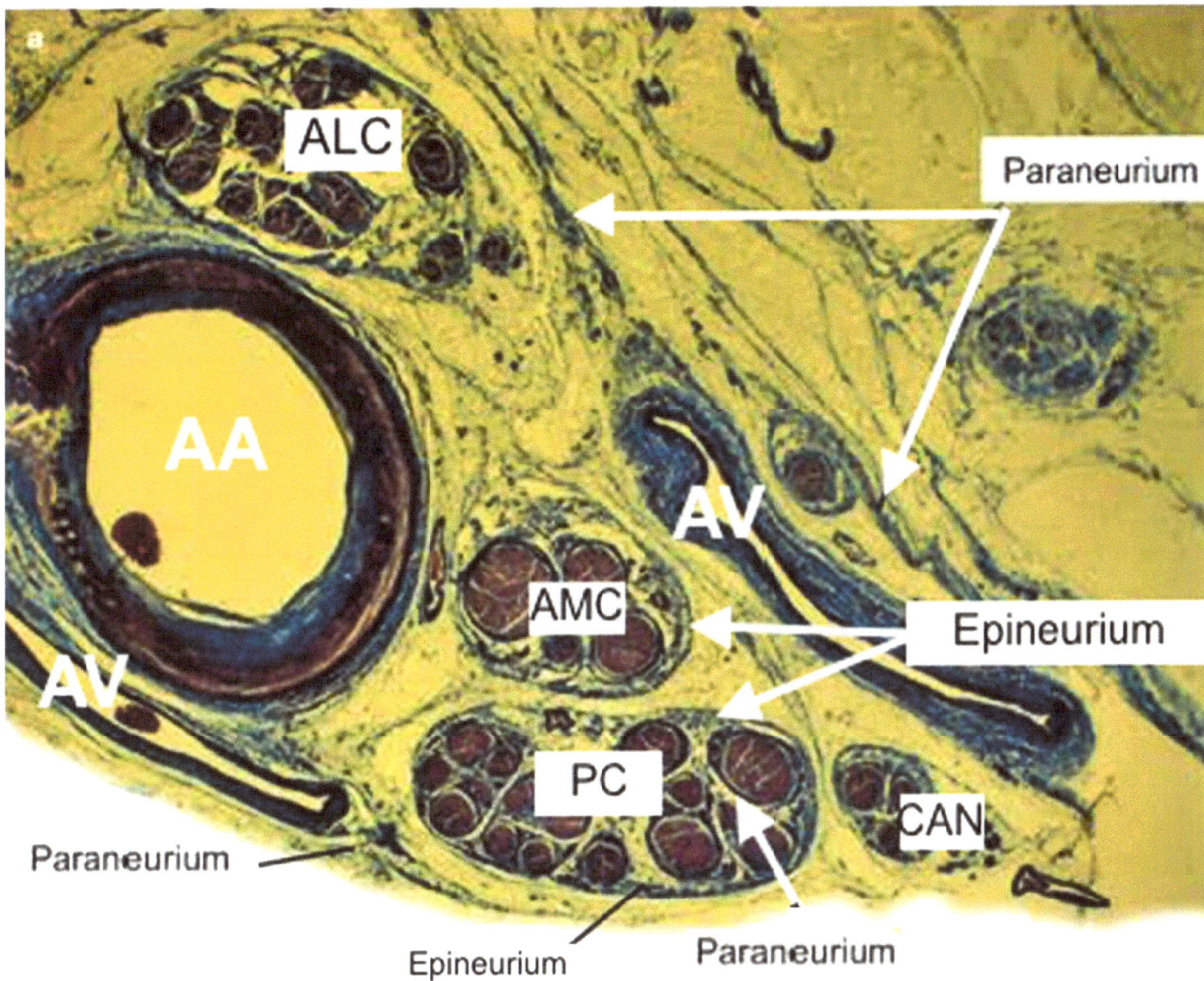

Figure 2-10: Brachial plexus cords in the proximal infraclavicular area.

Masson's trichrome stained histological section showing cauda-cranial view of the brachial plexus cords that are arranged to the lateral side of the axillary artery (AA) and vein and in a communal circumneural (AKA paraneural) sheath.

| | |
|---|---|
| AA | Axillary artery |
| ALC | Anterolateral cord |
| AMC | Anteromedial cord |
| AV | Branch of axillary vein |
| CAN | Cutaneous antebrachial nerve |
| PC | Posterior cord |

Reprinted with permission from: Reina MA, Sala-Blanch X. Cross-sectional microscopic anatomy of the brachial plexus and paraneural sheaths. In: Reina MA, editor. Atlas of Functional Anatomy For Regional Anesthesia And Pain Medicine. New York: Springer Science and Business Media, 2015: 187. (Some Annotations by author)

# The Proximal Infraclavicular Area

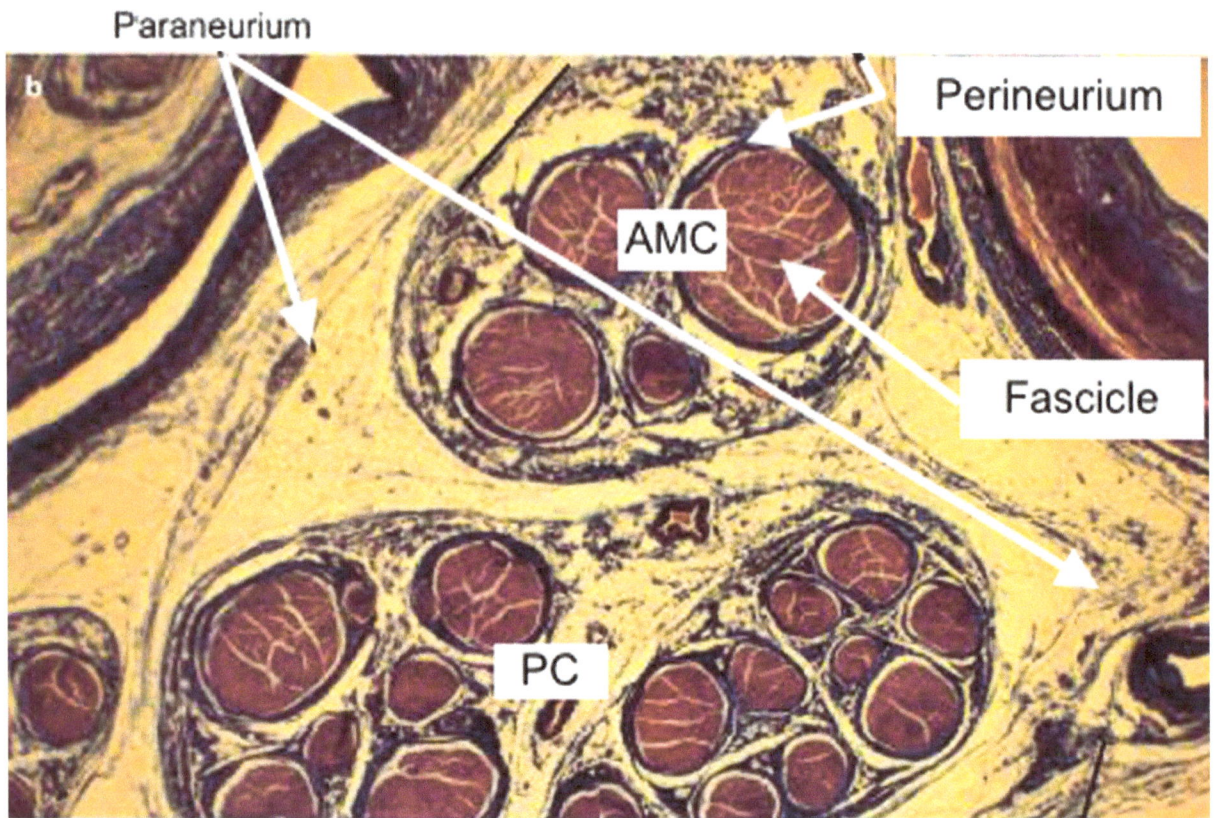

**Paraneurium**

**Perineurium**

**AMC**

**Fascicle**

**PC**

*Figure 2-11: Brachial plexus cords in the proximal infraclavicular area.*

Masson's trichrome stained histological section showing cauda-cranial view of the brachial plexus cords that are arranged to the lateral side of the axillary artery (AA) and vein and in a communal circumneural (AKA paraneural) sheath.

AMC  Anteromedial cord
PC    Posterior cord

*Reprinted with permission from: Reina MA, Sala-Blanch X. Cross-sectional microscopic anatomy of the brachial plexus and paraneural sheaths. In: Reina MA, editor. Atlas of Functional Anatomy For Regional Anesthesia And Pain Medicine. New York: Springer Science and Business Media, 2015: 187. (Some Annotations by author)*

# Circumneurium (aka Paraneurium)

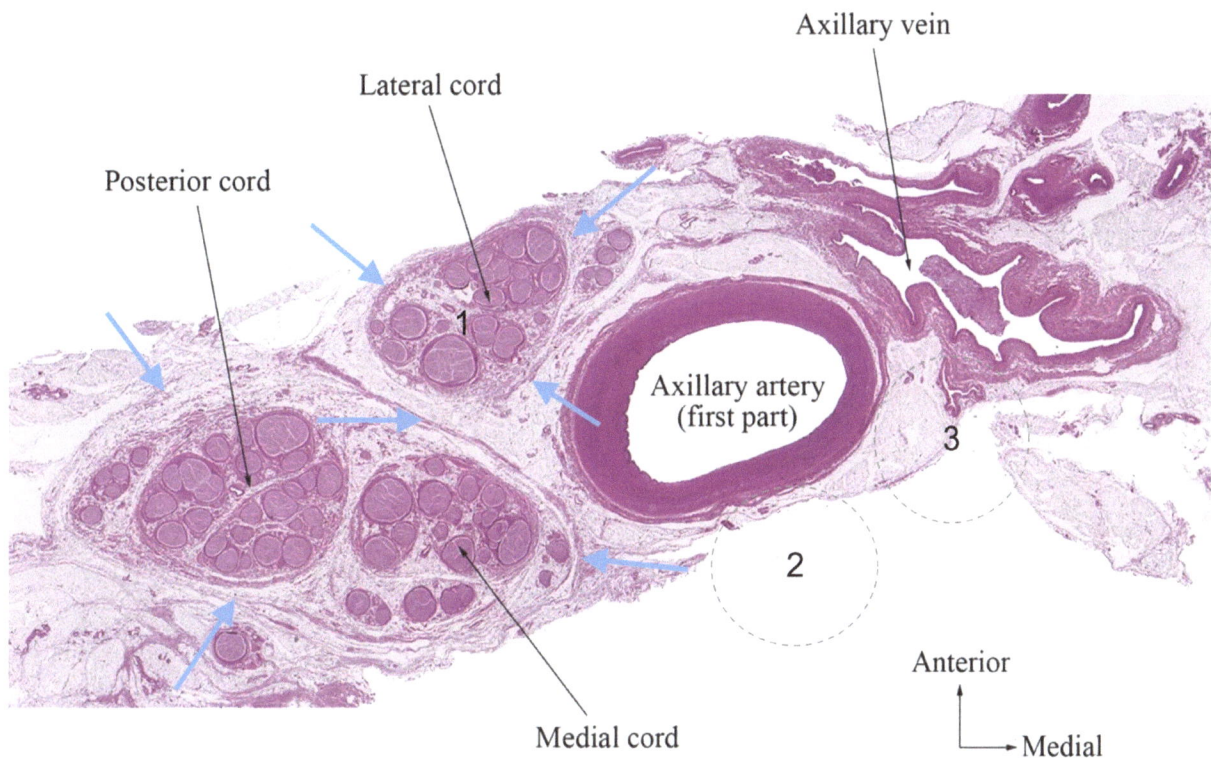

Figure 2-12: Histological section of the right costo-clavicular space (CCS).

The tissue in this section was stained with hematoxylin and eosin, showing the anatomic arrangement and relations of the cords of the brachial plexus (caudo-cranial view). It can be seen that the lateral cord is now in its own circumneural fascia sheath, while the medial and posterior cord still share the same common circumneural sheath.

Note: The red arrows again indicate the circumneurium. The lateral cord (LC) more distally starts to move antero-medially around the axillary artery to its final antero-lateral position. The posterior cord will move underneath, or posterior to the artery and the medial cord moves medially.

The lateral cord is now starting to form its own circumneurium and is no longer in the same circumneurium as the other two cords.

Further distally, the lateral cord remains lateral of the axillary artery while the posterior cord moves posterior to the artery to Position 2, and the medial cord moves to Position 3, medial to the artery. Each cord is now in its own circumneural fascia sheath.

*Reprinted with permission from: Sala-Blanch X, Reina MA, Pangthipampai P, Karmakar MK. Anatomic basis for brachial plexus block at the costoclavicular space: a cadaver anatomic study. Reg Anesth Pain Med 2016; 41: 387 - 391. Positions 1,2,3 and arrows added by author.*

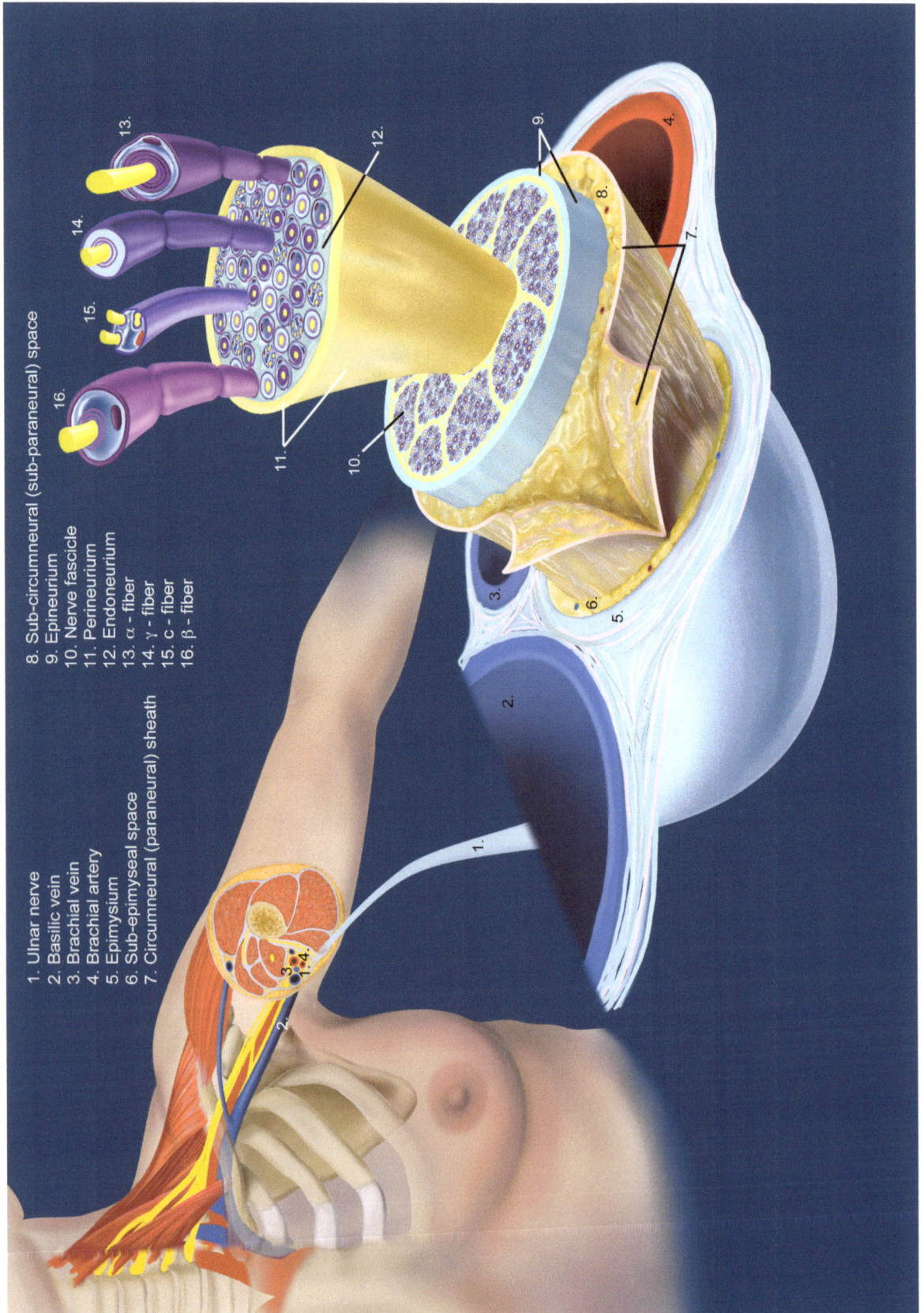

1. Ulnar nerve
2. Basilic vein
3. Brachial vein
4. Brachial artery
5. Epimysium
6. Sub-epimyseal space
7. Circumneural (paraneural) sheath
8. Sub-circumneural (sub-paraneural) space
9. Epineurium
10. Nerve fascicle
11. Perineurium
12. Endoneurium
13. α - fiber
14. γ - fiber
15. c - fiber
16. β - fiber

*Figure 2-13: Micro- structure of th e ulnar nerve.*

- The ulnar nerve (1), like all the peripheral nerves in the axilla, lies in its own circumneural sheath (7) (AKA paraneural sheath).

- Outside the circumneural sheath (7) is the sub-epimyseal space (6), which is surrounded by the epimysium (5), which is the fascia that surrounds the nerves, muscles, and blood vessels (4).

- Deep to the circumneural sheath (7) is the sub-circumneural space (8), which is the ideal space for the needle and catheter placement for single injection or continuous nerve blocks. Also referred to the "sweet spot" of the nerve.

- The next layer, which engulfs the bundle of nerve fascicles, is the epineurium (9). This is thought to originate from the paravertebral fascia (see Figures 1-16, 1-19 & 1-28b).

- Each individual fascicle is surrounded by its own perineurium (11), which is a continuation of the dura (see Figures 1-16 & 1-19). This is a tough layer and intrafascicular injection, unlike intra-root injection, needs high injection pressure.

- Inside the perineurium are the endoneurium and nerve axons (13-16).

- The fluid inside the fascicle is cerebrospinal fluid while the interstitial fluid outside the fascicles is lymph that drains to the lymph nodes.

Ref: Boezaart AP. The Sweet Spot of the Nerve: Is the "paraneural sheath" named correctly, and does it matter? Reg Anesth Pain Med 2014;39:557-8.

# Sonoanatomy
## The Proximal Infraclavicular Area

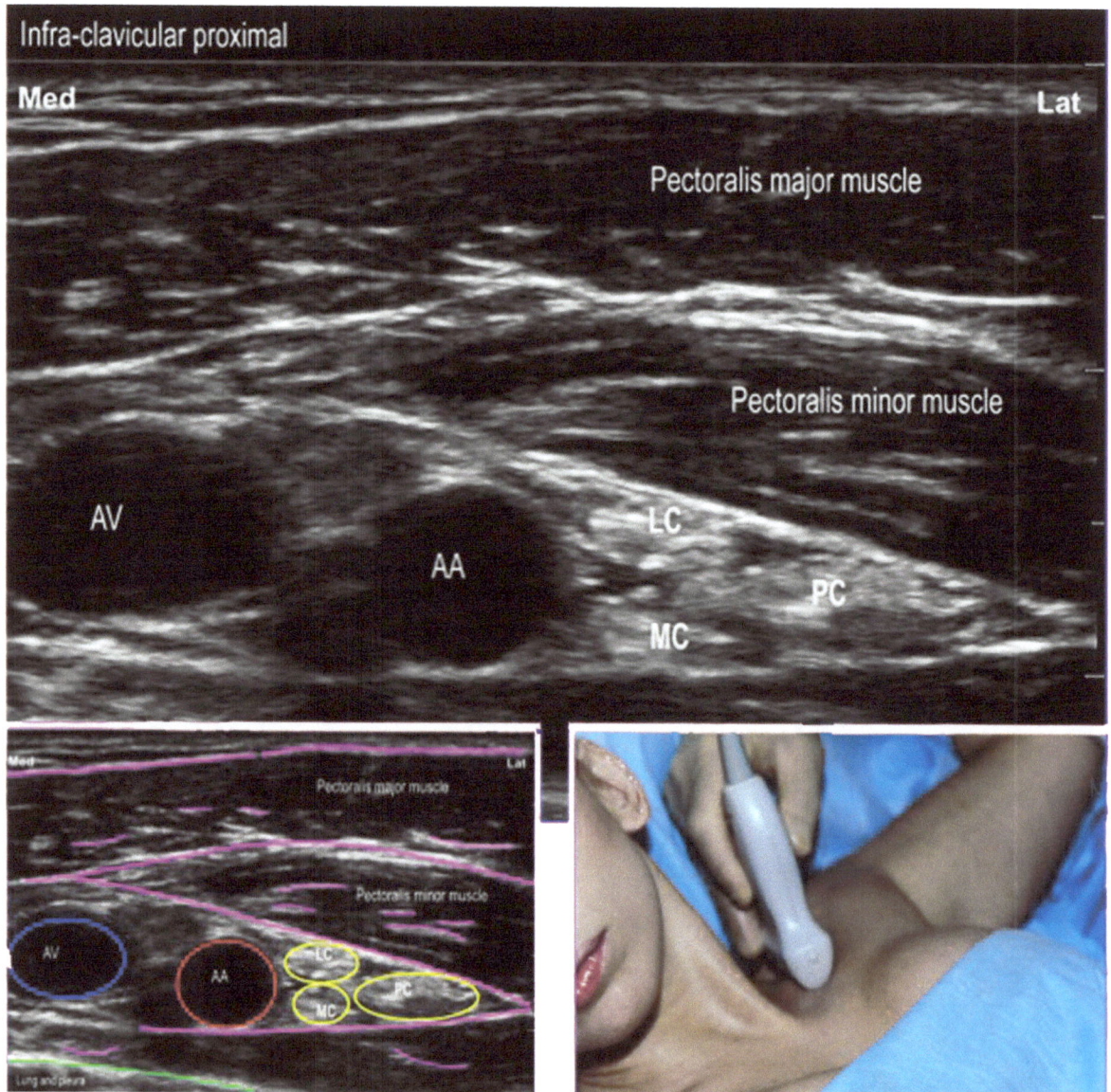

Figure 2-14: Sonoanatomy of the proximal brachial plexus below the clavicle.

AA      Axillary artery
AV      Axillary vein
Lat     Lateral
LC      Lateral cord of the brachial plexus
MC      Median cord of the brachial plexus
Med     Medial
PC      Posterior cord of the brachial plexus

View Video at RAEducation.com
Acute Pain Medicine - Anatomy -
Sonoanatomy: Brachial Plexus Cords

# The Distal Infraclavicular Area

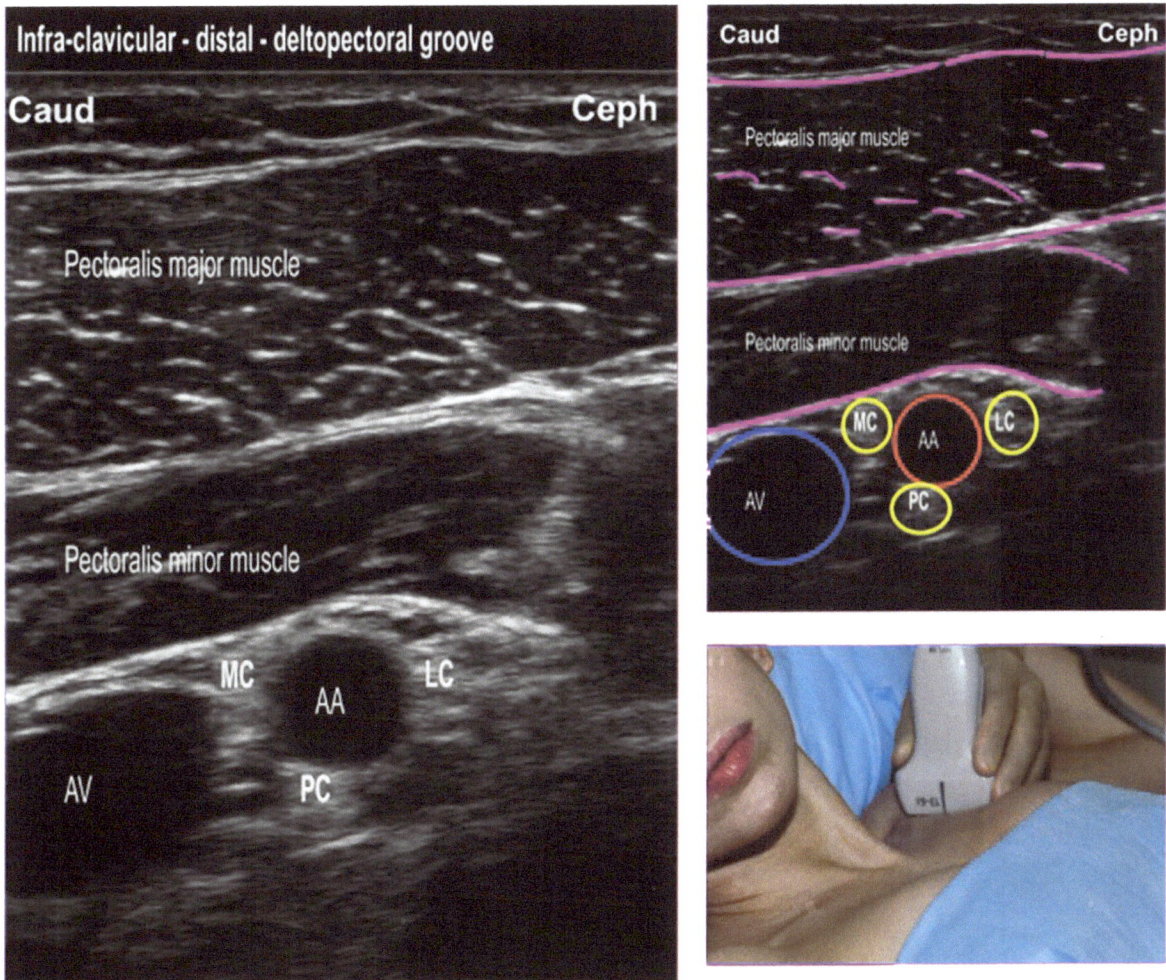

Figure 2-15: Sonoanatomy of the brachial plexus cords in the sagittal view through the deltopectoral groove.

| | |
|---|---|
| AA | Axillary artery |
| AV | Axillary vein |
| Caud | Caudad |
| Ceph | Cephalad |
| LC | Lateral cord of the brachial plexus |
| MC | Medial cord of the brachial plexus |
| PC | Posterior cord of the brachial plexus |

# Fascia between Major & Minor Pectoralis Muscles

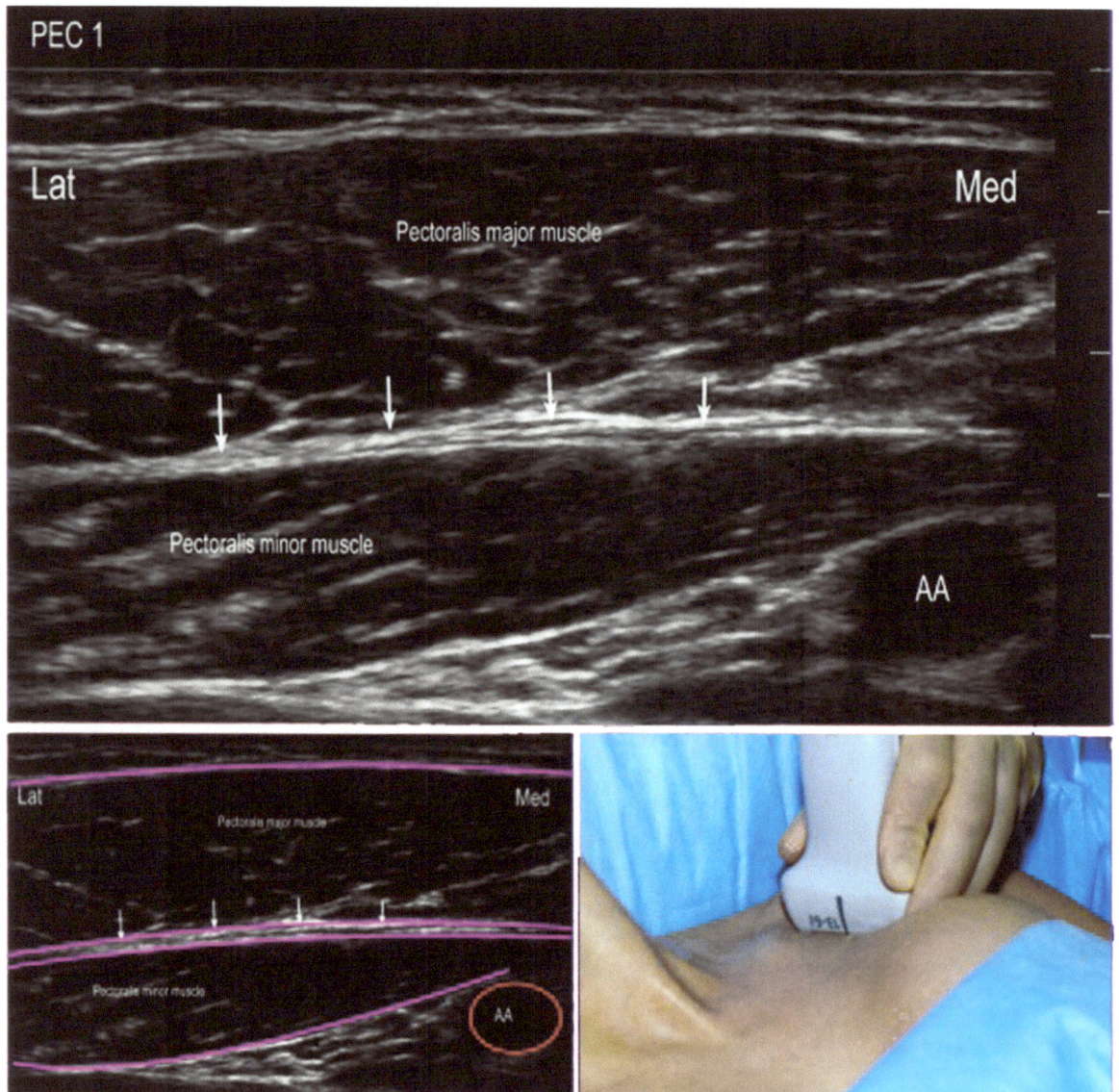

Figure 2-16: Sonoanatomy of the fascial plane between the major and minor pectoral muscles.

AA      Axillary artery
Lat     Lateral
Med   Medial

Arrows indicate the pectoralis fascia plane where the medial and lateral pectoral nerves are situated.

# The Axilla

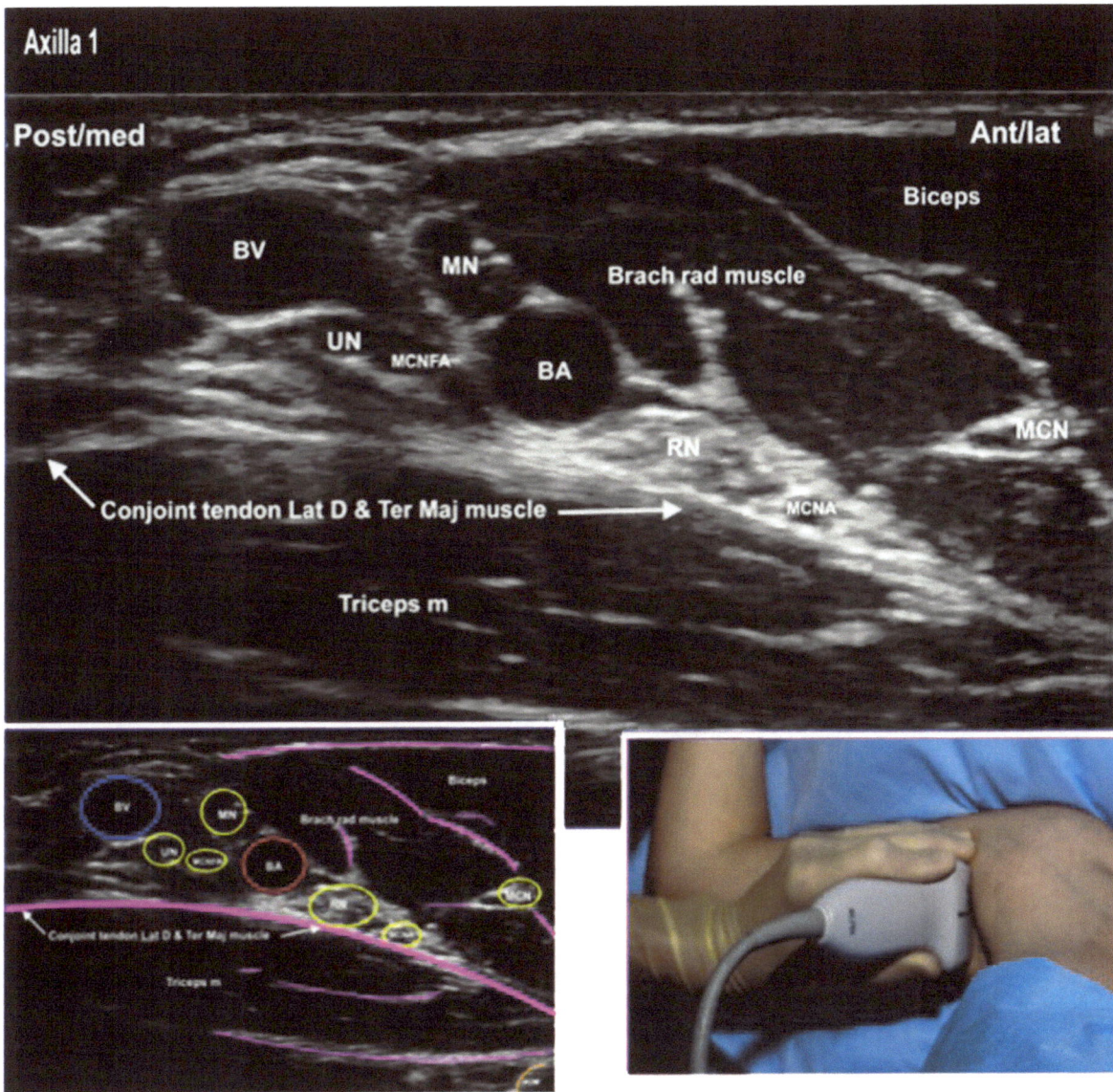

Figure 2-17: Sonoanatomy of the nerves in the axilla.

| | | | |
|---|---|---|---|
| Ant/lat | Anterolateral | RN | Radial nerve |
| BA | Brachial artery | Ter Maj muscle | Teres major muscle |
| Biceps | Biceps brachii muscle | Triceps m | Triceps brachii muscle |
| Brach rad muscle | Brachioradial muscle | UN | Ulnar nerve |
| BV | Brachial vein | | |
| Lat D | Latissimus dorsi muscle | | |
| MCN | Musculocutaneous nerve | | |
| MCNA | Medial cutaneous nerve of the arm | | |
| MCNFA | Medial cutaneous nerve of the forearm | | |
| Post/med | Posteromedial | | |

**View Video at RAEducation.com**

**Acute Pain Medicine - Anatomy -**

**Sonoanatomy: Nerves of the Axilla**

# Mid Humeral Area

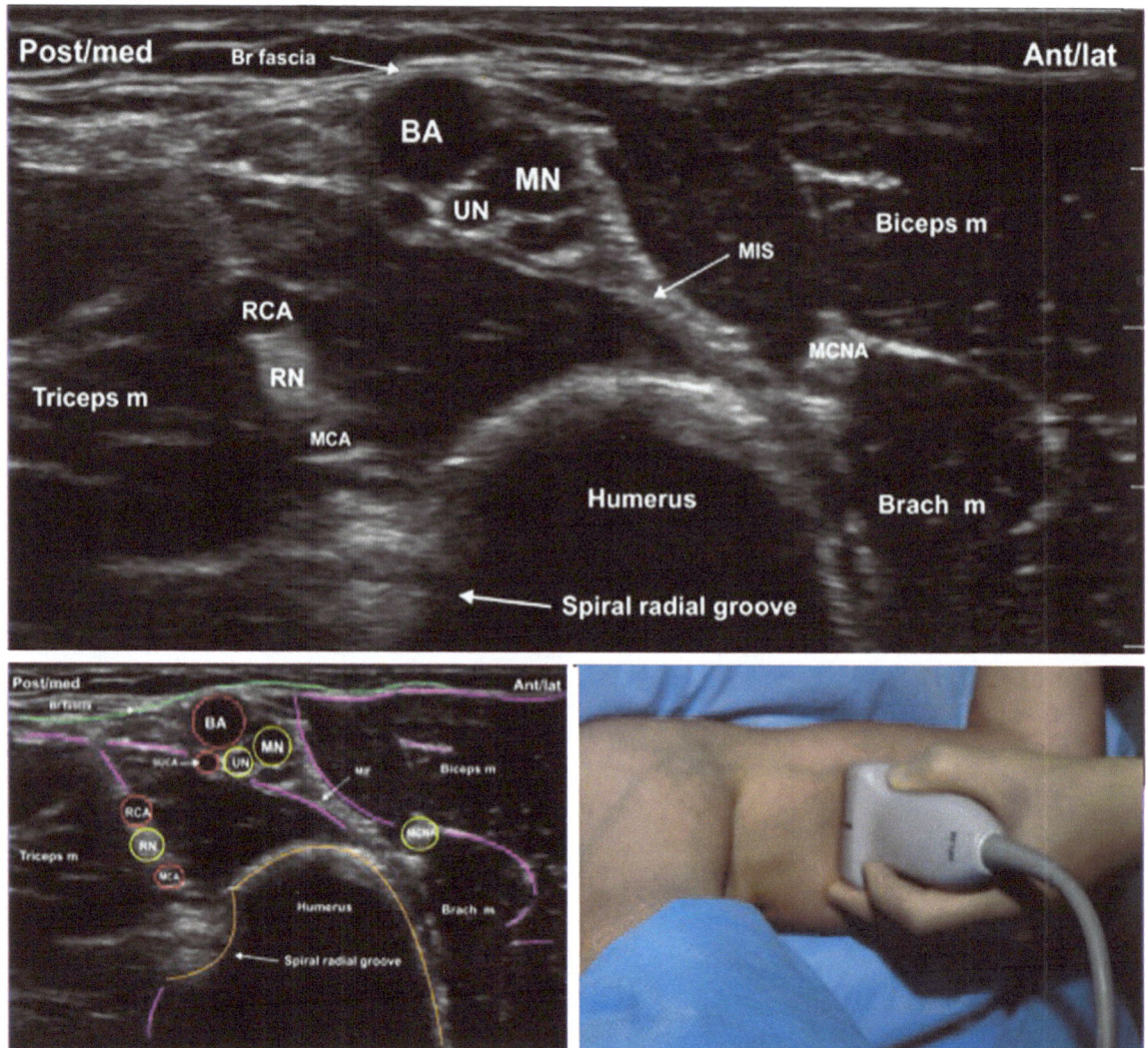

Figure 2-18: Sonoanatomy of the radial nerve as it courses around the humerus through the spiral radial groove.

| | | | |
|---|---|---|---|
| Ant/lat | Anterolateral | RCA | Radial collateral artery |
| BA | Brachial artery | RN | Radial nerve |
| Biceps m | Biceps brachii muscle | Triceps m | Triceps brachii muscle |
| Br fascia | Brachial fascia | UN | Ulnar nerve |
| Brach m | Brachialis muscle | | |
| MCA | Middle collateral artery | | |
| MCNA | Medial cutaneous nerve of the arm | | |
| MIS | Medial intermuscular septum | | |
| MN | Median nerve | | |
| Post/med | Posteromedial | | |

Please note: Above the elbow, the radial nerve is usually a solitary nerve that splits into a deep and a superficial branch at or below the elbow.

# Above the Elbow (Medial)

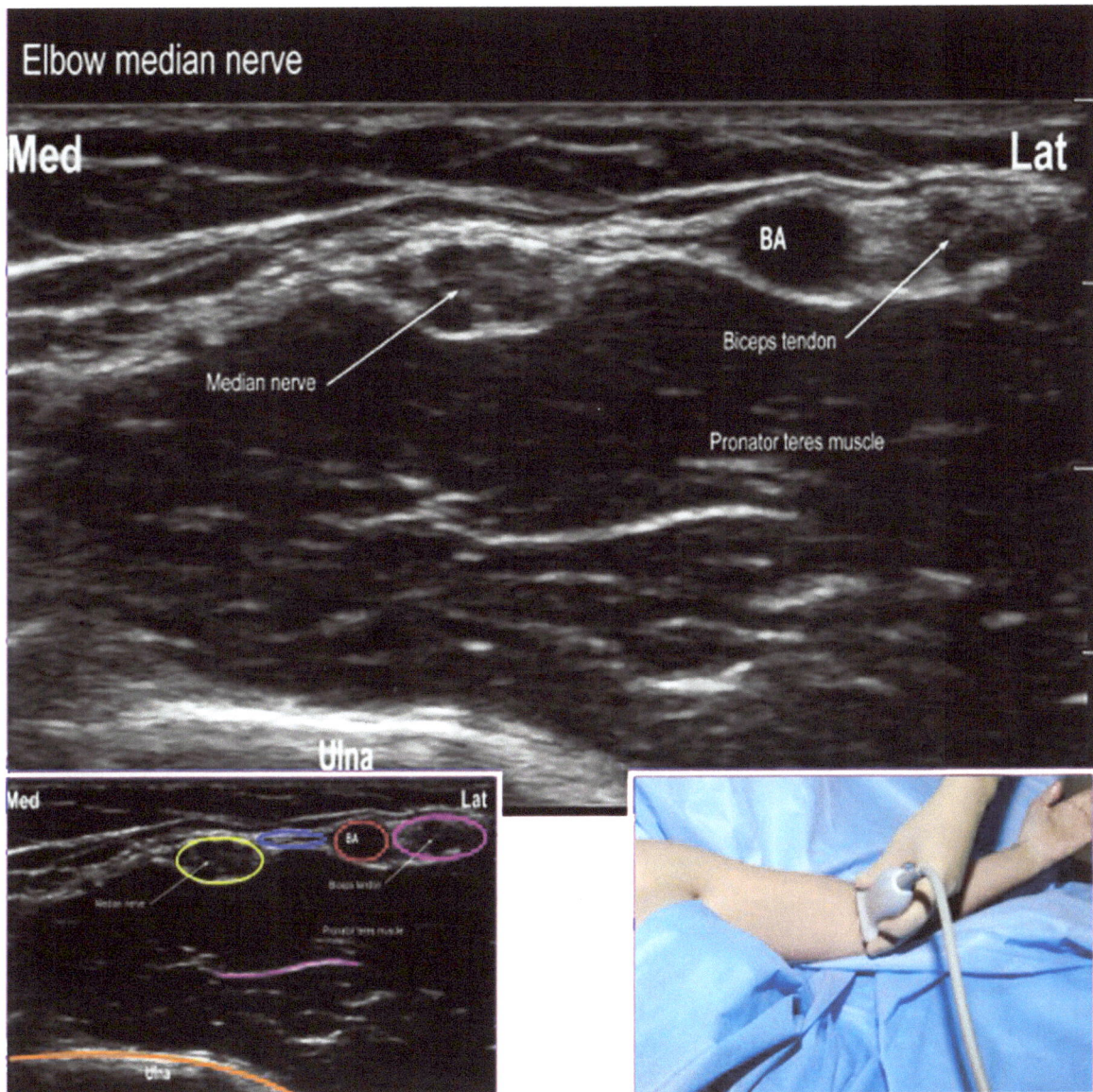

Figure 2-19: The sonoanatomy of the median nerve at the elbow.

BA     Brachial artery
Lat     Lateral
Med    Medial

Please note: The brachial vein, situated in this image between the brachial artery (BA) and the median nerve, has been compressed by the external pressure of the ultrasound probe.

# Above the Elbow (Lateral)

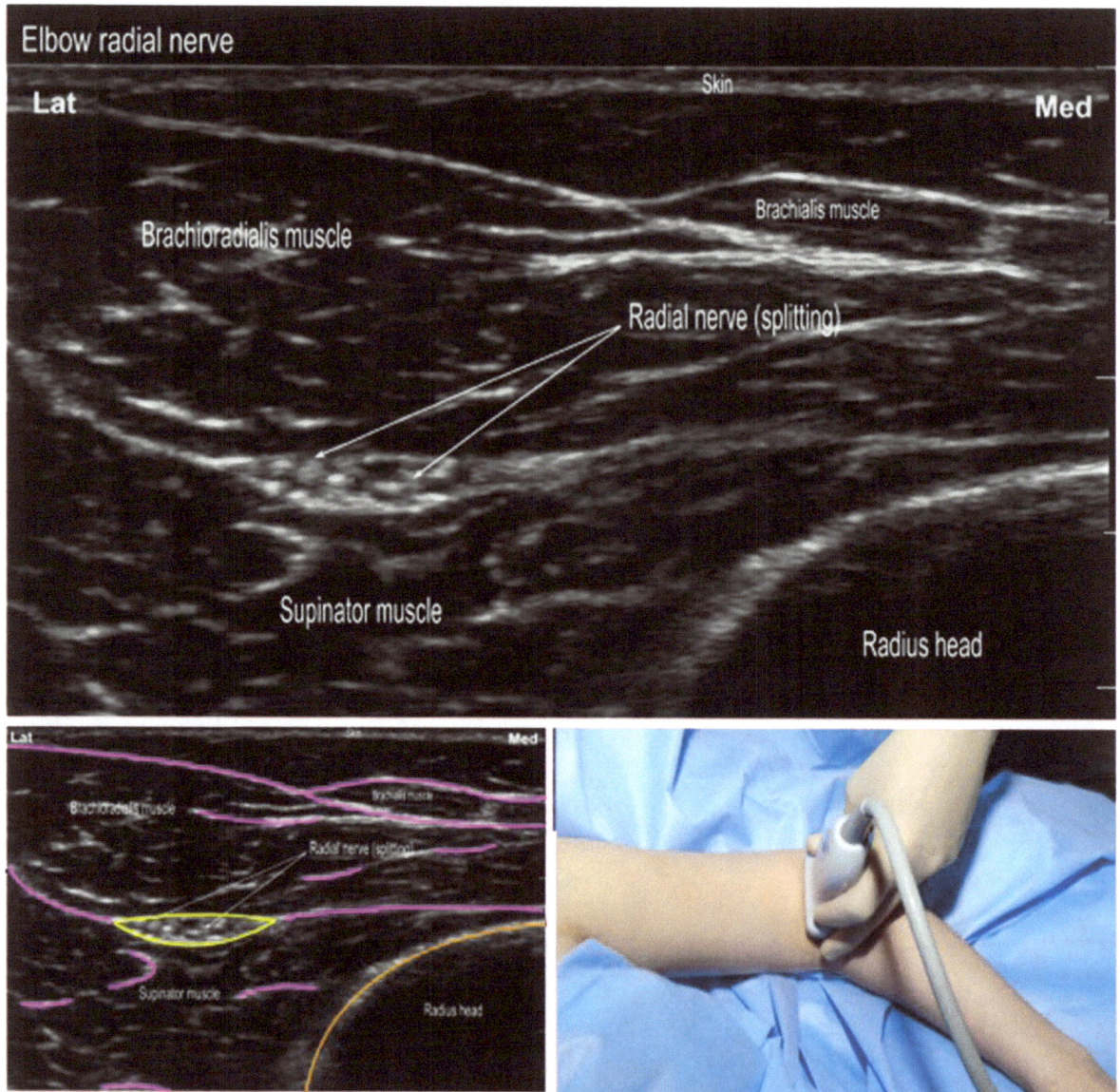

*Figure 2-20: The sonoanatomy of the radial nerve at the elbow.*

Lat    Lateral
Med   Medial

Please note: In this image, the radial nerve is in the process of splitting. Each branch can be followed further distally.

# Above the Elbow (Posterior)

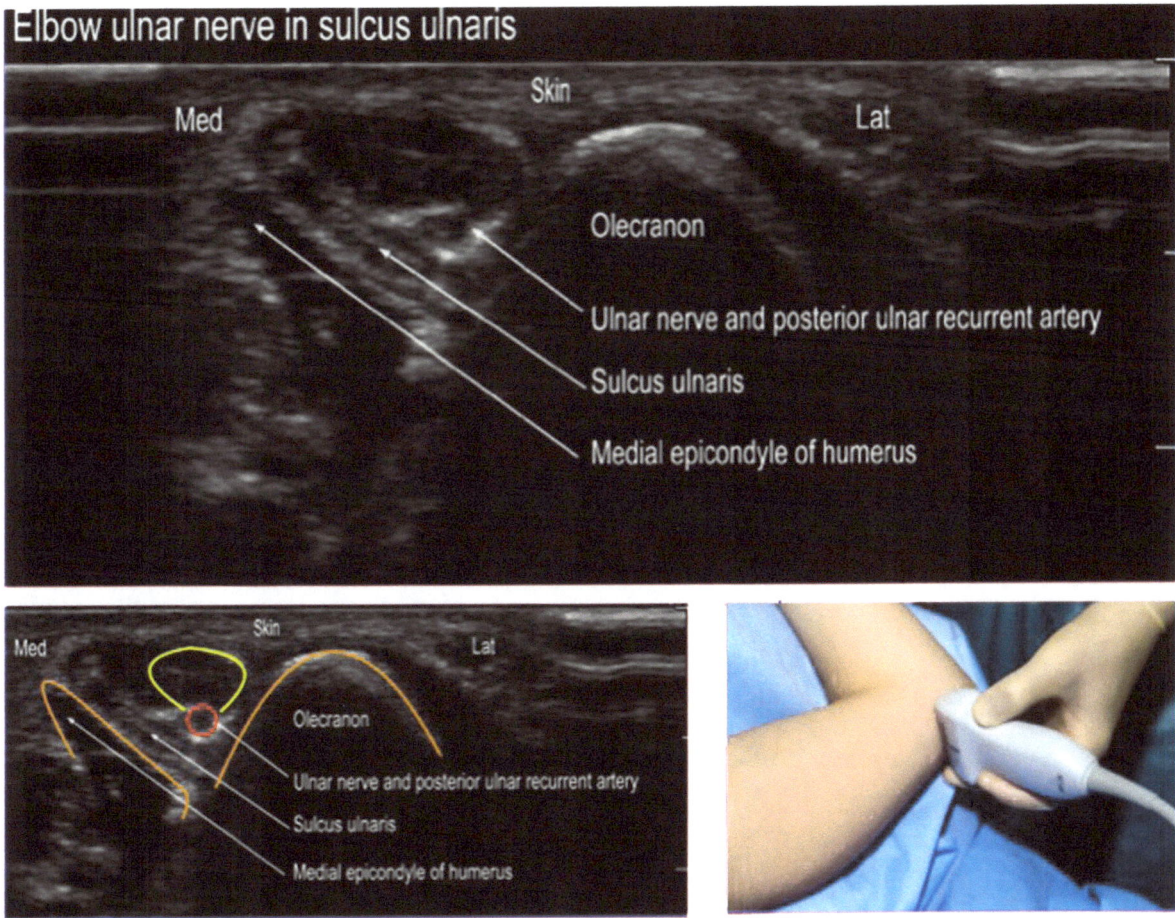

Elbow ulnar nerve in sulcus ulnaris

Med — Skin — Lat

Olecranon

Ulnar nerve and posterior ulnar recurrent artery

Sulcus ulnaris

Medial epicondyle of humerus

Figure 2-21: The sonoanatomy of the ulnar nerve and posterior ulnar recurrent artery in the sulcus ulnaris behind the elbow.

Lat   Lateral
Med   Medial

Please note: The ulnar nerve is in a tight compartment and does not lend itself to a safe nerve block at this level.

# Above the Elbow (Proximal Lateral)

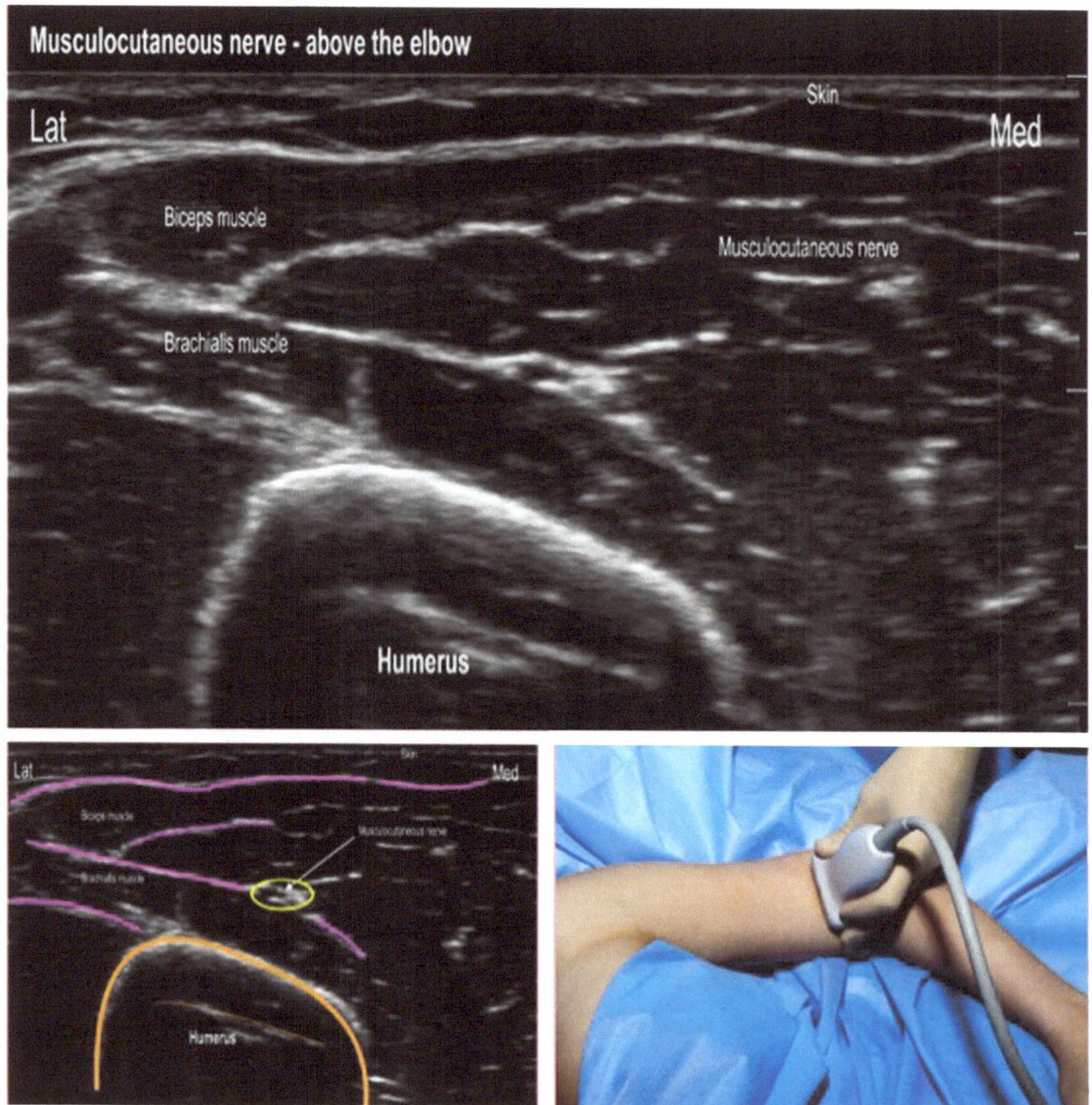

Figure 2-22: *The sonoanatomy of the musculocutaneous nerve in the distal upper arm just above the elbow.*

Lat      Lateral
Med      Medial

# The Wrist (Volar)

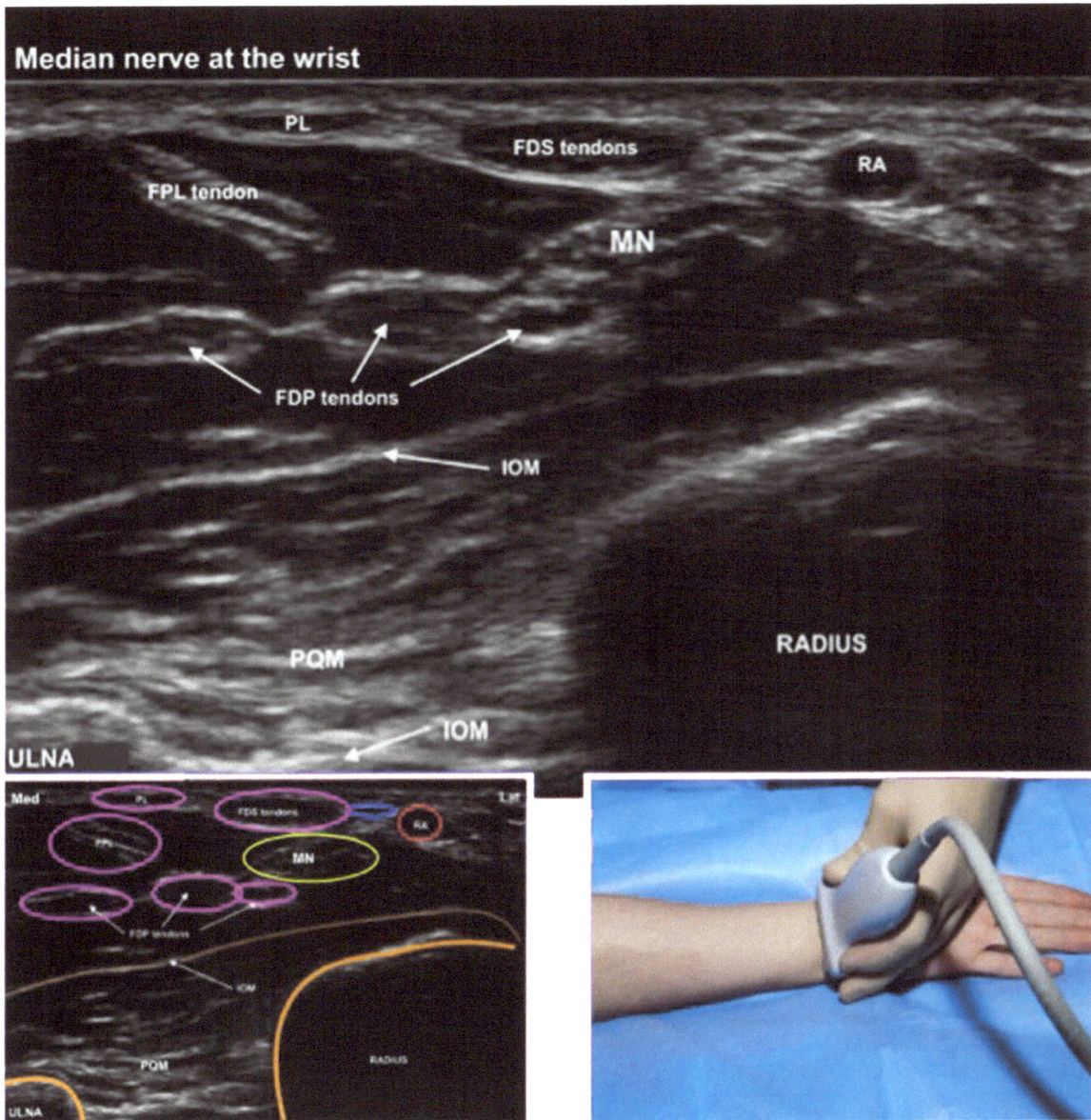

Figure 2-23: Sonoanatomy of the median nerve at the wrist.

| | | | |
|---|---|---|---|
| FDP | Flexor digitorum profundus muscle and tendons | MN | Median nerve |
| FDS tend | Flexor digitorum superficialis tendon | Pl | Palmaris longus muscle |
| FPL | Flexor pollicis longus muscle | PQM | Pronator quadratus muscle |
| IOM | Interosseous membrane | RA | Radial artery |
| Lat | Lateral | | |
| Med | Medial | | |

If the median nerve is followed further distally, it goes under the thick transverse carpal ligament or flexor retinaculum.

# The Wrist (Dorsal)

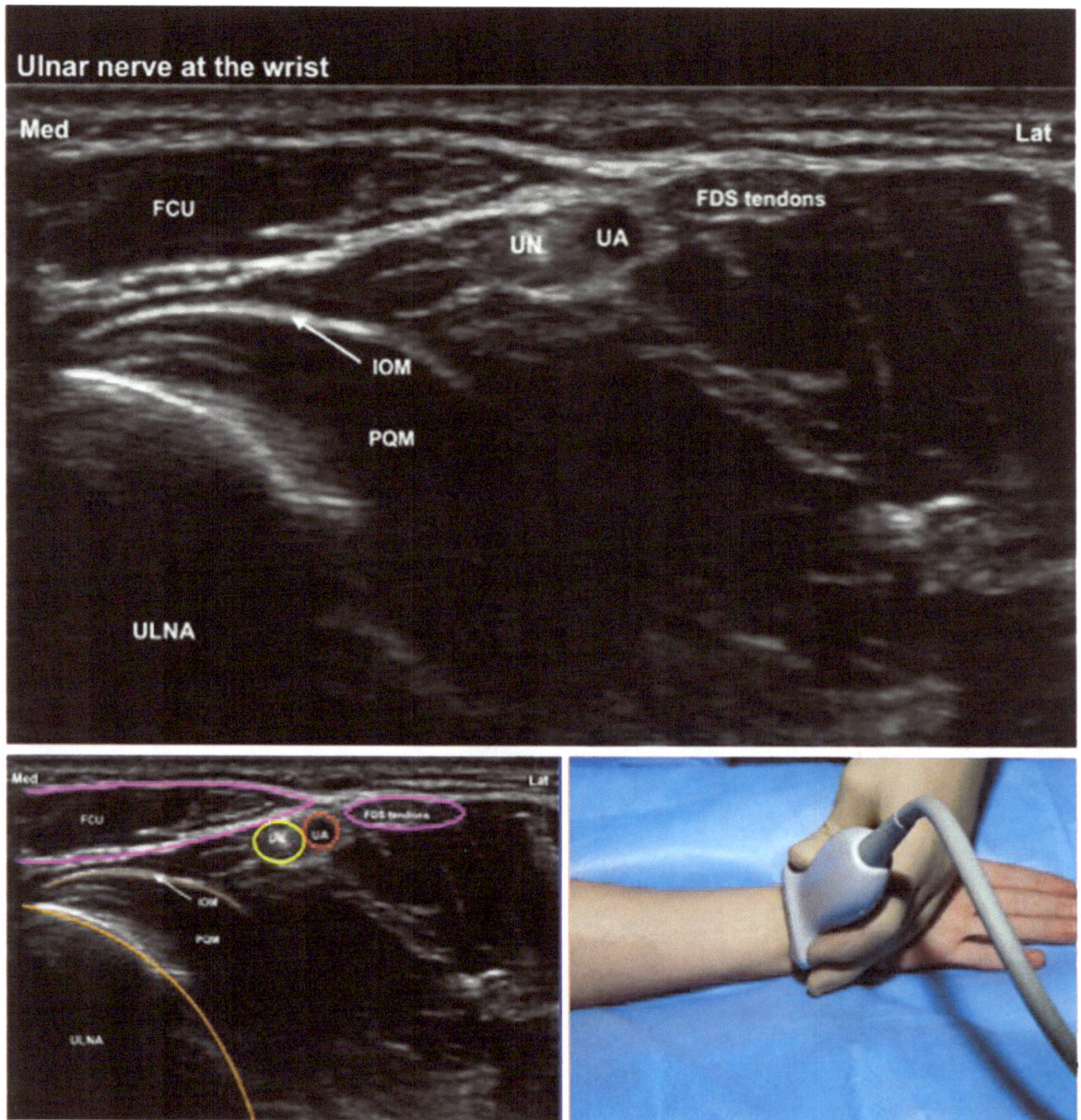

Figure 2-24: Sonoanatomy of the ulnar nerve at the wrist.

| | | | |
|---|---|---|---|
| FCU | Flexor carpi ulnaris tendon | Med | Medial |
| FDS | Flexor digitorum superficialis tendons | PQM | Pronator quadratus muscle |
| | | UA | Ulnar artery |
| IOM | Interosseous membrane | UN | Ulnar nerve |
| Lat | Lateral | | |

# Functional Anatomy

## Neurotomes around the Shoulder

■ Superficial cervical plexus (C3, C4)

■ Intercosto-brachail nerve (T1)

■

■ Axillary nerve (C5, C6)

■

■

■

■

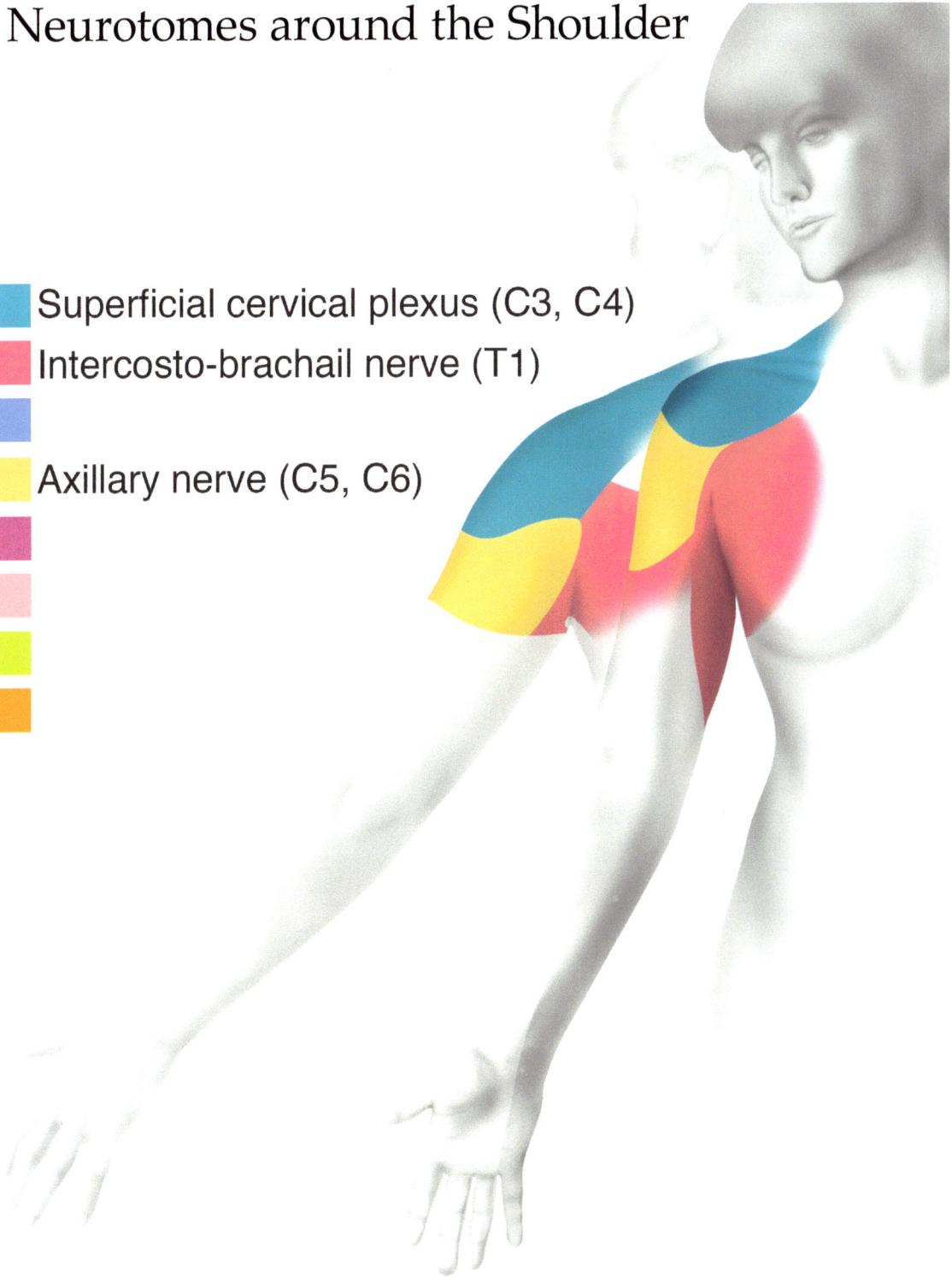

*Figure 2-25: Neurotomes of the superficial cervical plexus, the axillary nerve, and the intercosto-brachial nerve (with their corresponding dermatomal origins).*

# Radial Nerve Neurotome

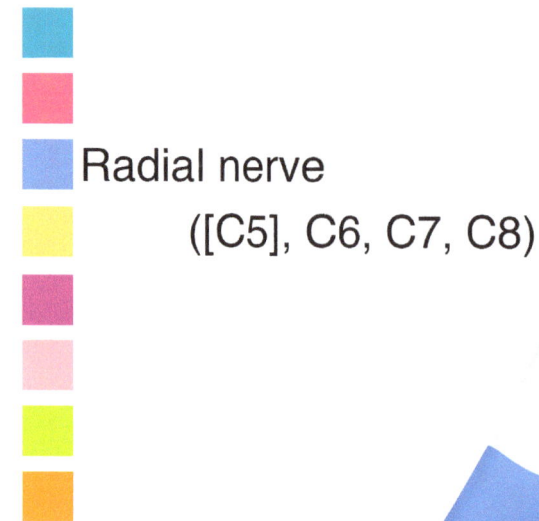

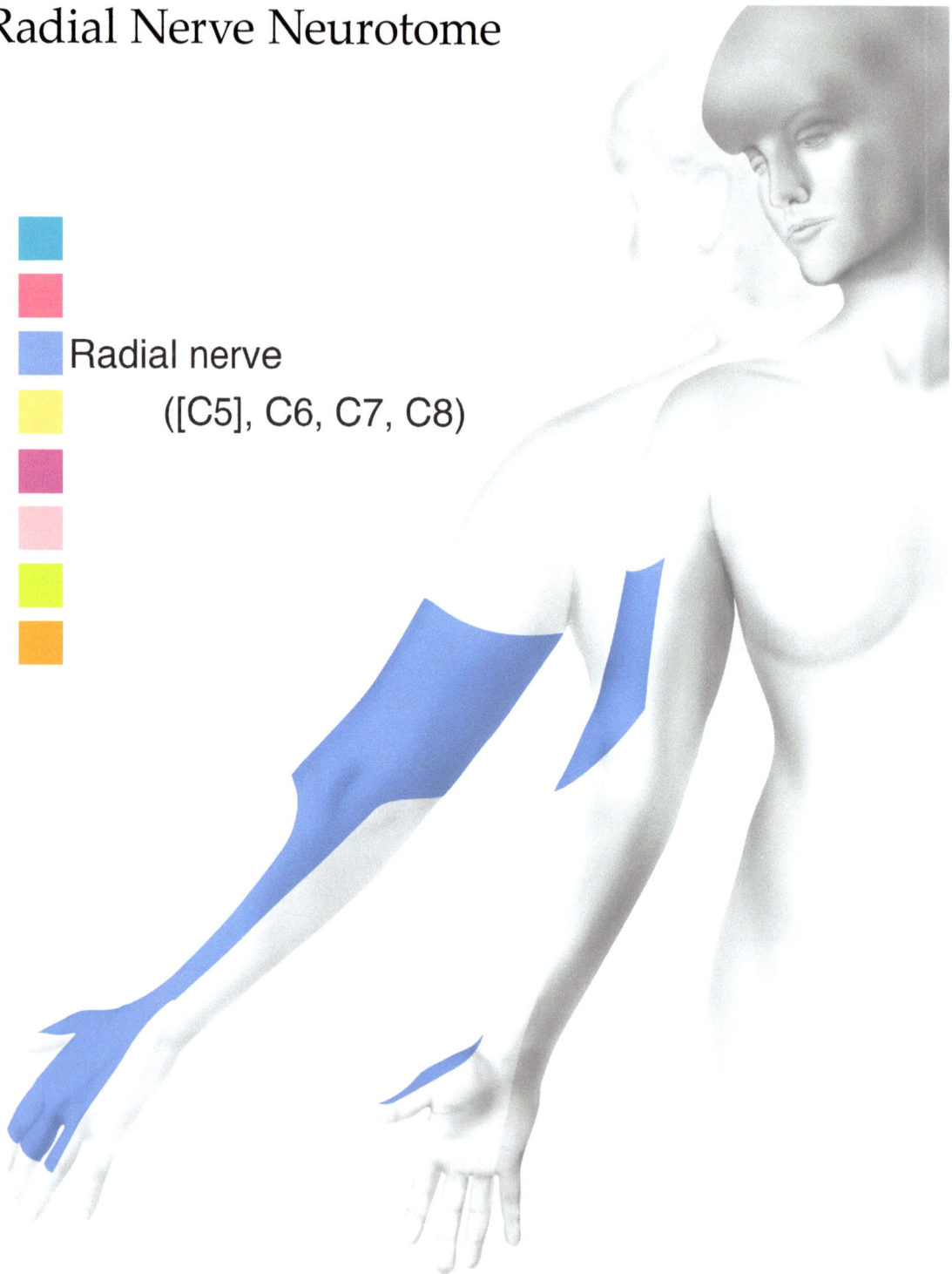

Radial nerve

([C5], C6, C7, C8)

*Figure 2-26: Neurotomes of the radial nerve (with its corresponding dermatomal origins).*

# Musculotaneous Nerve Nuerotome

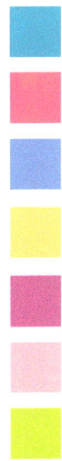

Musculocutaneous nerve (C5, C6, [C7])

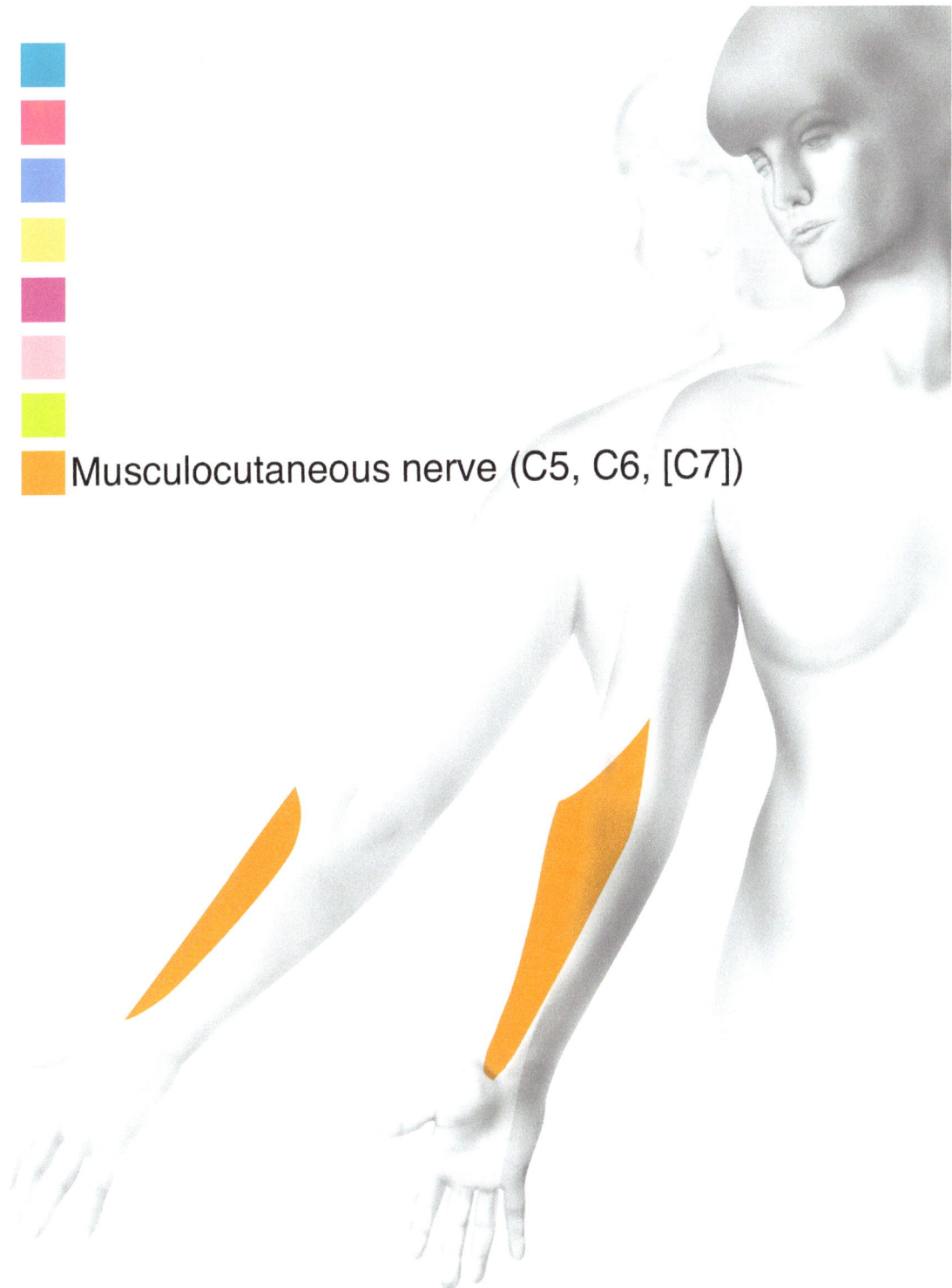

*Figure 2-27: Neurotomes of the musculocutaneous nerve (with its corresponding dermatomal origins).*

# Median Cutaneous Nerve Neurotome

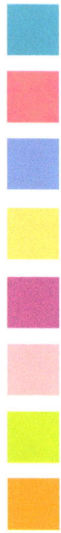

Med. cutaneous n. of forearm (C8, T1)

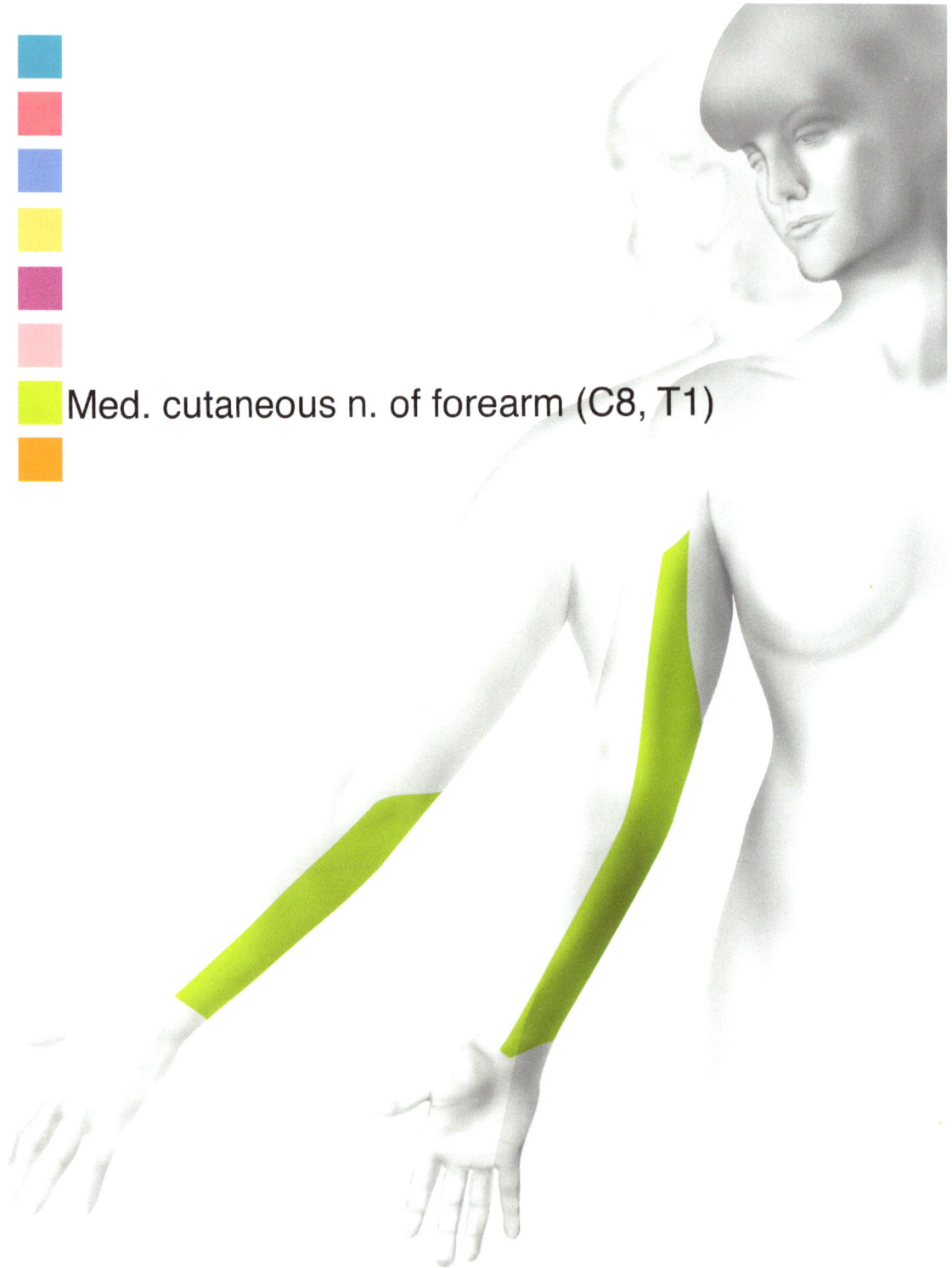

*Figure 2-28: Neurotomes of the median cutaneous nerve of the forearm (with its corresponding dermatomal origins).*

# Median Nerve & Ulnar Nerve Neurotomes

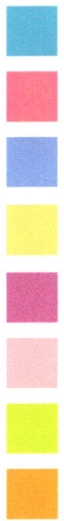

■ Ulnar nerve (C8, T1)
■ Median nerve
     (C6, C7, C8)

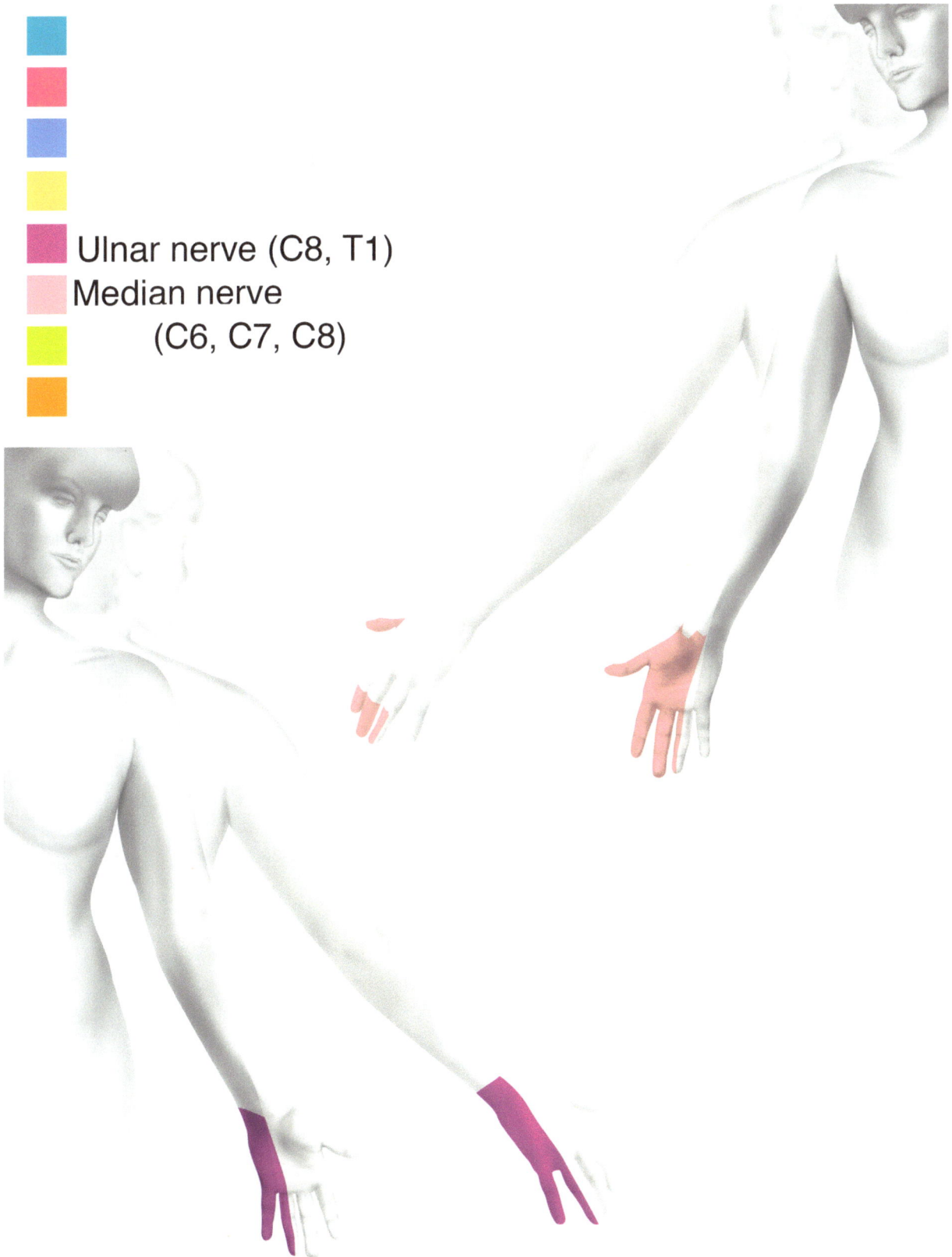

*Figure 2-29: The right figure shows the neurotomes of the median nerve.and the left figure shows the neurotomes of the ulnar nerve (both with corresponding dermatomal origins).*

# Myotomes of Median & Musculocutaneous Nerves
# The Lateral Cord

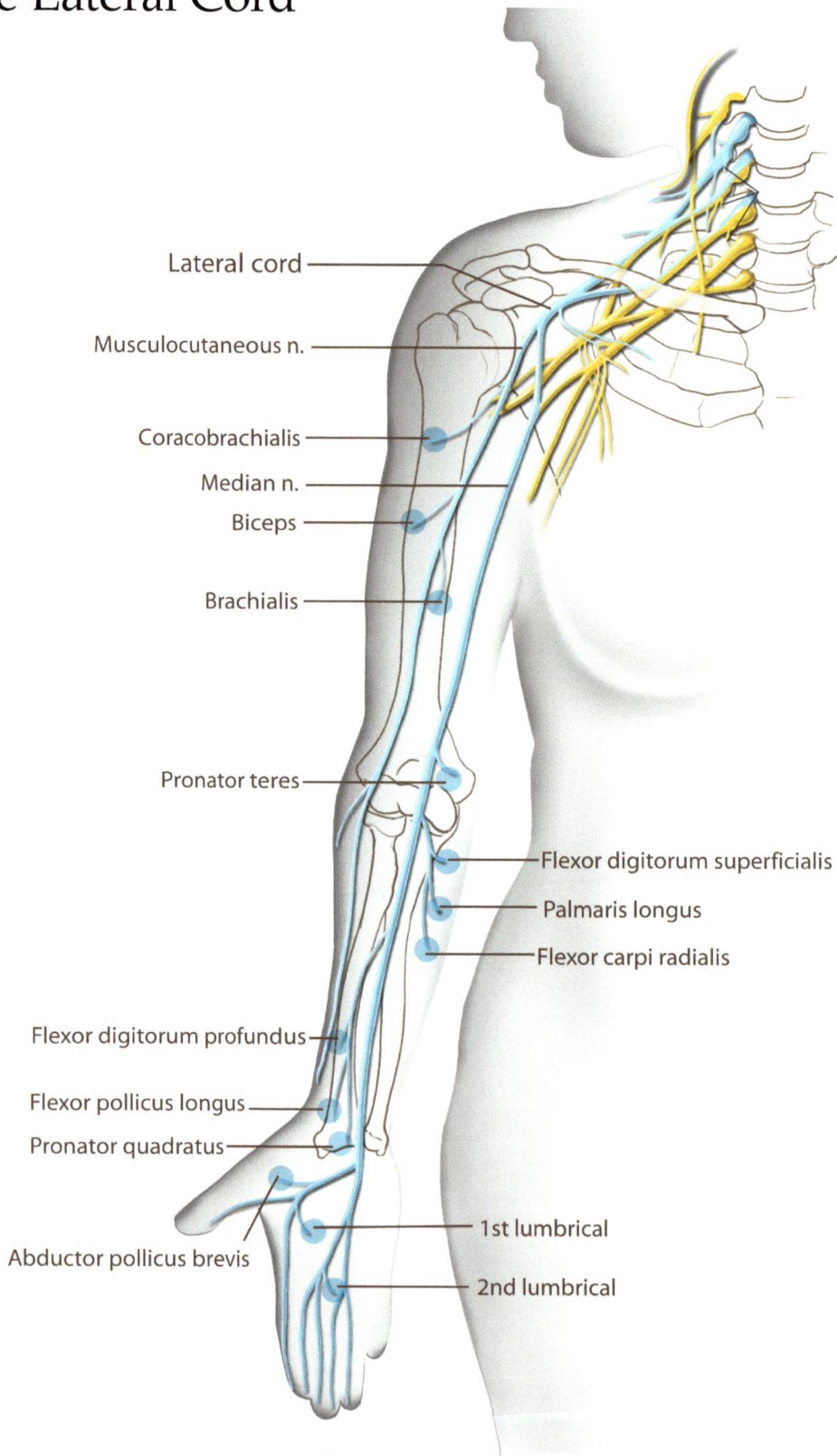

Lateral cord

Musculocutaneous n.

Coracobrachialis

Median n.

Biceps

Brachialis

Pronator teres

Flexor digitorum superficialis

Palmaris longus

Flexor carpi radialis

Flexor digitorum profundus

Flexor pollicus longus

Pronator quadratus

1st lumbrical

Abductor pollicus brevis

2nd lumbrical

*Figure 2-30: Functional anatomy of the musculocutaneous and median nerves (lateral cord).*

The musculocutaneous nerve innervates the coracobrachialis and biceps and brachialis muscles – all flexors of the upper arm. The median nerve has no branches in the upper arm and, in the forearm, innervates the pronator of the forearm and superficial flexor of the medial two fingers and deep flexors of the lateral fingers. It finally supplies motor innervation to the abductor of the thumb and the first and second lumbrical muscles. One, therefore, expects that electrical stimulation of the lateral cord will result in flexion at the elbow, pronation of the forearm, and flexion in the hand. The net effect of this will be that the fifth digit, the pinkie, will move laterally – toward the cord being stimulated, i.e., the lateral cord.

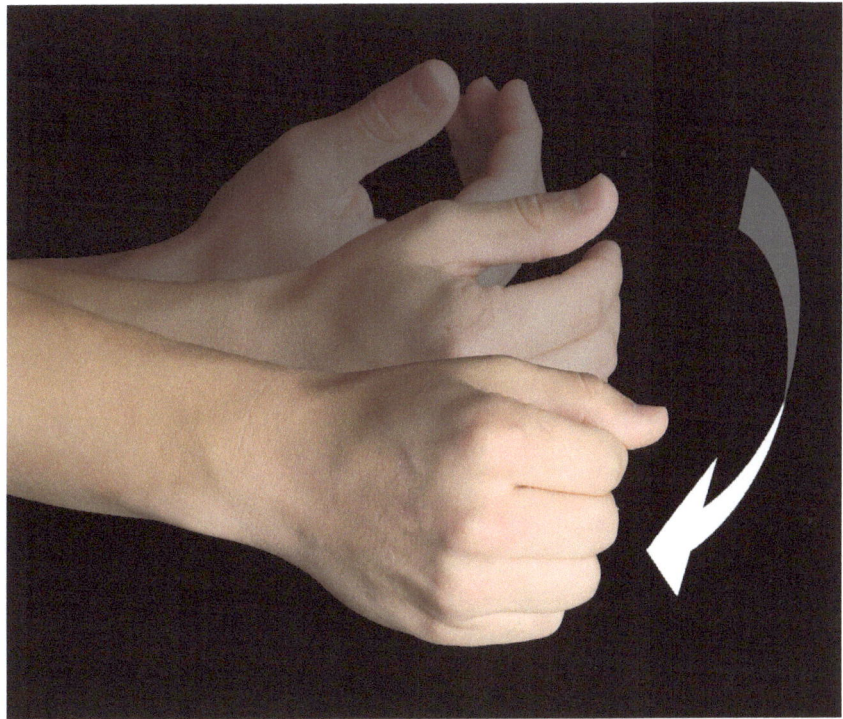

*Figure 2-31: Functional anatomy of the brachial plexus cords – the lateral cord.*

**View Video at RAEducation.com**
**Acute Pain Medicine - Anatomy -**
**Functional Anatomy: Upper extremity**

*Ref: Borene SC, Edwards JN, Boezaart AP. At the cords, the pinkie towards: Interpreting infraclavicular motor responses to neurostimulation. Reg Anesth Pain Med 2004;29:125-129.*

# Myotomes of Axillary & Radial Nerves
# The Posterior Cord

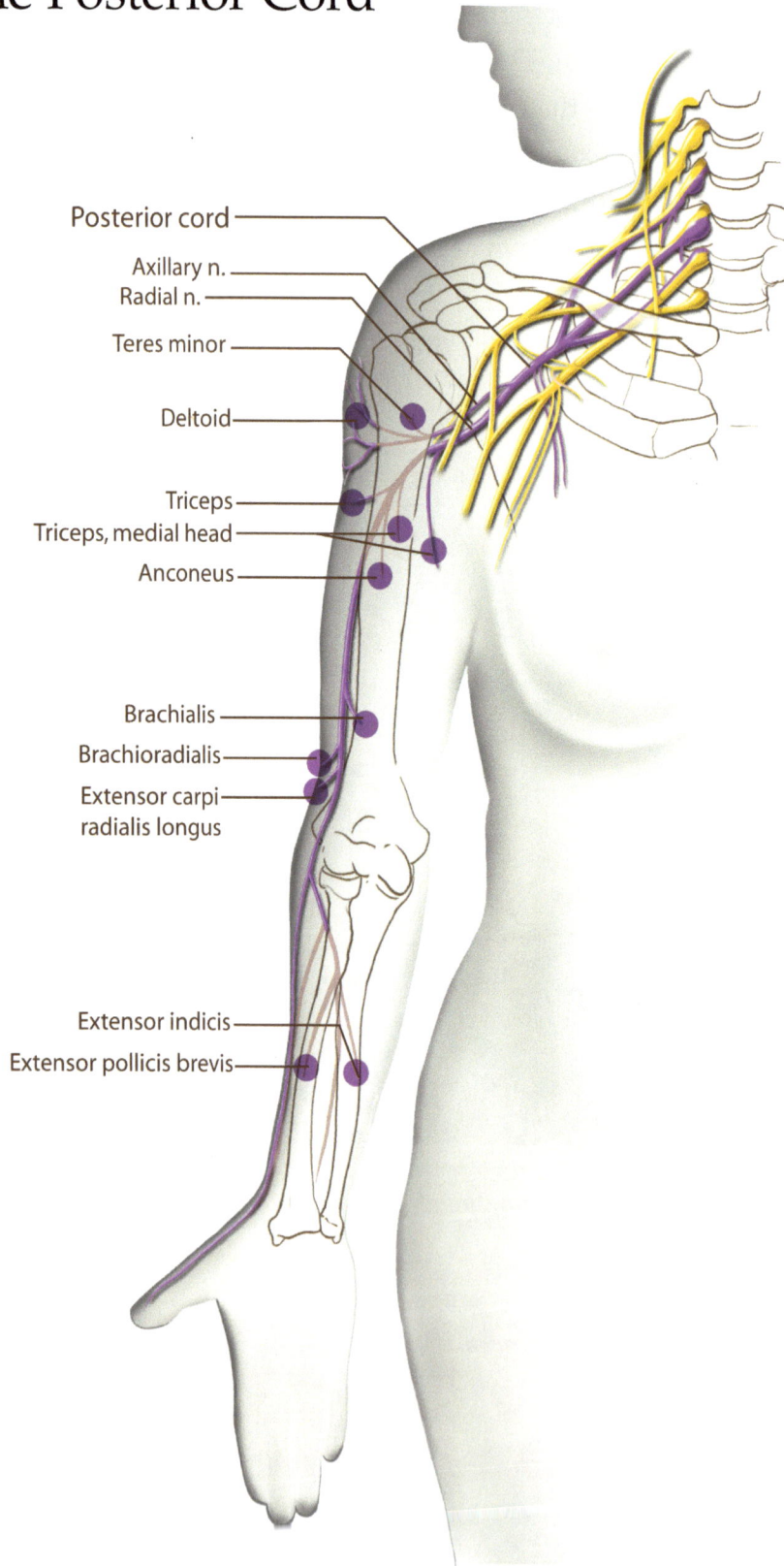

Posterior cord

Axillary n.

Radial n.

Teres minor

Deltoid

Triceps

Triceps, medial head

Anconeus

Brachialis

Brachioradialis

Extensor carpi
radialis longus

Extensor indicis

Extensor pollicis brevis

Figure 2-32: Functional anatomy of the axillary and radial nerves  (posterior cord).

The axillary nerve supplies motor innervation to the deltoid muscle, whereas the radial nerve innervates the extensor muscles of the arm, forearm, wrist, and hand. One, therefore, expects that electrical stimulation of the posterior cord will result in extension of the elbow, wrist and hand. The pinkie moves posterior, due to extension of the elbow and fingers when the posterior cord is stimulated. It should now be obvious that the fifth digit, or pinkie, moves "toward" the cord that is being stimulated.

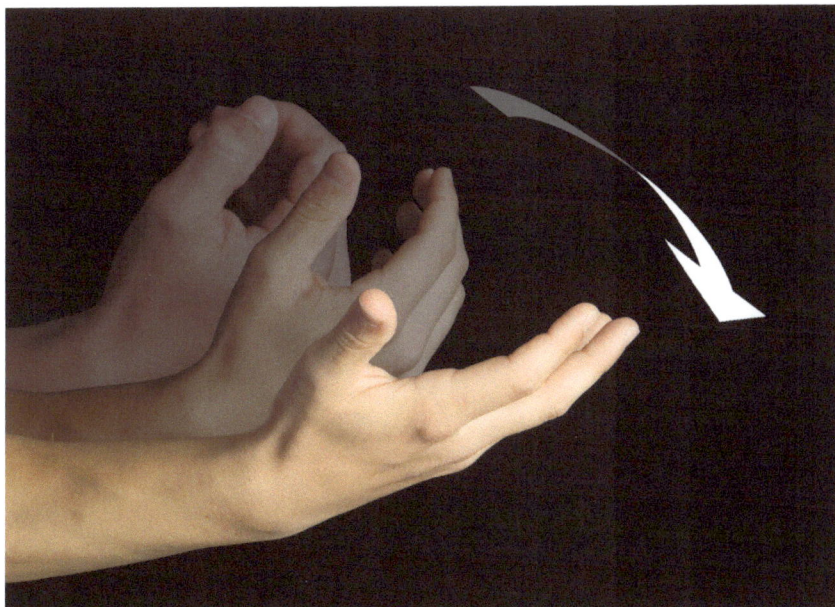

Figure 2-33: Functional anatomy of the brachial plexus cords – the posterior cord.

Ref: Borene SC, Edwards JN, Boezaart AP. At the cords, the pinkie towards: Interpreting infraclavicular motor responses to neurostimulation. Reg Anesth Pain Med 2004;29:125-129.

# Myotomes of Ulnar Nerve
## The Medial Cord

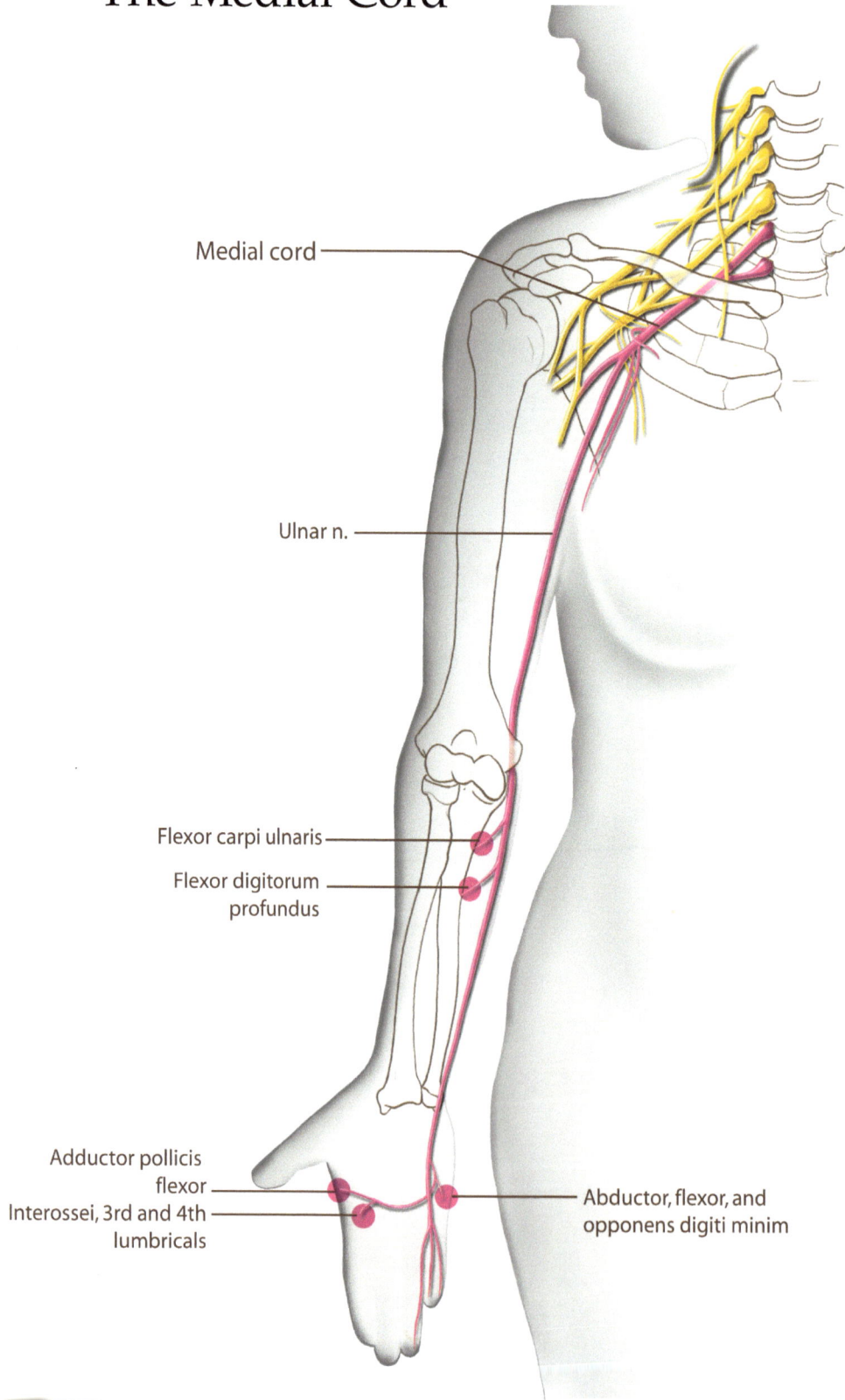

Medial cord

Ulnar n.

Flexor carpi ulnaris

Flexor digitorum profundus

Adductor pollicis flexor

Interossei, 3rd and 4th lumbricals

Abductor, flexor, and opponens digiti minim

*Figure 2-34: Functional anatomy of the ulnar nerve (medial cord).*

The ulnar nerve supplies motor innervation to the deep flexors of the forearm, the abductor, the flexor and opponens of the fifth digit, and the abductor of the thumb and 3rd and 4th lumbrical muscles in the hand. The median nerve has no branches in the upper arm. It innervates the pronator of the forearm, superficial flexors of the medial two fingers, and deep flexors of the lateral fingers. It also innervates the abductor of the thumb and the first and second lumbrical muscles. One, therefore, expects that electrical stimulation of the medial cord will result in flexion of the fingers and flexion and ulnar deviation of the wrist. With the arm in the anatomical position, the fifth digit moves medially when the medial cord is stimulated. This is because of flexion of the fingers and ulnar deviation of the wrist.

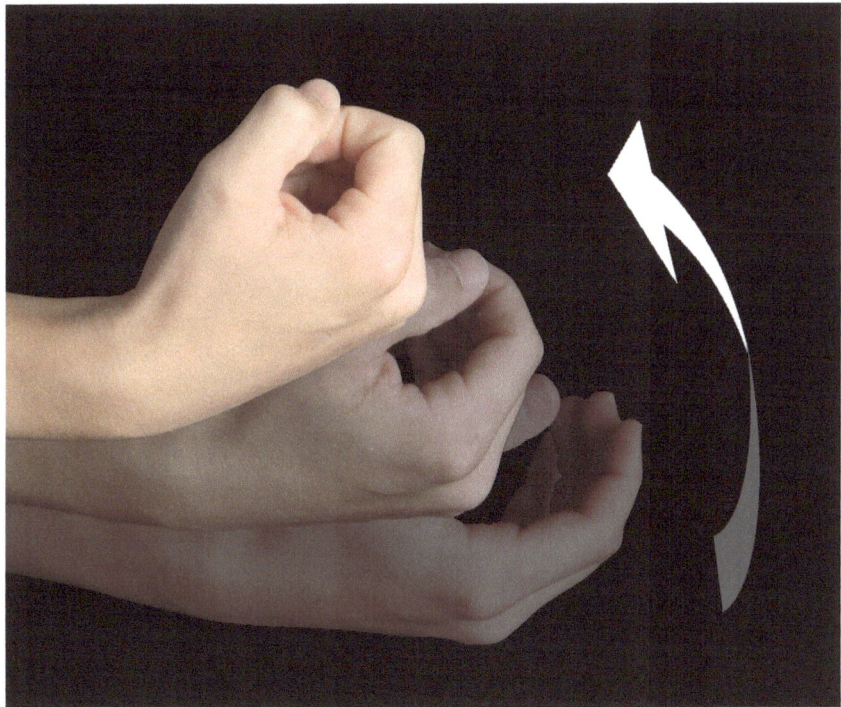

*Figure 2-35: Functional anatomy of the brachial plexus cords – the medial cord cuases flexion of tje fingers and wrist.*

*Ref: Borene SC, Edwards JN, Boezaart AP. At the cords, the pinkie towards: Interpreting infraclavicular motor responses to neurostimulatio). Reg Anesth Pain Med 2004;29:125-129.*

## Videos & more information available at RAEducation.com

Learn more about the effects of electrical stimulation of the:
1. C5/6 root
2. The brachial plexus upper trunk
3. The cervical accessory nerve
4. The dorsal scapular nerve
5. The nerve to levator scapulae
6. The phrenic nerve
7. The suprascapular nerve
8. The radial nerve
9. The ulnar nerve
10. The median nerve
11. The musculocutaneous nerve

References:

Borene SC, Edwards JN, Boezaart AP. At the cords, the pinkie towards: Interpreting infraclavicular motor responses to neurostimulation. Reg Anesth Pain Med 2004;29:125-129.

Boezaart AP, Franco CD. Blocks above the clavicle. In: Boezaart AP, Ed. Anesthesia and orthopaedic surgery. New York: McGraw-Hill, 2006: 291-309.

Bösenberg AT, Raw R, Boezaart AP. Surface mapping of peripheral nerves in children with a nerve stimulator. Paediatr Anaest 2002;12:398-403.

Leis AA, Trapani VC. Atlas of Electromyography. Cambridge, UK: Oxford University Press 2000: 95-105.

# Chapter 3

## The Anterior Thigh

*Macroanatomy*
*Microanatomy*
*Sonoanatomy*
*Functional Anatomy*

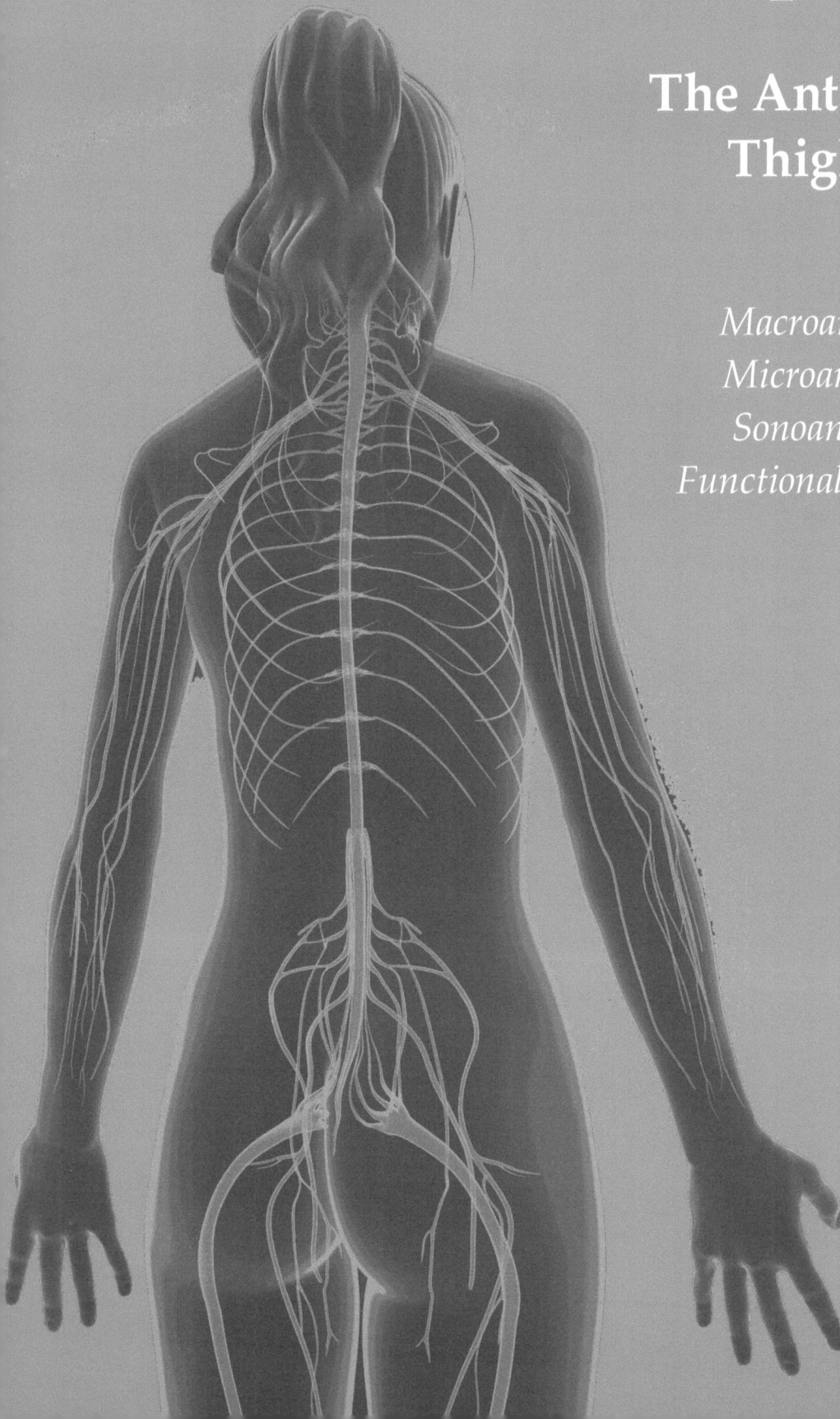

# Macroanatomy

## The Lumbosacral Plexus

### Nerves

1. Subcostal nerve (T12)
2. Iliohypogastric nerve (L1)
3. Ilioinguinal nerve (L1)
4. Lateral femoral cutaneous nerve (L2,3)
5. Femoral branch of genitofemoral nerve (L1,2)
6. Genital branch of genitofemoral nerve (L1,2)
7. Femoral nerve (L2,3,4)
8. Sciatic nerve
   a. Common peroneal nerve (L4,5,S1,2)
   b. Tibial nerve (L4,5,S1,2,3)
9. Posterior femoral cutaneous nerve (S1,2,3)
10. Nerve to Sartorius muscle (L2,3,4)
11. Saphenous branch of the Femoral nerve
12. Obturator nerve (L2,3,4)
13. Pudendal nerve (S1,2,3)
14. Sympathetic trunk
15. Lumbosacral trunk

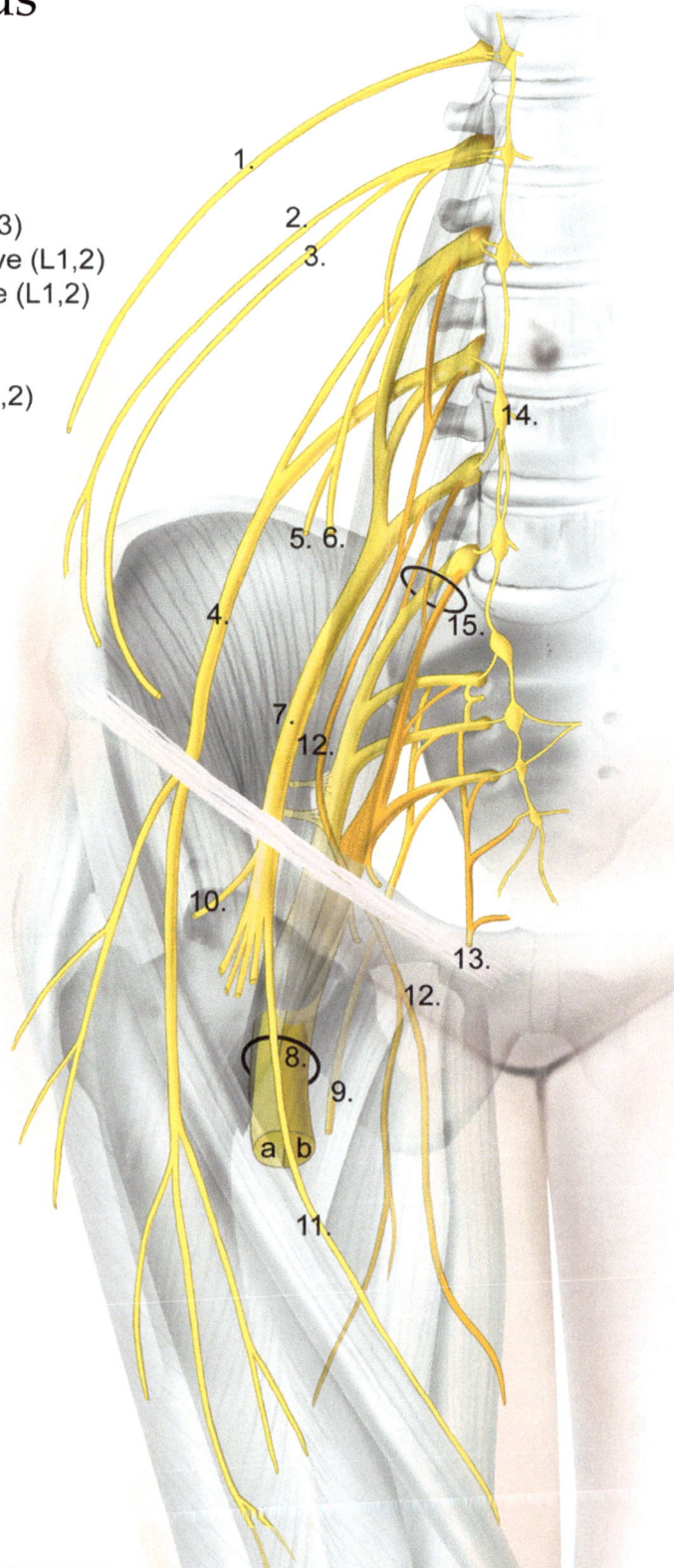

*Figure 3-1: Schematic representation of the lumbosacral plexus and its nerves.*

- The subcostal (1) and the ilioinguinal and iliohypogastric nerves (2, 3) originate from the 12th thoracic (T12) and 1st lumbar (L1) vertebra, respectively.
- The lateral cutaneous nerve of the thigh (4) and the genitofemoral nerve originate from the ventral rami of the 1st and 2nd lumbar vertebrae (L1 & L2), whereas the femoral nerve (7) stems from the dorsal rami of L2, L3, and L4.
- The 5th lumbar spinal root also gives of a branch to the lumbosacral trunk (15) at the level of L5.
- The anterior rami of L2 to L4 form the obturator nerve (12), whereas L5 and the first three sacral roots (S1, S2, and S3) form the sciatic nerve (8).
- The pudendal nerve (13) also originates from these roots.

# Dissection of Anterior Nerves of Leg - Pelvic View

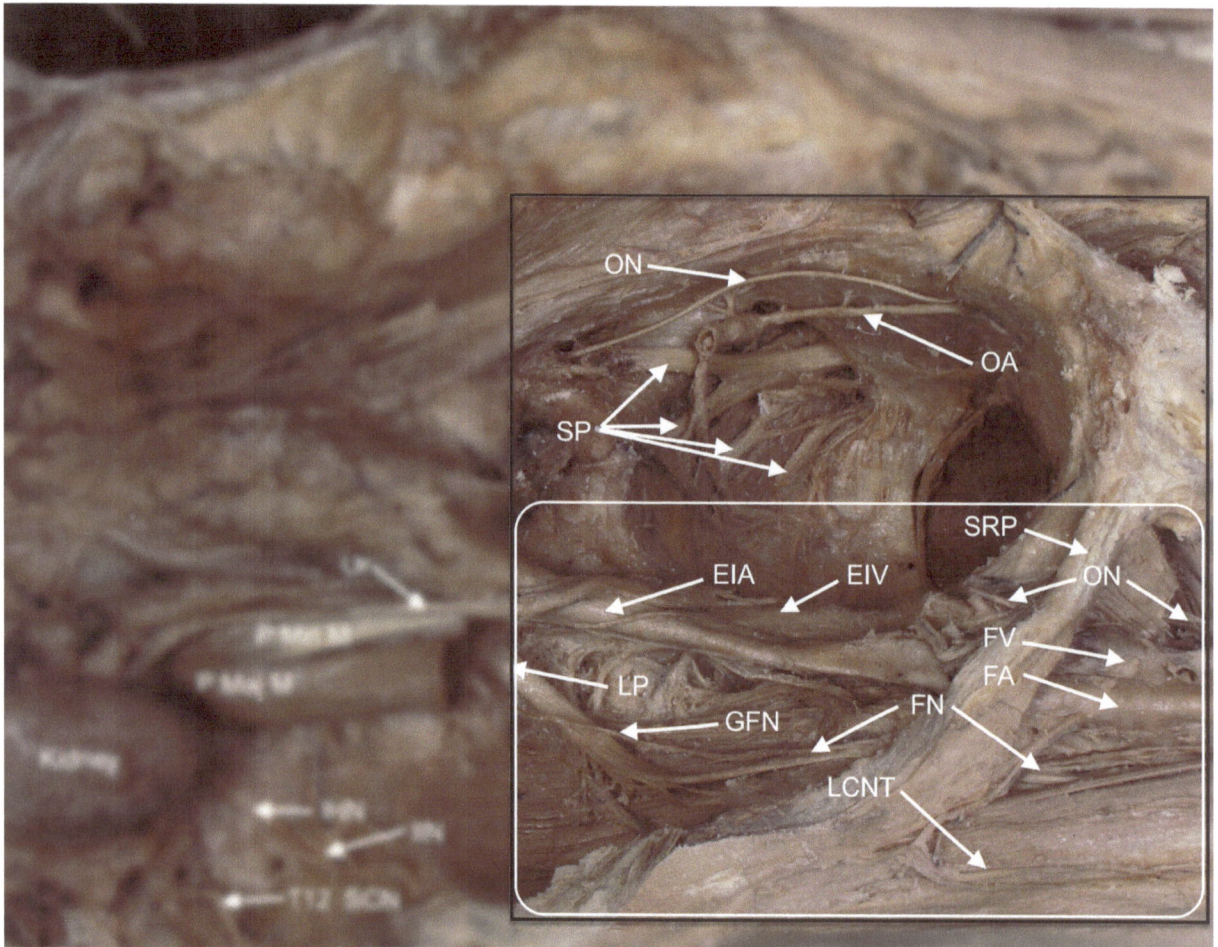

Figure 3-2: Anatomical dissection of femoral, obturator, and lateral cutaneous nerves of the thigh: abdominal view.

| | | | |
|---|---|---|---|
| EIA | External iliac artery | LCNT | Lateral cutaneous nerve of the thigh |
| EIV | External iliac vein | LP | Lumbar plexus |
| FA | Femoral artery | OA | Obturator artery |
| FN | Femoral nerve | ON | Obturator nerve |
| FV | Femoral vein | SP | Sacral plexus |
| GFN | Genitofemoral nerve | SRP | Superior ramus of the pubis. |

# Dissection of the Anterior Thigh

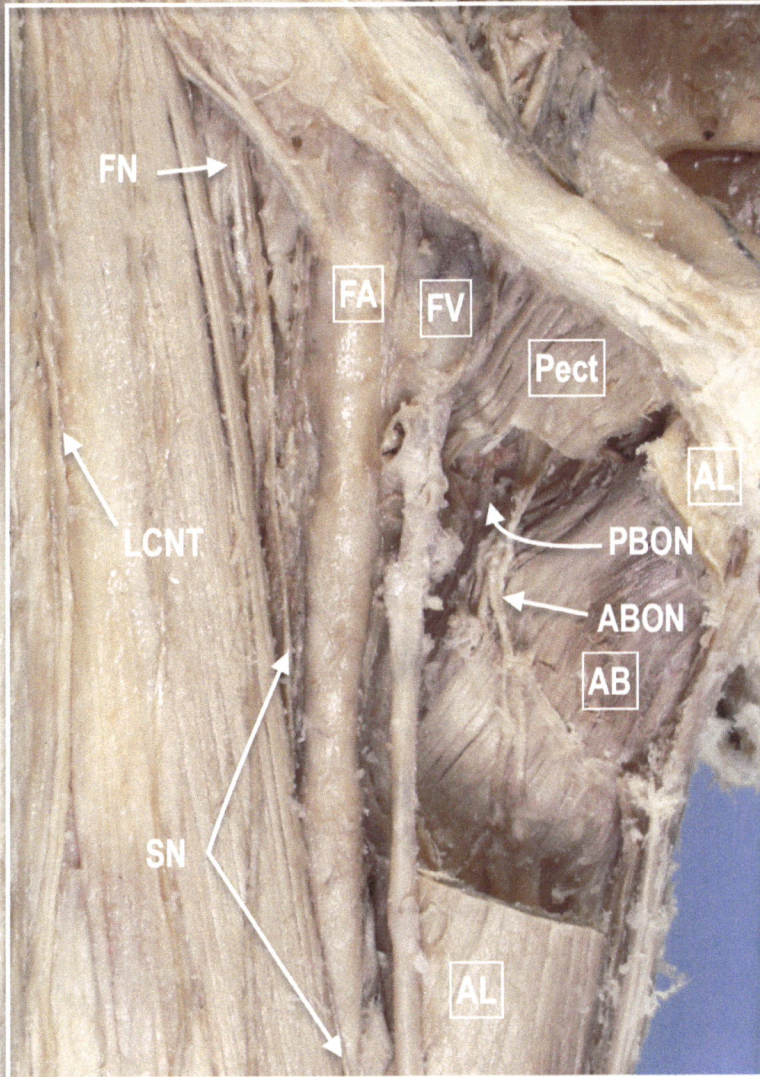

*Figure 3-3: Dissection of the upper thigh depicting the femoral and obturator nerves.*

AB        Adductor brevis muscle
ABON    Anterior branch of obturator nerve
AL        Adductor longus muscle (cut)
FA        Femoral artery
FN        Femoral nerve
FV        Femoral vein
LCNT    Lateral cutaneous nerve of the thigh
PBON    Posterior branch of obturator nerve
Pect      Pectinius muscle
SN        Saphenous nerve

The obturator nerve exits the obturator foramen and splits into an anterior (ABON) and posterior (PBON) branch. The anterior branch descends anterior to the adductor brevis muscle (AB), whereas the posterior branch descends between the adductor brevis and magnus muscles.

# Transection through the Superior Anterior Thigh

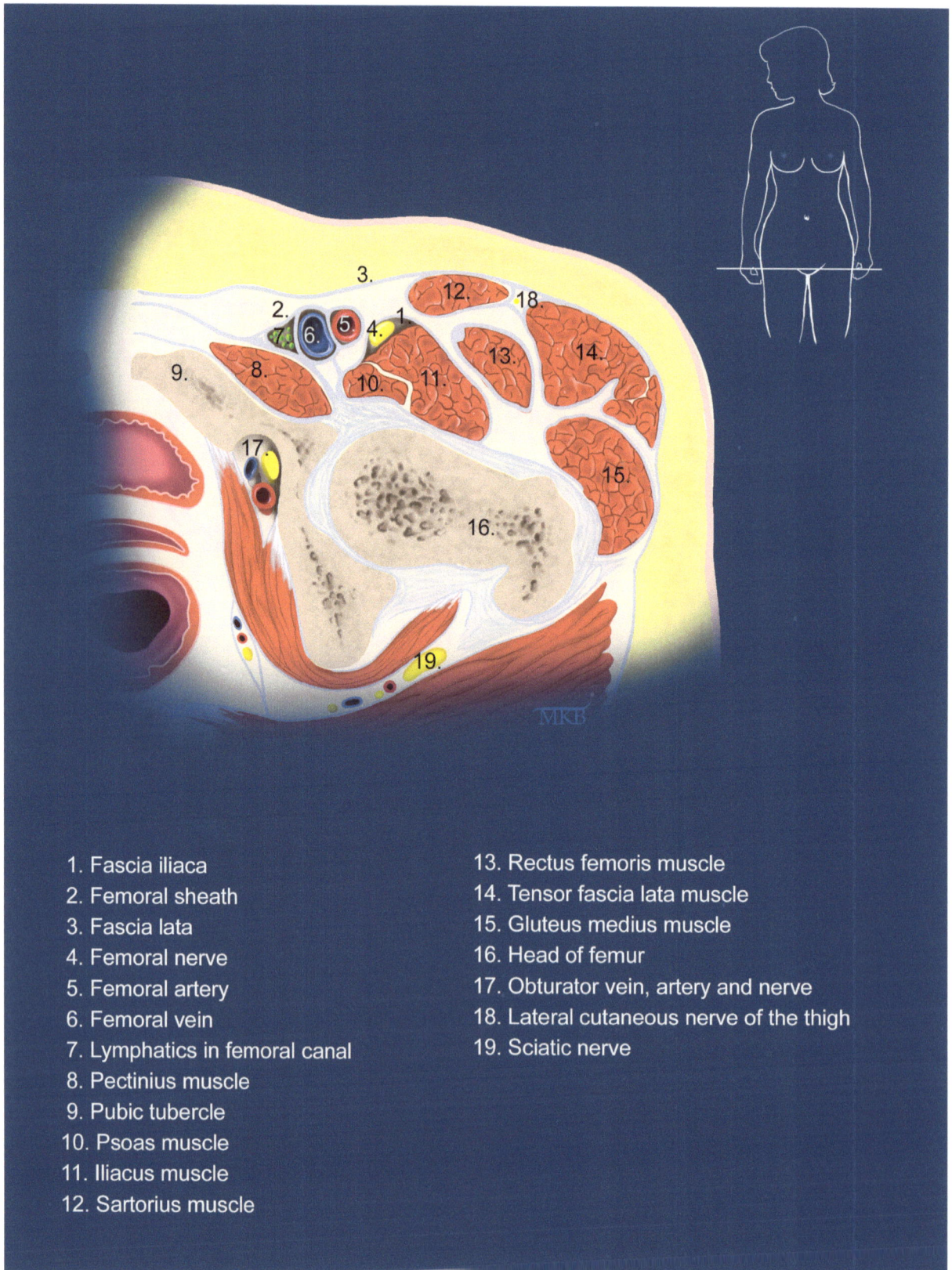

1. Fascia iliaca
2. Femoral sheath
3. Fascia lata
4. Femoral nerve
5. Femoral artery
6. Femoral vein
7. Lymphatics in femoral canal
8. Pectinius muscle
9. Pubic tubercle
10. Psoas muscle
11. Iliacus muscle
12. Sartorius muscle
13. Rectus femoris muscle
14. Tensor fascia lata muscle
15. Gluteus medius muscle
16. Head of femur
17. Obturator vein, artery and nerve
18. Lateral cutaneous nerve of the thigh
19. Sciatic nerve

Figure 3-4: Trans-sectional view at the level of the inguinal groove.

# Surface Anatomy of the Femoral Nerve

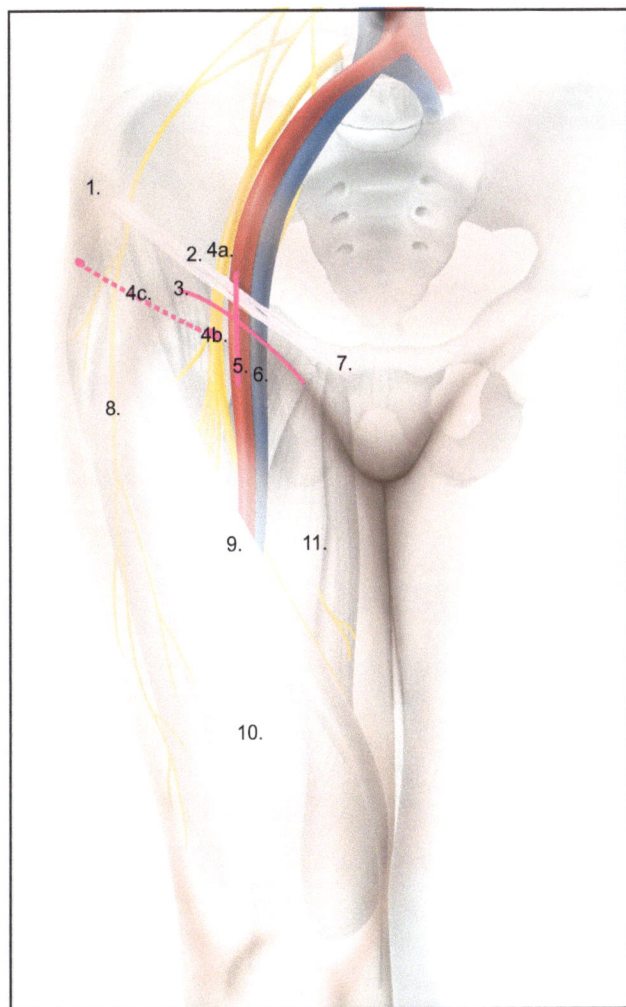

1. Anterior superior iliac spine
2. Inguinal ligament
3. Inguinal crease
4a. Femoral nerve
4b. Point of needle entry
4c. Intended catheter tunneling
5. Femoral artery
6. Femoral vein
7. Pubic tubercle
8. Lateral cutaneous nerve
9. Sartorius muscle
10. Quadriceps femoris muscles
11. Adductor muscles

The femoral crease (3) and the femoral artery (5) are marked. A point approximately 1 cm caudad and 1 cm lateral of where these lines cross marks the position of the femoral nerve (4a & 4b).

*Figure 3-5: Surface anatomy of the femoral nerve.*

**Please refer to standard textbooks for indications for and techniques of performing any of the blocks referred to in this book.**

# Microanatomy

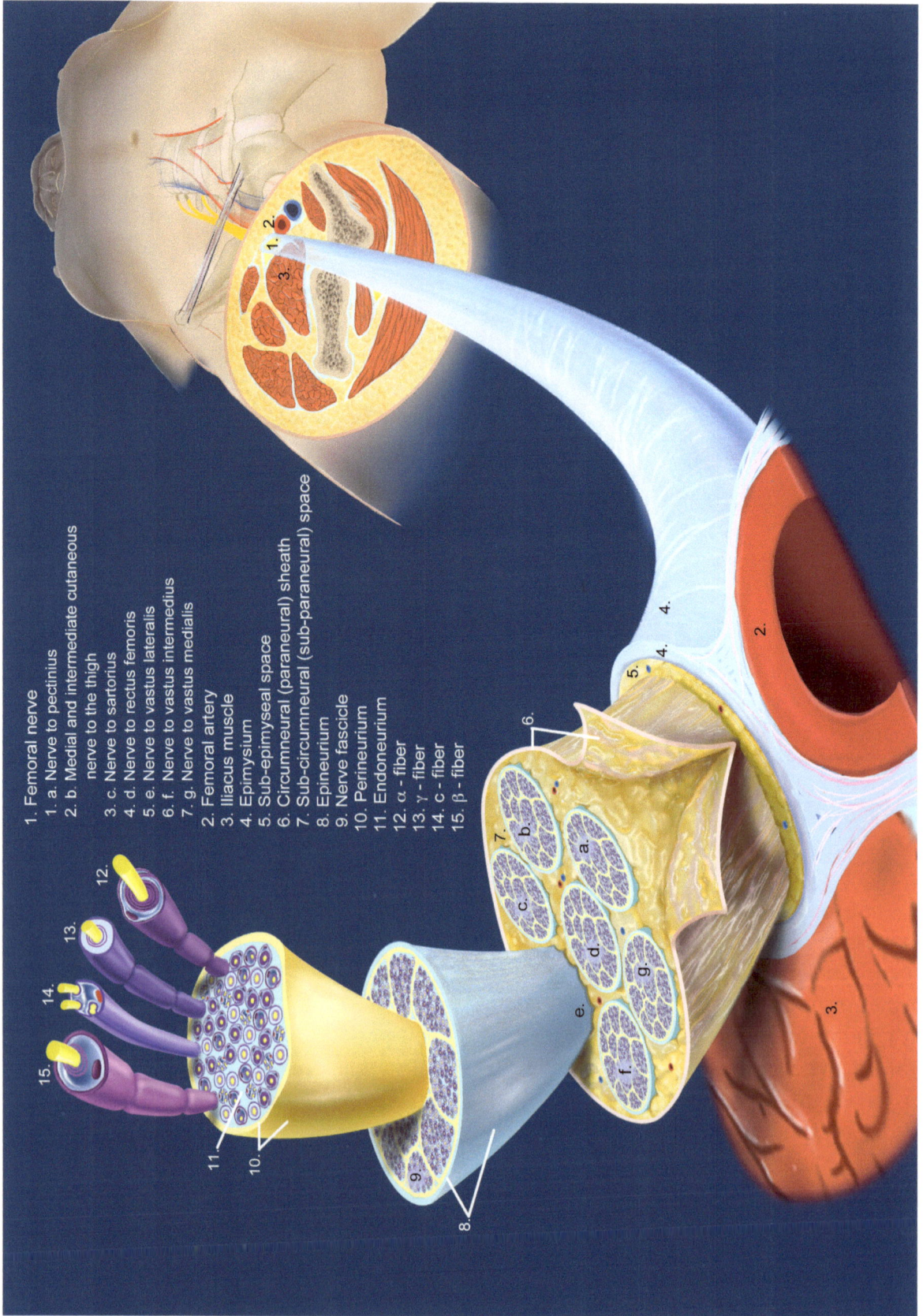

1. Femoral nerve
1. a. Nerve to pectinius
2. b. Medial and intermediate cutaneous
   nerve to the thigh
3. c. Nerve to sartorius
4. d. Nerve to rectus femoris
5. e. Nerve to vastus lateralis
6. f. Nerve to vastus intermedius
7. g. Nerve to vastus medialis
2. Femoral artery
3. Iliacus muscle
4. Epimysium
5. Sub-epimyseal space
6. Circumneural (paraneural) sheath
7. Sub-circumneural (sub-paraneural) space
8. Epineurium
9. Nerve fascicle
10. Perineurium
11. Endoneurium
12. α - fiber
13. γ - fiber
14. c - fiber
15. β - fiber

*Figure 3-5: Microstructure of the femoral nerve.*

- Please note:
- The branches of the femoral nerve are enclosed in a common circumneural sheath (6); also known as paraneural sheath).
- There are eight branches inside the femoral nerve (seven are shown here): the nerve to the pectinius, which usually comes off higher up, just above or below the inguinal ligament, the medial and intermediate cutaneous nerves to the thigh, and the nerves to the sartorius, rectus femoris, vastus lateralis, vastus intermedius, and vastus medialis muscles.
- Outside the circumneural sheath is the sub-epimyseal space (5), which is surrounded by the epimysium (4) – the fascia that surrounds the nerves, muscles, and blood vessels. Injection into this space forms the so-called doughnut sign on ultrasound.
- Deep to the circumneural sheath (6); AKA the paraneural sheath) is the sub-circumneural space (7), which is thought to be the ideal space for the needle in catheter placement for a continuous nerve block.
- The next layer, which encloses each individual branch, is the epineurium (8), surrounding the fascicles of each branch, thought to originate from the paravertebral fascia.
- In turn, each fascicle is surrounded by its own perineurium (10), which originates from the dura.
- Inside the perineurium are endoneurium and nerve axons (12-15).
- The fluid inside the fascicle is CSF, while the tissue fluid outside the fascicle is lymph.

References:

Reina MA, Navarro RA, Mateos EMD. Ultrastructure of myelinated and unmyelinated axons. In: Reina MA, Ed. Atlas of Functional Anatomy For Regional Anesthesia And Pain Medicine. New York: Springer, 2015; 3-126.

Andrerson HL, Anderson SL, Tranun-Jensen J. Injecting inside the paraneural sheath or the sciatic nerve: Direct comparison among ultrasound imaging, macroscopic anatomy and histologic analysis. Reg Anesth Pain Med 2012;37:410-4.

Karmakar MK, Shariat AN, Pangthipampai P, Chen J. High-definition ultrasound imaging defines the paraneural sheath and the fascial compartments surrounding the sciatic nerve at the popliteal fossa. Reg Anesth Pain Med 2013;38:447-51.

Millesi H, Zoch G, Rath T. The gliding apparatus of peripheral nerve and its clinical significance. Ann Chir Main Memb Super 1990;9:87-97.

Boezaart AP. The sweet spot of the nerve: Is the "paraneural sheath" named correctly, and does it matter? Reg Anesth Pain Med 2014;39:557-8.

# Sonoanatomy
## The Proximal Femoral Nerve

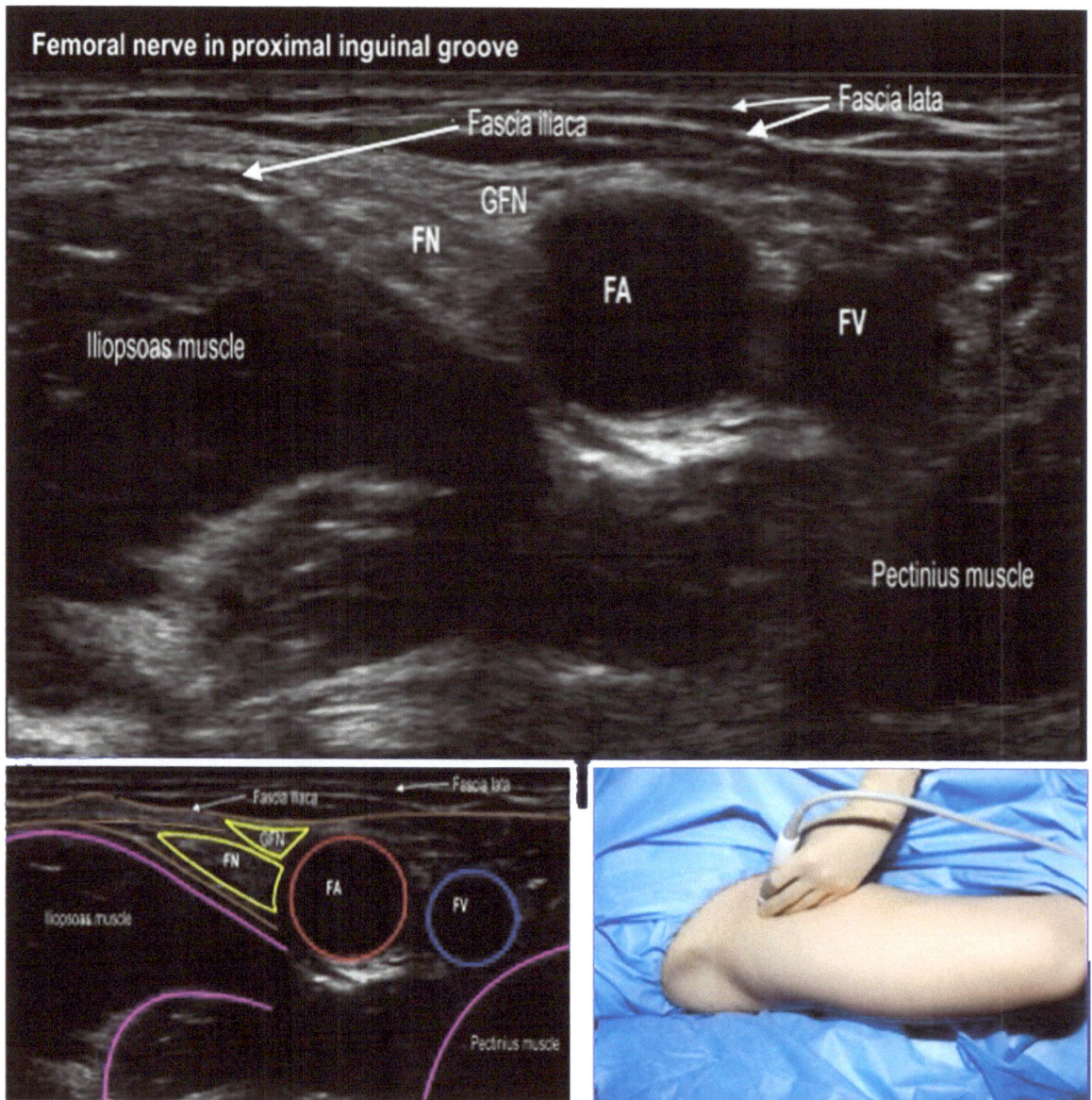

*Figure 3-7: Sonoanatomy of the femoral nerve as viewed in the inguinal crease.*

FA     Femoral artery
FN     Femoral nerve
FV     Femoral vein
GFN   Femoral branch of the
          genitofemoral nerve

**View Video at RAEducation.com**
**Acute Pain Medicine - Anatomy -**
**Sonoanatomy: Femoral Nerve**

The left side of the image is the lateral side of the model.

# The Distal Femoral Nerve

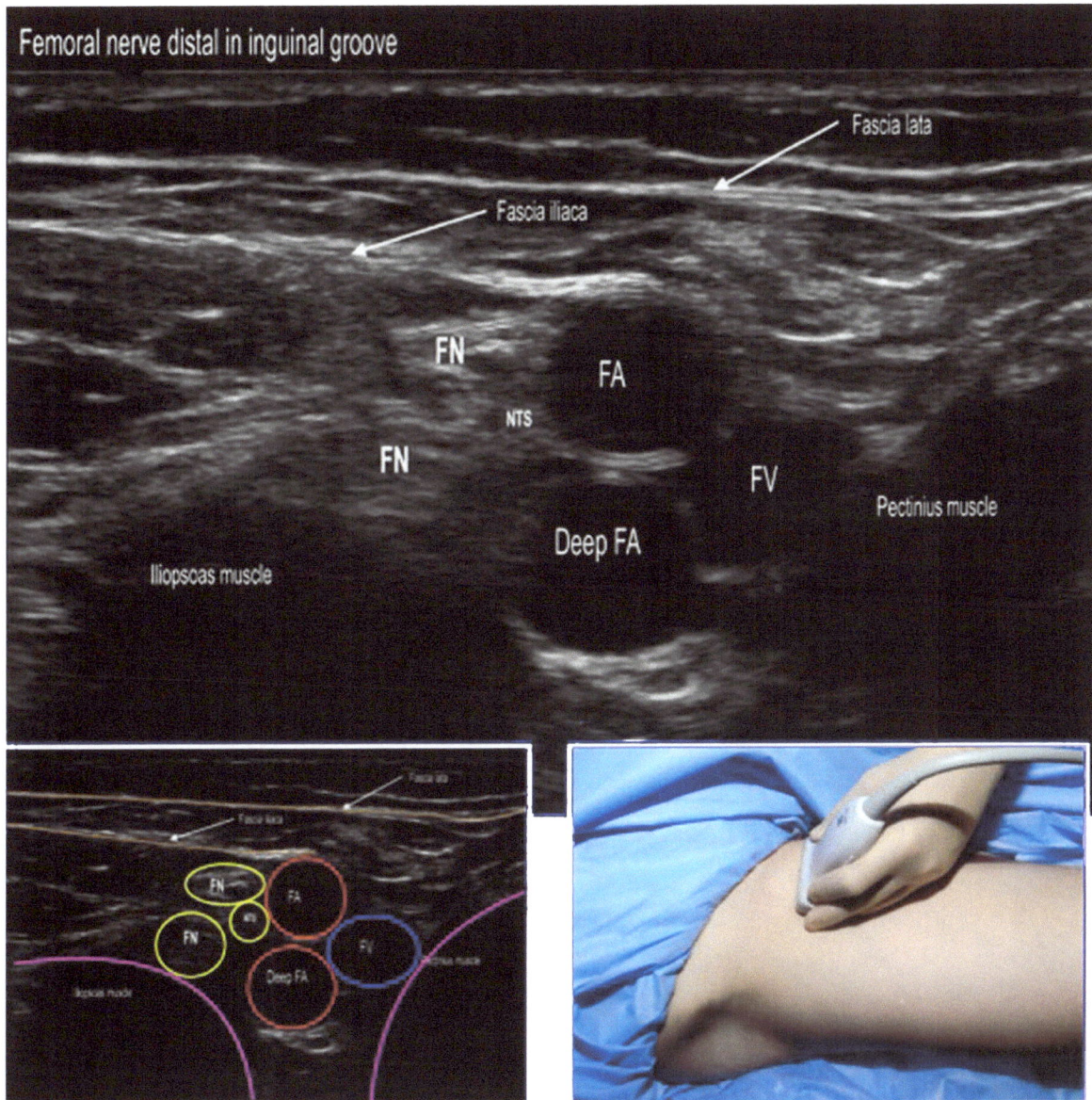

*Figure 3-8: More distal view of the femoral nerve below the inguinal crease.*

FA        Femoral artery
FN        Femoral nerve
FV        Femoral vein
NTS       Nerve to sartorius

The left side of the image is the lateral side
of the model.

# The Proximal Obturator Nerve

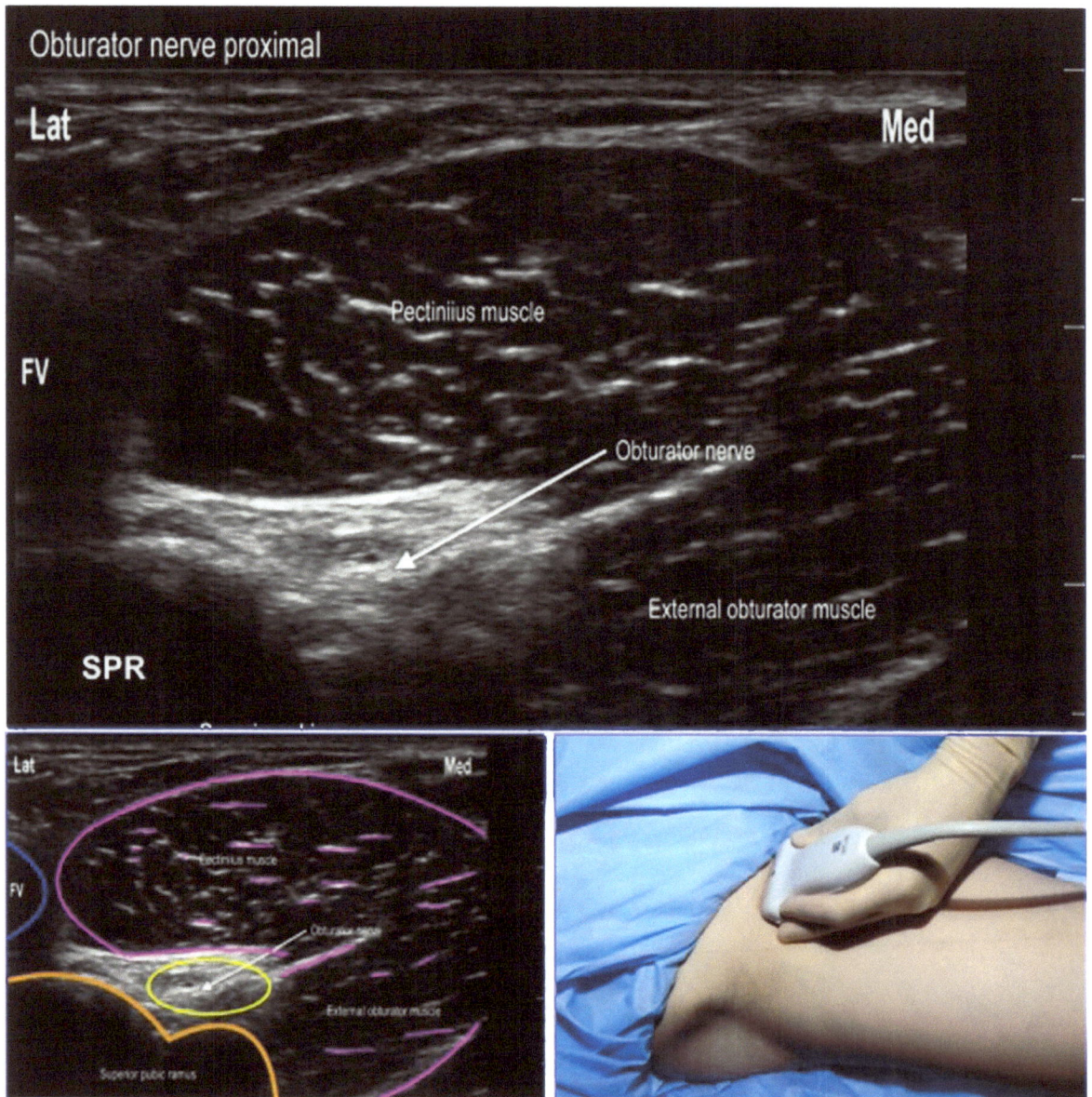

*Figure 3-9: Sonoanatomy of the obturator nerve.*

FV    Femoral vein
Lat   Lateral
Med   Medial
SPR   Superior pelvic ramus

View Video at RAEducation.com
Acute Pain Medicine - Anatomy -
Sonnanatomy: Obturator Nerve

# The Distal Obturator Nerve

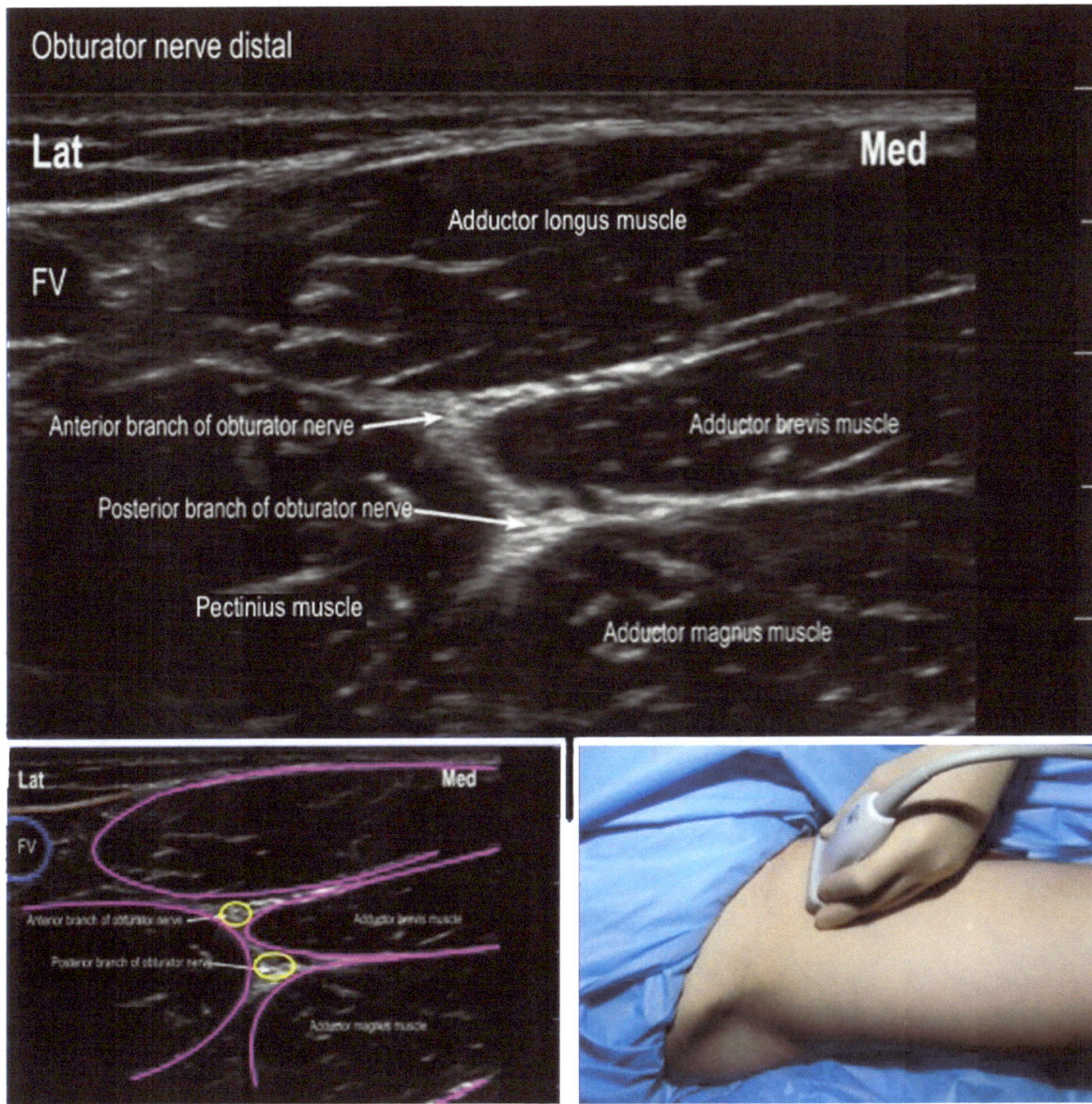

*Figure 3-10: Sonoanatomy of the anterior and posterior branches of the obturator nerve.*

FV      Femoral vein
Lat     Lateral
Med   Medial

# The Lateral Cutaneous Nerve of the Thigh

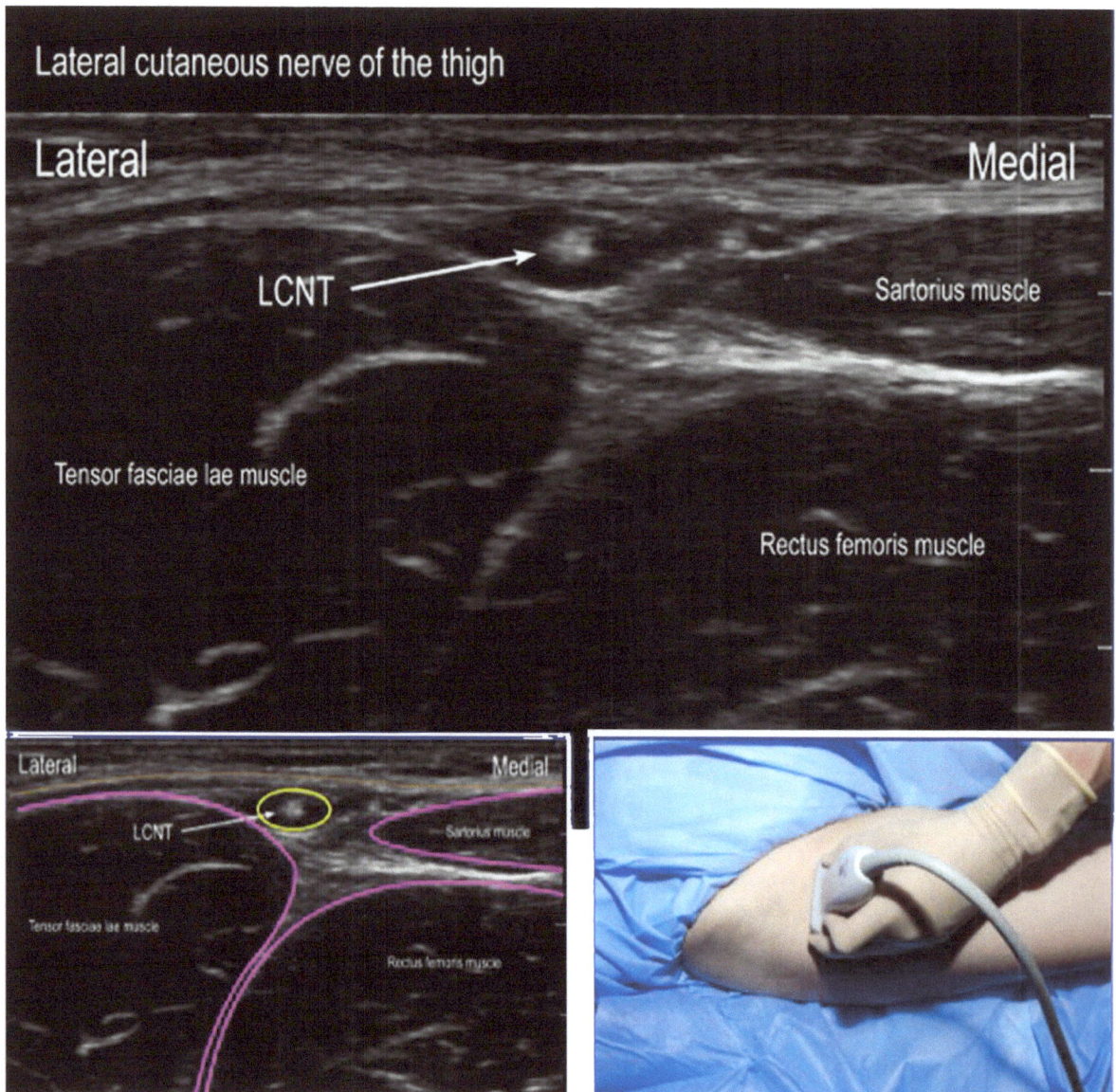

*Figure 3-11: Sonoanatomy of the lateral cutaneous nerve of the thigh.*

LCNT     Lateral cutaneous nerve of thigh

View Video at RAEducation.com
Acute Pain Medicine - Anatomy -
Sonoanatomy; Lateral Cutaneous Nerve

# The Saphenous Nerve

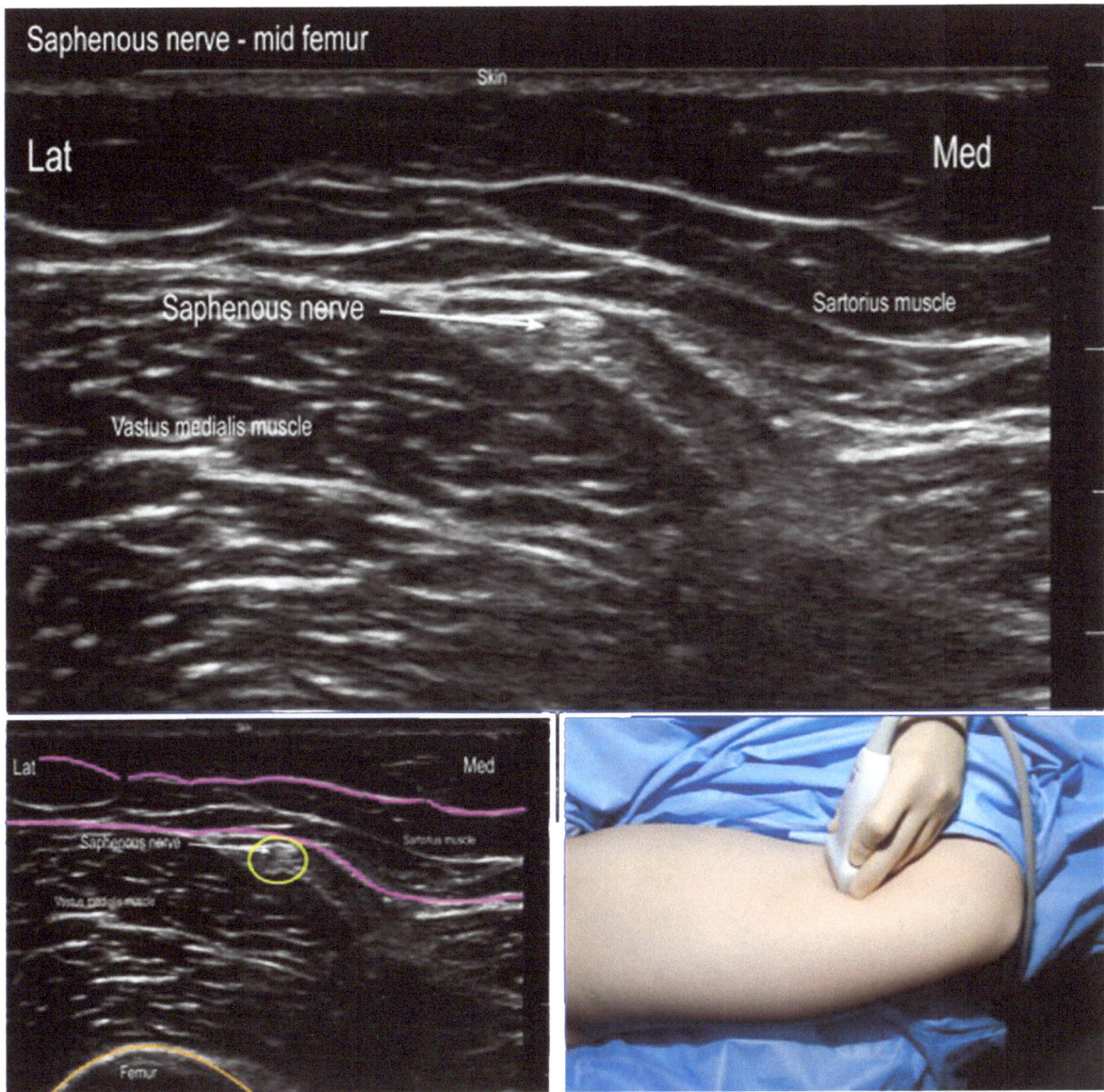

Figure 3-12: Sonoanatomy of the saphenous nerve in the thig

Lat     Lateral
Med    Medial

Please note: What is annotated here as "Saphenous nerve" may well be the patellar branch of the saphenous nerve, which usually lies more medially in this same fascial layer.

# The Adductor Canal

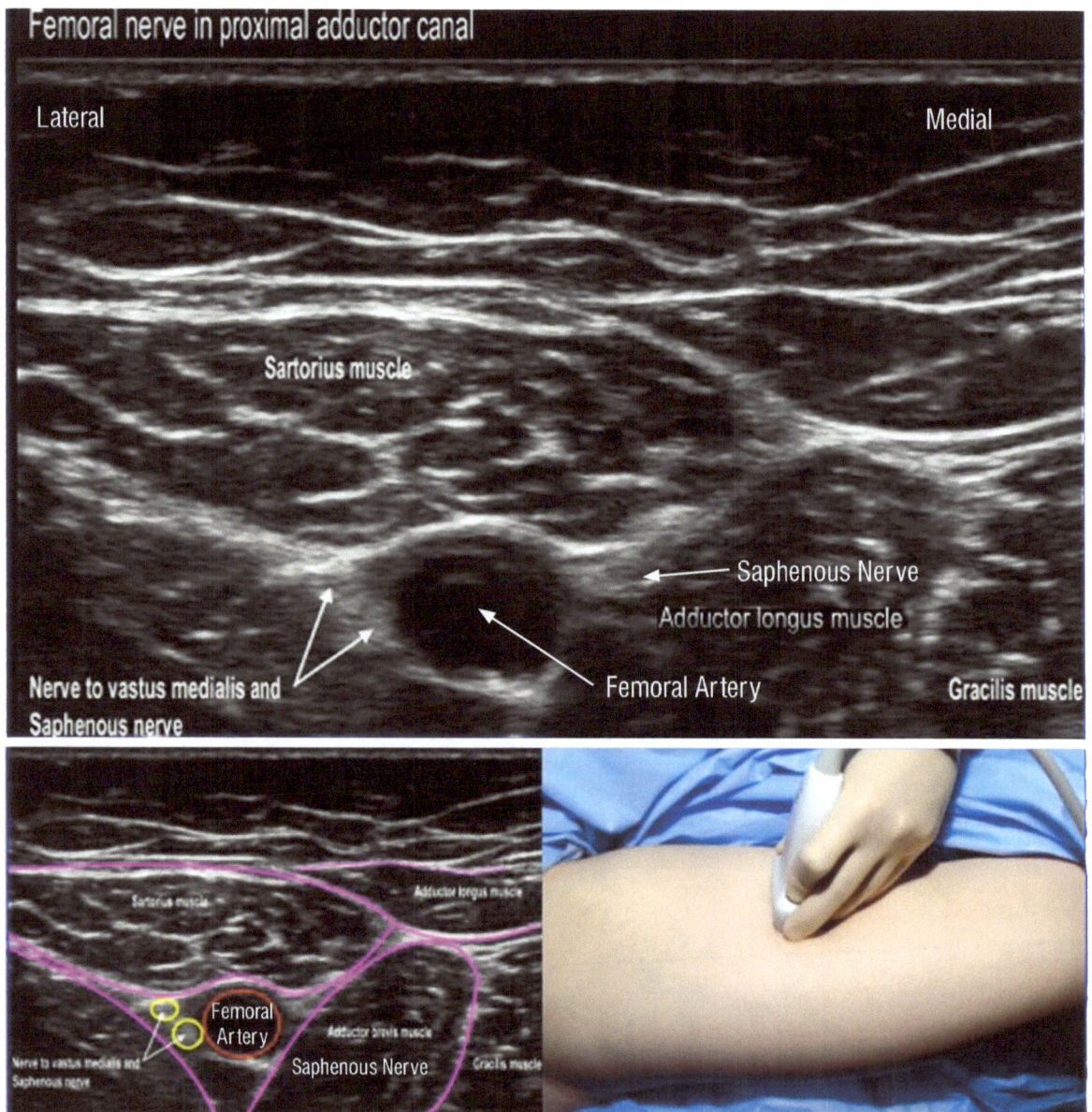

Figure 3-13: Sonoanatomy of the distal adductor canal. The left side of the image is anterior.

Please note: The femoral vein is posterior and medial of the artery and is usually compressed. The saphanous nerve is medial of the artery originally but more distal it is lateral.

**View Video at RAEducation.com**
**Acute Pain Medicine - Anatomy -**
**Sonoanatomy: Adductor Canal**

Ref: Boezaart AP, Parvataneni HK. Adductor canal block may just be an (unreliable) indirect femoral nerve block. Reg Anesth Pain Med 2014;39:556. • Chen J, Lesse J, Hadzic A, ReissW. Resta-Florer F. Adductor canal block can result in motor block of the quadriceps muscle. Reg Anesth Pain Med 2014;39:170–1 • Davies JJ, Bond TS, Swenson JD. Adductor canal block more than just the saphenous nerve. Reg Anesth Pain Med 2009;34:618–9 • Veal C, Auyong DB, Hanson NA, Allen CJ, Strodtbeck W. Delayed quadriceps weakness after continuous adductor canal block for total knee arthroplasty: a case report. Acta Anaesth Scan 2013;58:362-4.

# Functional Anatomy

## Dermatomes of the Leg

- L1
- L2
- L3
- L4
- L5
- S1
- S2
- S3
- S4
- S5
- Co

| | |
|---|---|
| Co | coccyx |
| L1,-L5 | lumbar roots L2 to L5 |
| S1-S5 | sacral spinal roots |

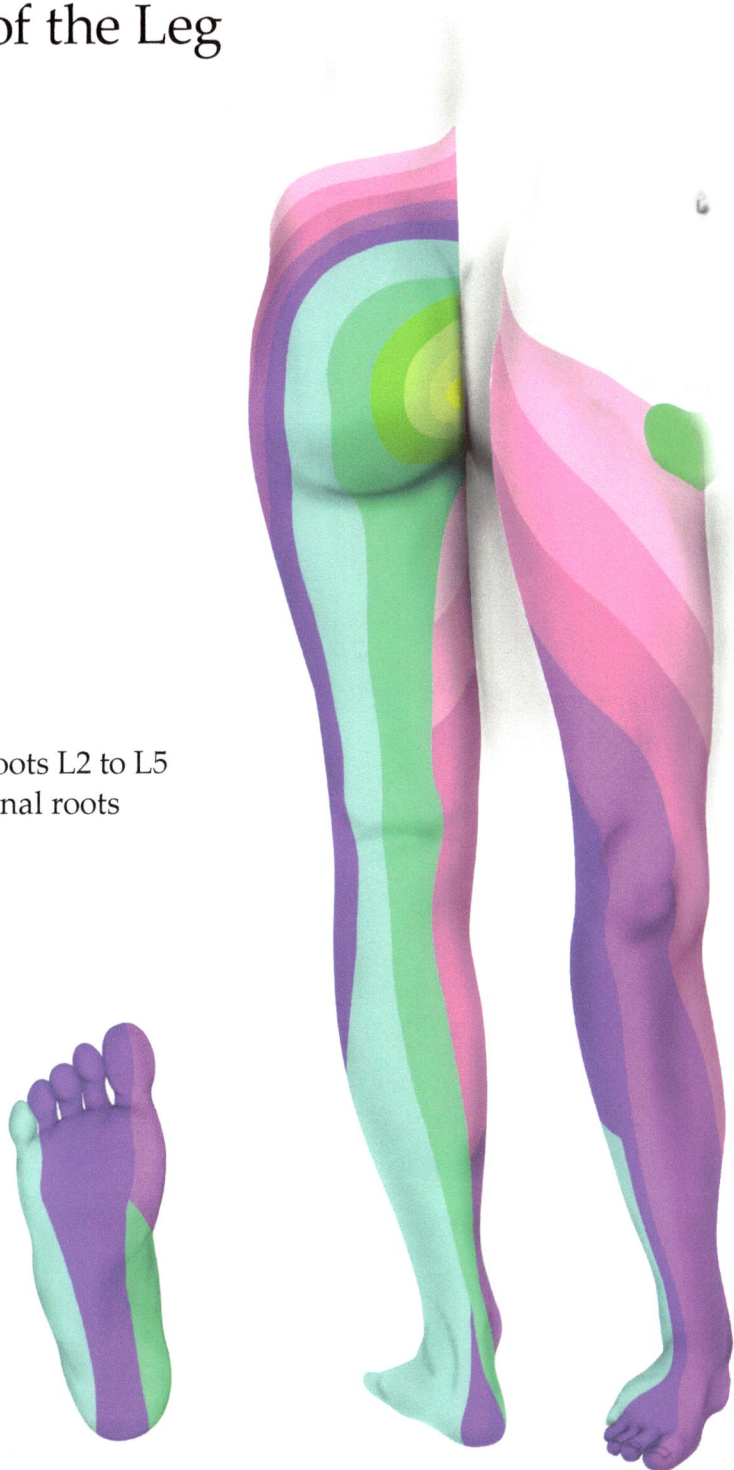

*Figure 3-14: Schematic demarcation of the dermatomes of the lower limb.*

These demarcations are not distinct segments as depicted here because there is significant overlap between adjacent dermatomes.

# Osteotomes of the Leg

L2
L3
L4
L5
S1
S2

L1,-L5     lumbar roots L2 to L5
S1-S5      sacral spinal roots

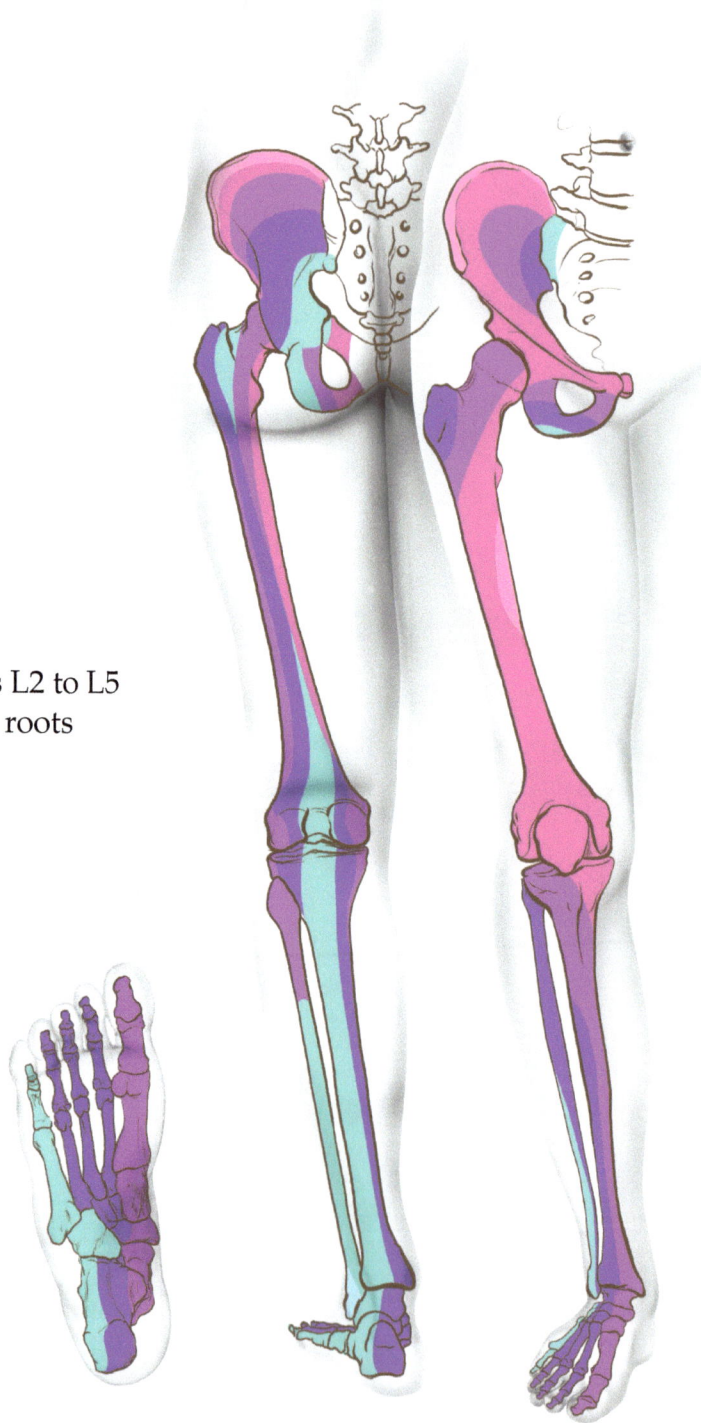

*Figure 3-15: Schematic demarcation of the osteotomes of the lower limb.*

These demarcations are not distinct segments as depicted here because there is significant overlap between adjacent osteotomes.

# Neurotomes of the Leg

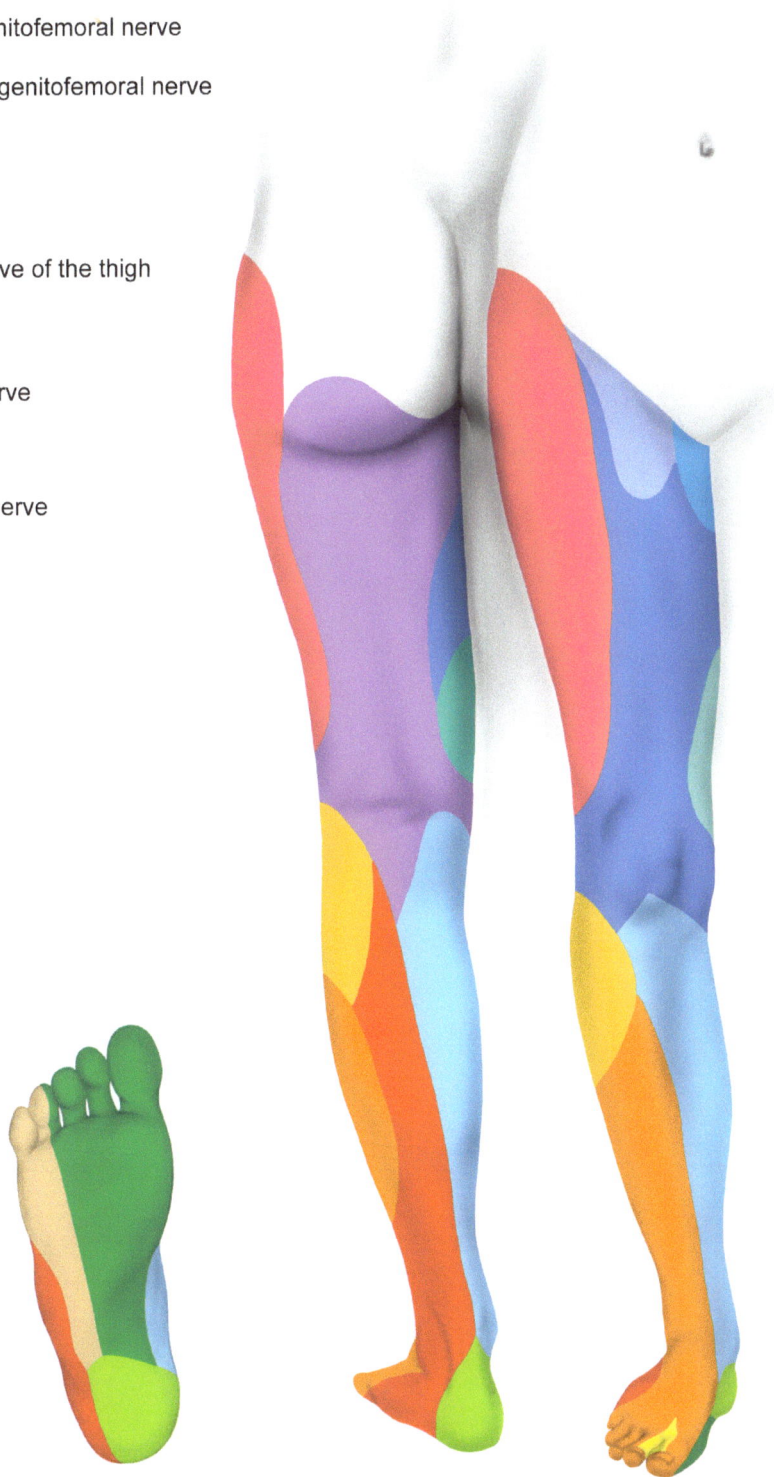

- Posterior femoral cutaneous nerve
- Femoral branch of genitofemoral nerve
- Genital branch of the genitofemoral nerve
- Femoral nerve
- Saphenous nerve
- Lateral cutaneous nerve of the thigh
- Obturator nerve
- Common peroneal nerve
- Deep peroneal nerve
- Superficial peroneal nerve
- Sural nerve
- Lateral plantar nerve
- Calcaneal nerve
- Medial plantar nerve

*Figure 3-16: Schematic demarcation of the neurotomes of the upper limb.*

These demarcations are not distinct areas as depicted here because there is significant overlap between adjacent neurotomes.

# Dermatomes of the Femoral & Saphenous Nerves

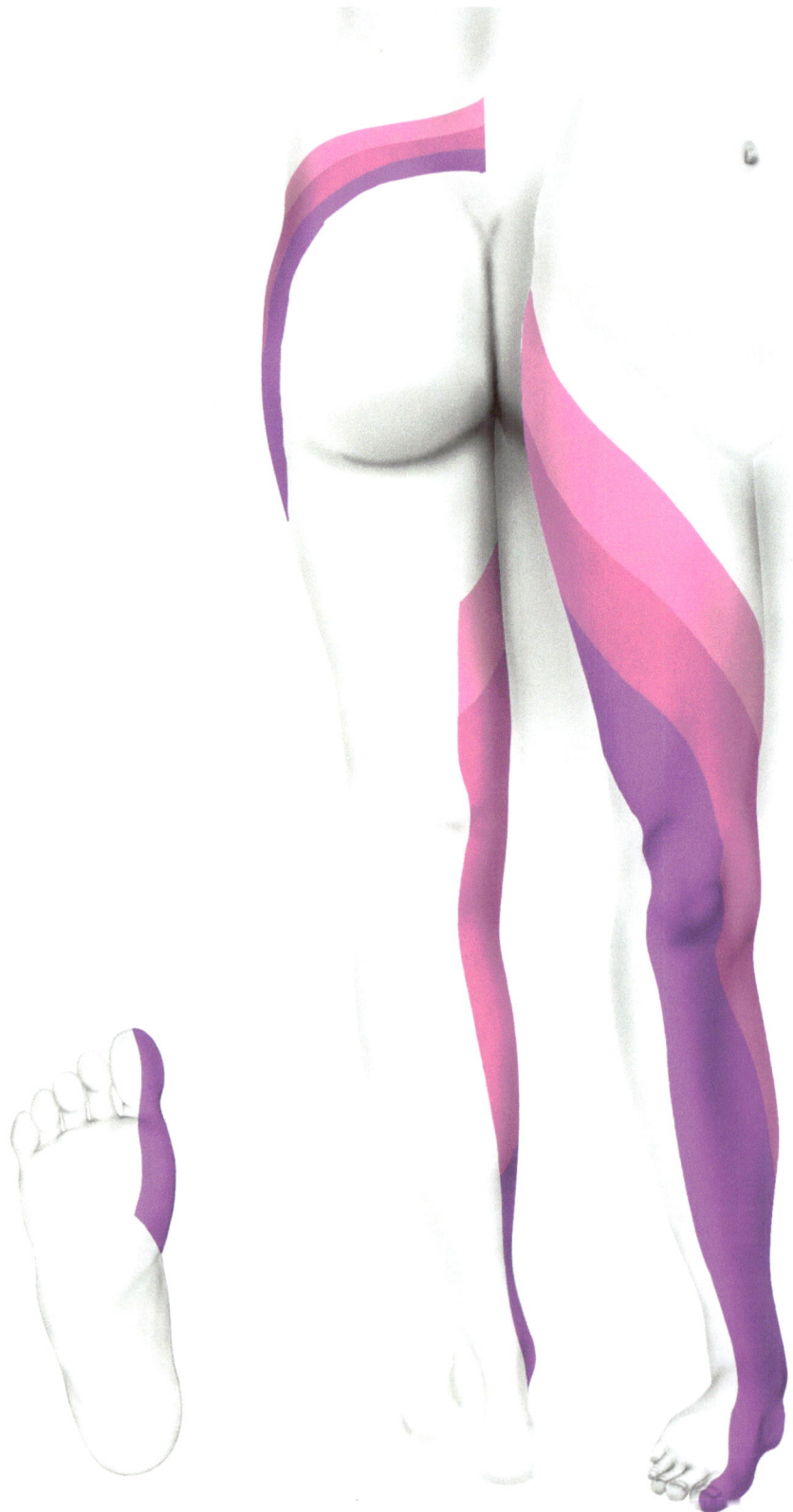

L2

L3

L4

Figure 3-17: Schematic demarcation of the dermatomes of the lower limb innervated by the femoral nerve and its branches.

# Osteotomes of the Femoral & Saphenous Nerves

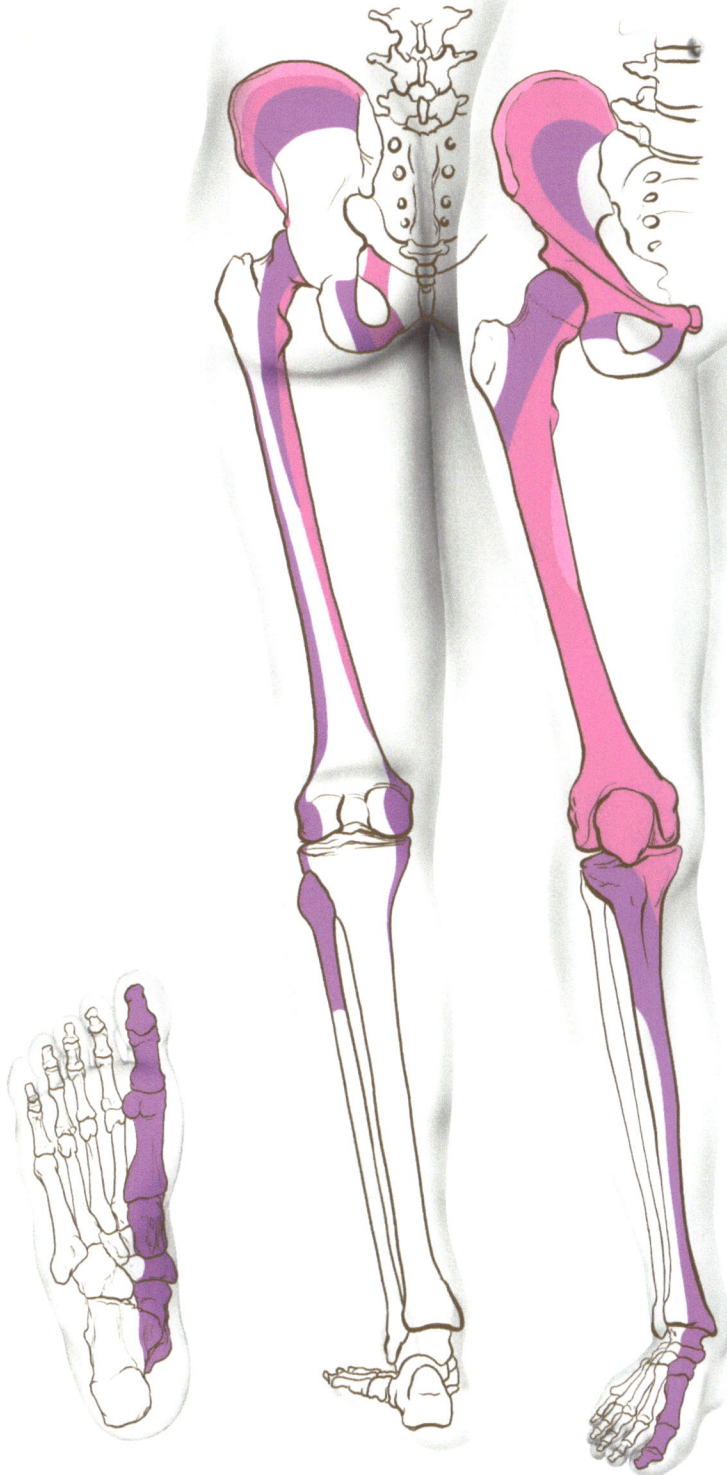

L2
L3
L4

Figure 3-18: Schematic demarcation of the osteotomes of the lower limb innervated by the femoral nerve and its branches.

# Neurotomes of the Femoral & Saphenous Nerves

branch of femoral nerve

Femoral nerve

Saphenous nerve

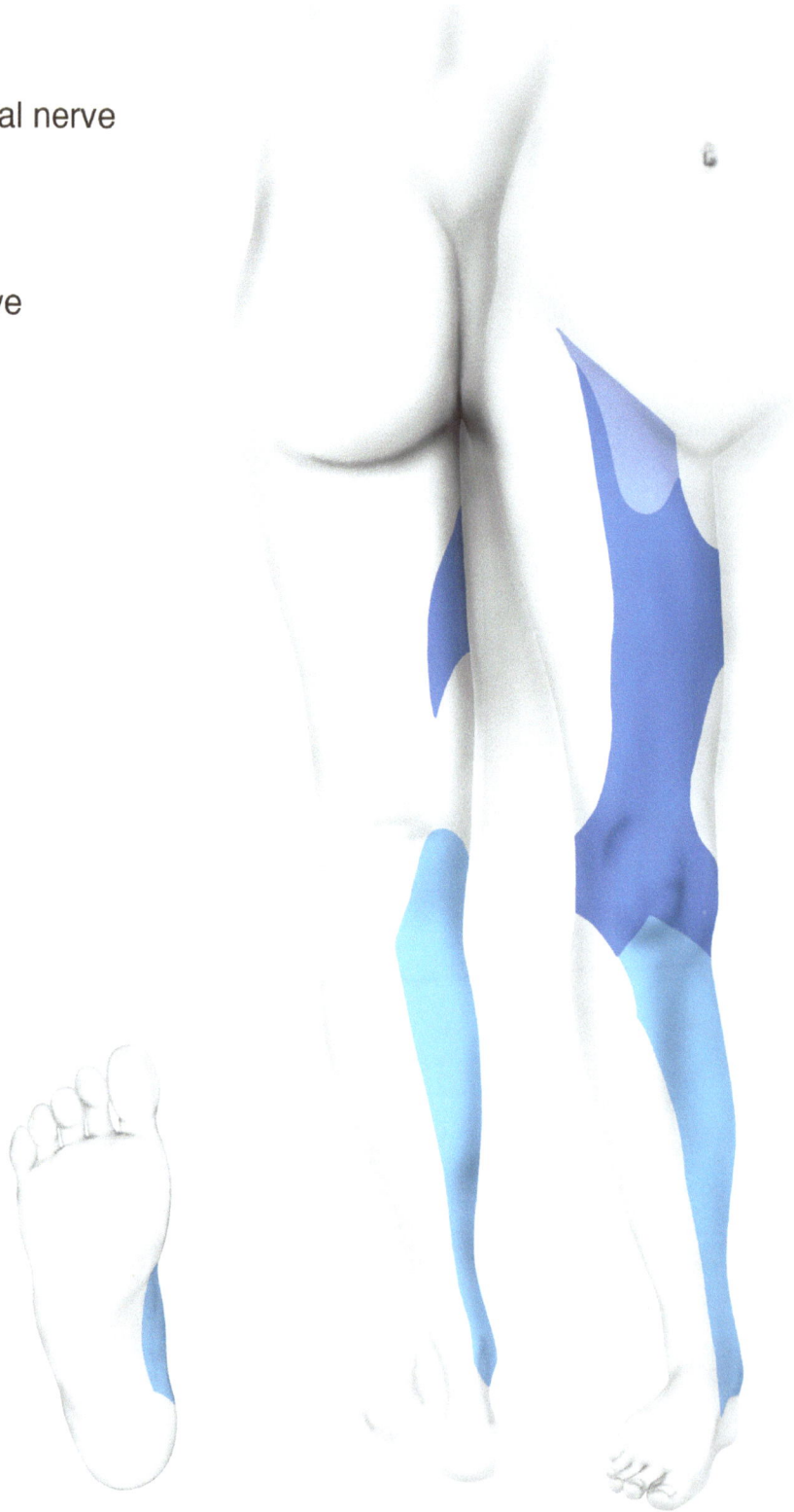

*Figure 3-19: Schematic demarcation of the neurotomes of the lower limb innervated by the femoral nerve and its branches.*

# Neurotomes of the Obturator Nerve

**Obturator Nerve**

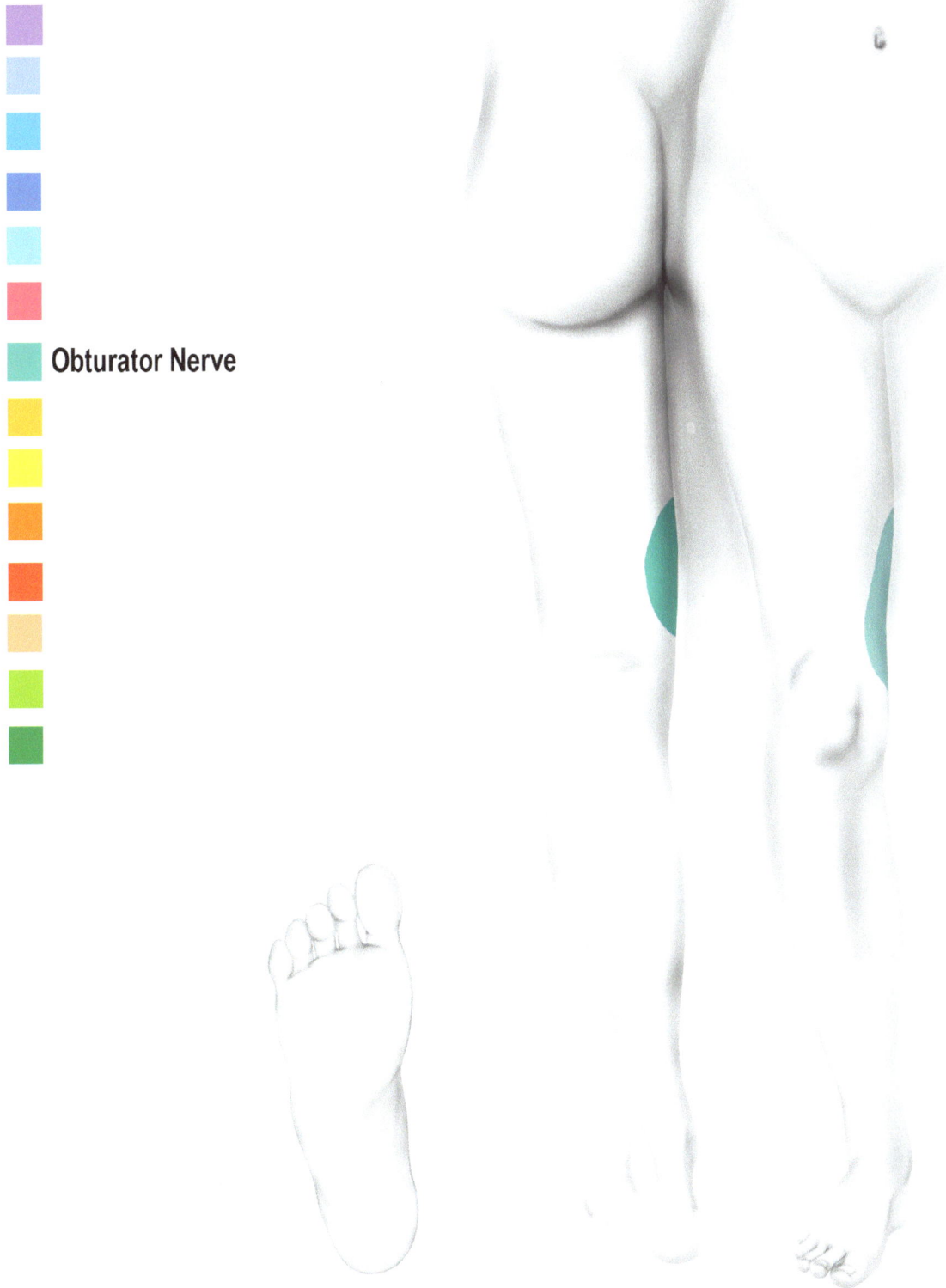

*Figure 3-20: Schematic demarcation of the neurotome of the lower limb innervated by the obturator nerve*

# Neurotomes of the Lateral Cutaneous Nerve

Lateral femoral cutaneous nerve

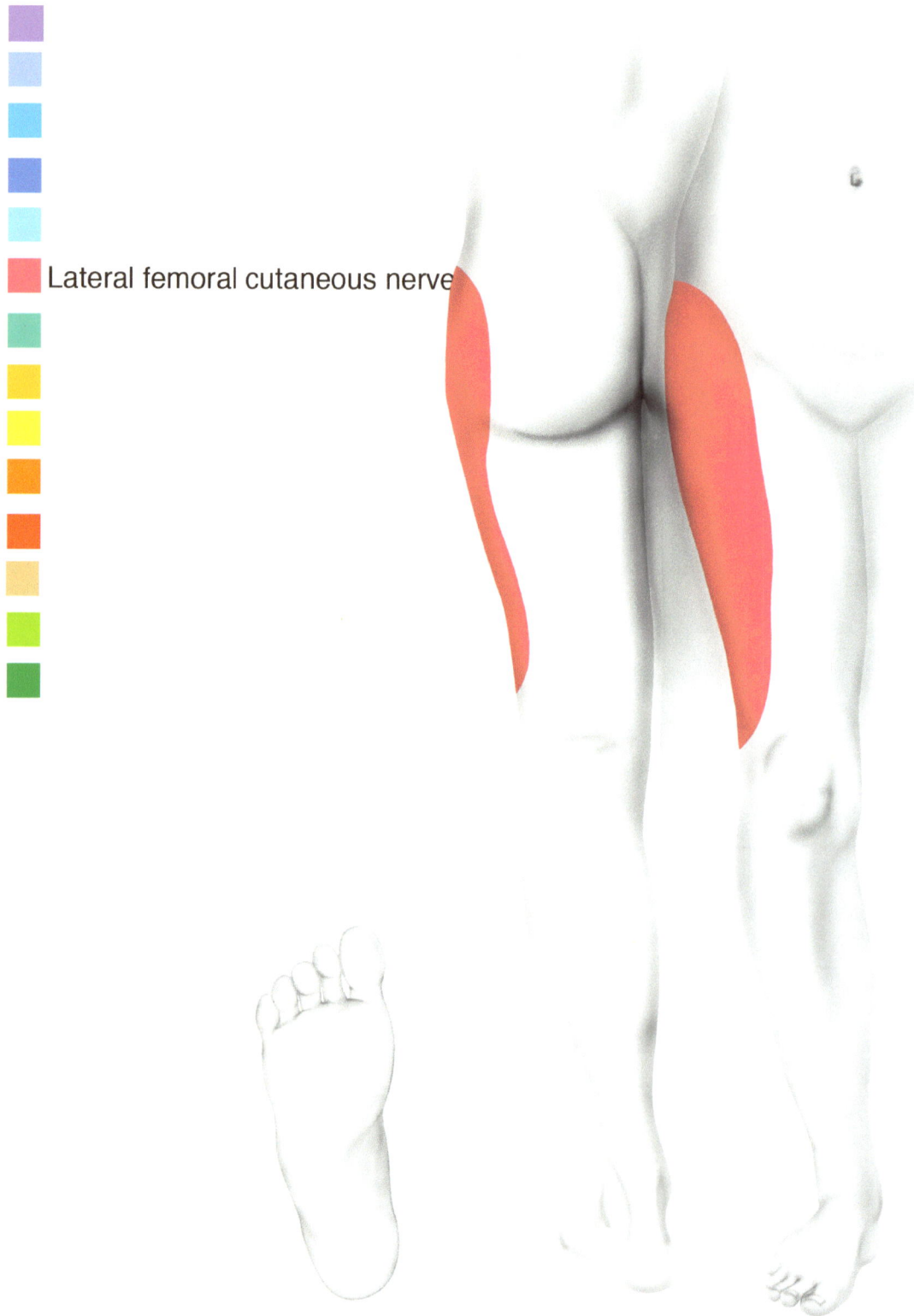

Figure 3-21: Schematic demarcation of the neurotome of the lower limb innervated by the lateral cutaneous nerve of the thigh.

# Chapter 4

## The Posterior Thigh

*Macroanatomy*
*Microanatomy*
*Sonoanatomy*
*Functional Anatomy*

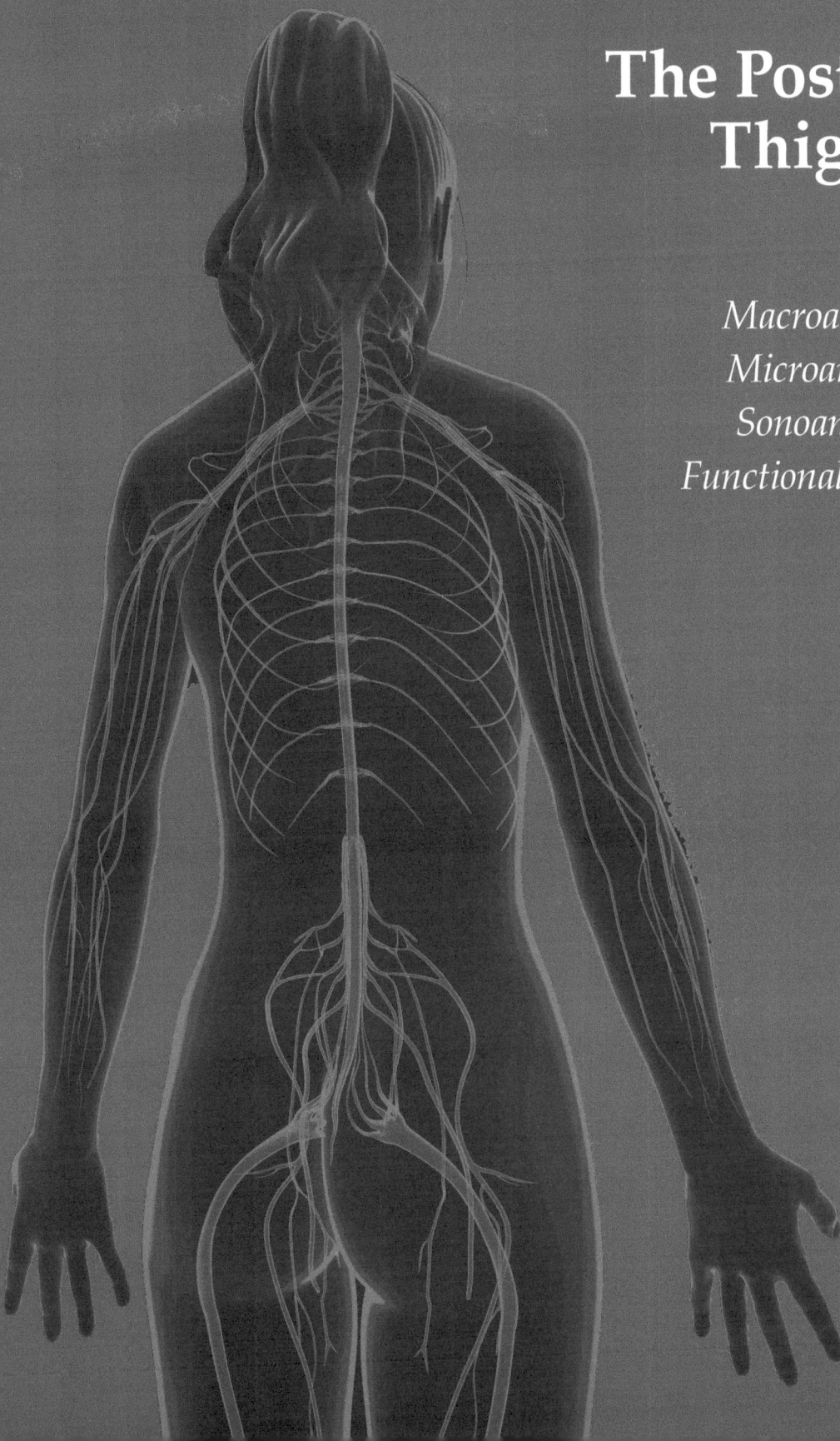

# Macroanatomy

## The Lumbosacral Plexus

### Nerves
1. Subcostal nerve (T12)
2. Iliohypogastric nerve (L1)
3. Ilioinguinal nerve (L1)
4. Lateral femoral cutaneous nerve (L2,3)
5. Femoral branch of genitofemoral nerve (L1,2)
6. Genital branch of genitofemoral nerve (L1,2)
7. Femoral nerve (L2,3,4)
8. Sciatic nerve
    a. Common peroneal nerve (L4,5,S1,2)
    b. Tibial nerve (L4,5,S1,2,3)
9. Posterior femoral cutaneous nerve (S1,2,3)
10. Nerve to Sartorius muscle (L2,3,4)
11. Saphenous branch of the Femoral nerve
12. Obturator nerve (L2,3,4)
13. Pudendal nerve (S1,2,3)
14. Sympathetic trunk
15. Lumbosacral trunk

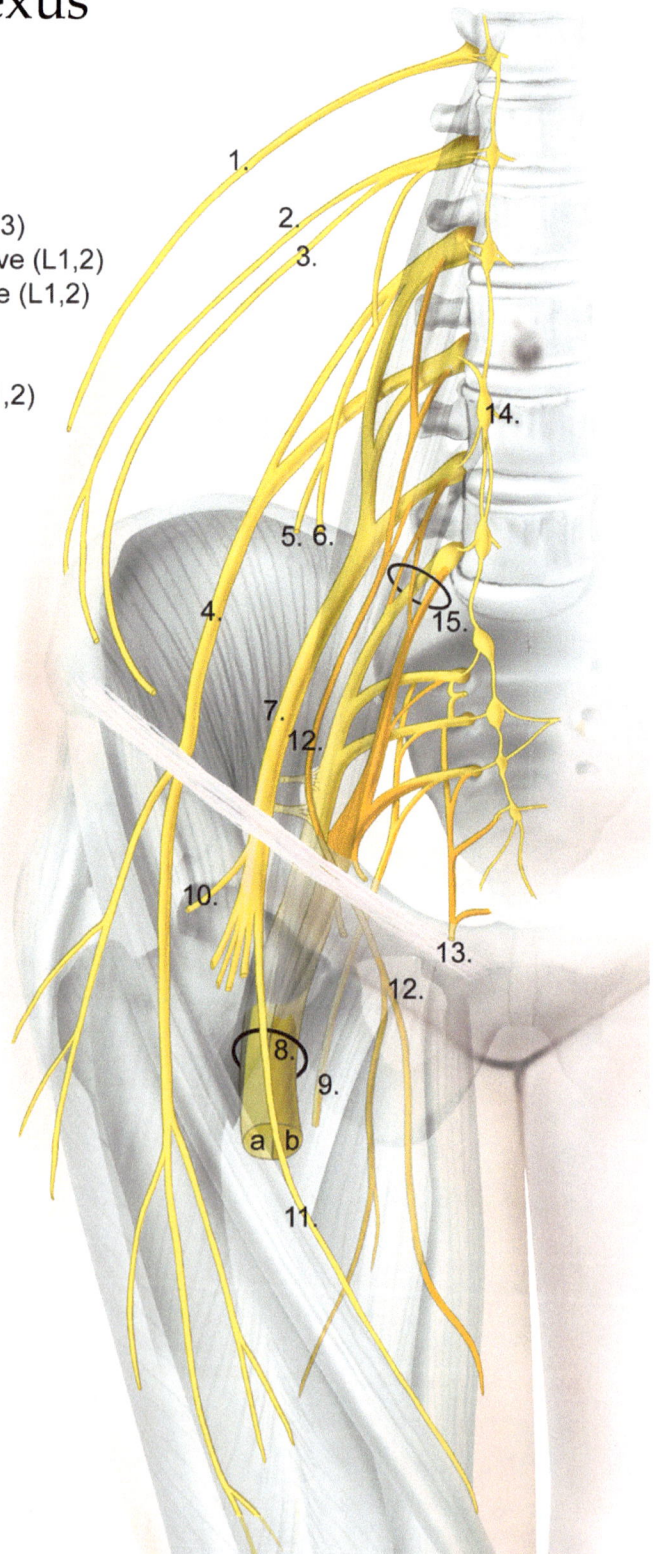

*Figure 4-1: Schematic representation of the lumbosacral plexus and its nerves.*

Please note:

The subcostal (1), ilioinguinal, and iliohypogastric nerves (2, 3) originate from the 12th thoracic (T12) and 1st lumbar (L1) vertebra, respectively.

The lateral cutaneous nerve of the thigh (4) and the genitofemoral nerve originate from the ventral rami of the 1st and 2nd lumbar vertebrae (L1 & L2), whereas the femoral nerve (7) stems from the dorsal rami of L2, L3, and L4.

The 5th lumbar spinal root also gives off a branch to the lumbosacral trunk (15) at the level of L5.

The anterior rami of L2 to L4 form the obturator nerve (12), while L5 and the first three sacral roots (S1, S2, and S3) form the sciatic nerve (8).

The pudendal nerve (13) also arises from these roots.

# Dissection of the Pelvic Sciatic Plexus

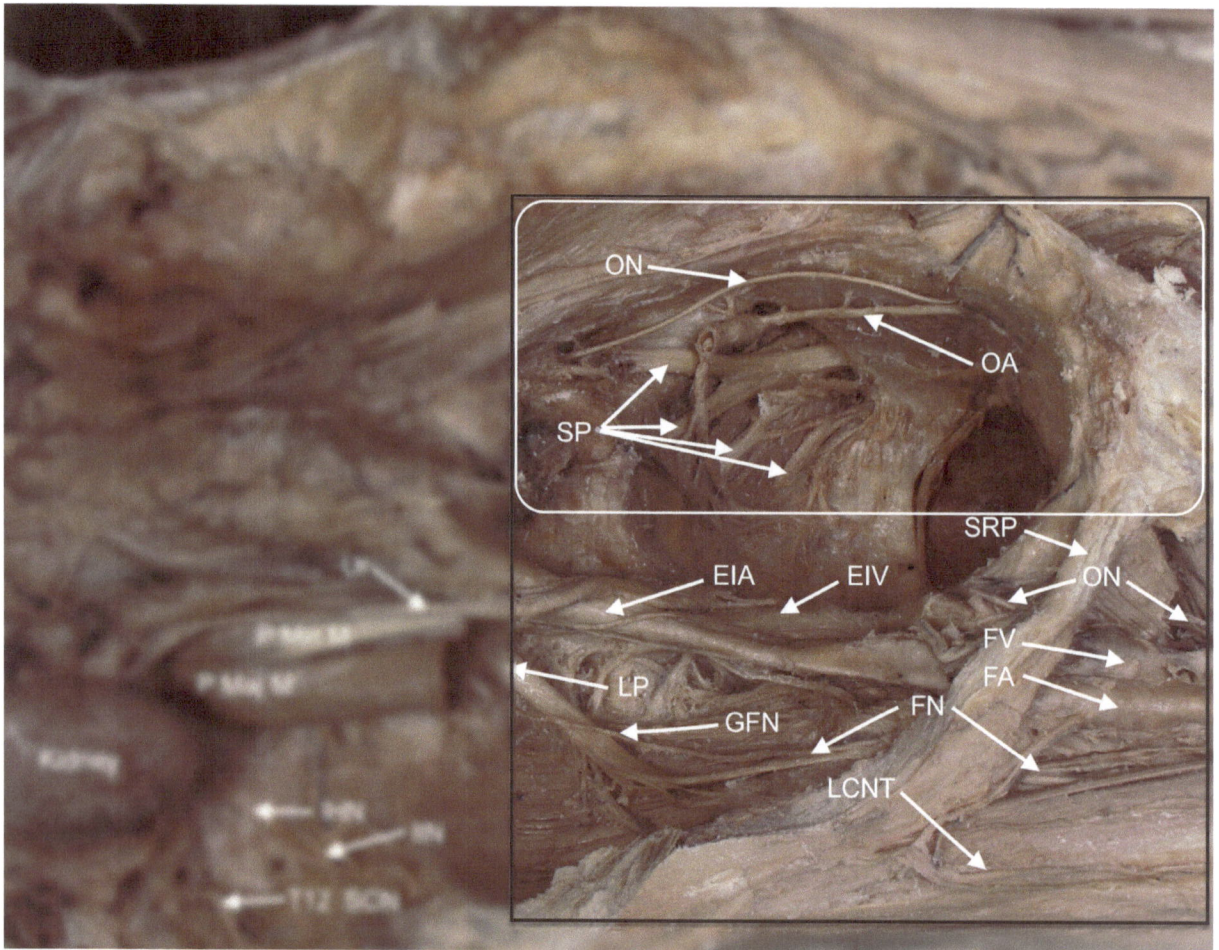

*Figure 4-2: Anatomical dissection of sciatic plexus (SP): abdominal view.*

| | | | |
|---|---|---|---|
| EIA | External iliac artery | LP | Lumbar plexus |
| EIV | External iliac vein | OA | Obturator artery |
| FA | Femoral artery | ON | Obturator nerve |
| FN | Femoral nerve | SP | Sacral plexus |
| FV | Femoral vein | SRP | Superior ramus of the pubis. |
| GFN | Genitofemoral nerve | | |
| LCNT | Lateral cutaneous nerve of the thigh | | |

# Dissection of the Sciatic Nerve

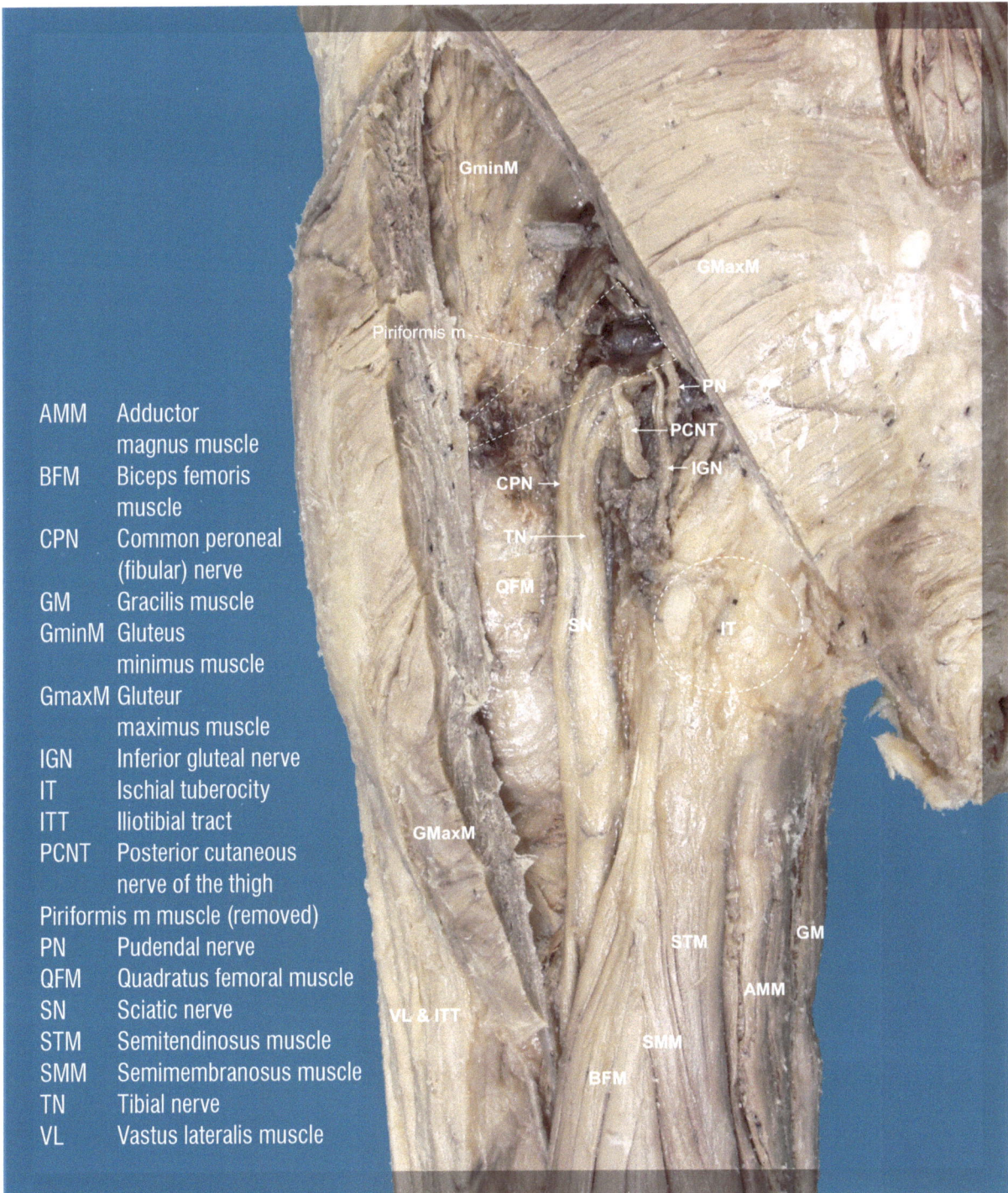

| | |
|---|---|
| AMM | Adductor magnus muscle |
| BFM | Biceps femoris muscle |
| CPN | Common peroneal (fibular) nerve |
| GM | Gracilis muscle |
| GminM | Gluteus minimus muscle |
| GmaxM | Gluteur maximus muscle |
| IGN | Inferior gluteal nerve |
| IT | Ischial tuberocity |
| ITT | Iliotibial tract |
| PCNT | Posterior cutaneous nerve of the thigh |
| Piriformis m | muscle (removed) |
| PN | Pudendal nerve |
| QFM | Quadratus femoral muscle |
| SN | Sciatic nerve |
| STM | Semitendinosus muscle |
| SMM | Semimembranosus muscle |
| TN | Tibial nerve |
| VL | Vastus lateralis muscle |

Figure 4-3: Anatomy of the sciatic nerve.

# Dissection of the Popliteal Fossa

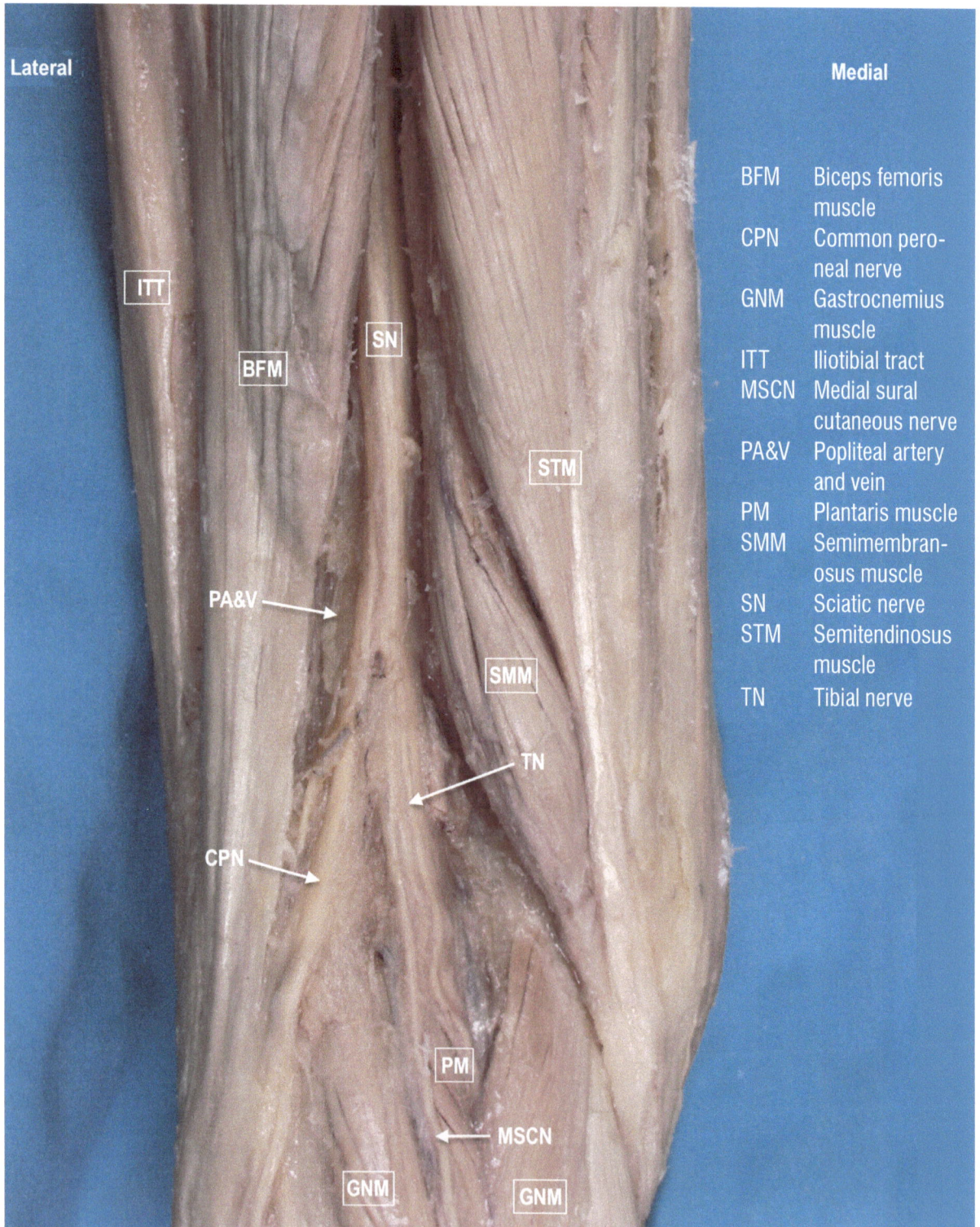

**Lateral**

**Medial**

ITT

SN

BFM

STM

PA&V

SMM

TN

CPN

PM

MSCN

GNM

GNM

| | |
|---|---|
| BFM | Biceps femoris muscle |
| CPN | Common peroneal nerve |
| GNM | Gastrocnemius muscle |
| ITT | Iliotibial tract |
| MSCN | Medial sural cutaneous nerve |
| PA&V | Popliteal artery and vein |
| PM | Plantaris muscle |
| SMM | Semimembranosus muscle |
| SN | Sciatic nerve |
| STM | Semitendinosus muscle |
| TN | Tibial nerve |

*Figure 4-4: Anatomic dissection of the popliteal fossa.*

This view in the region of the subgluteal groove is where a subgluteal sciatic nerve block is usually performed. Note the two parts of the sciatic nerve, the tibial part and the common peroneal part. The pudendal nerve is prominent.

# Transection at the Infragluteal Level

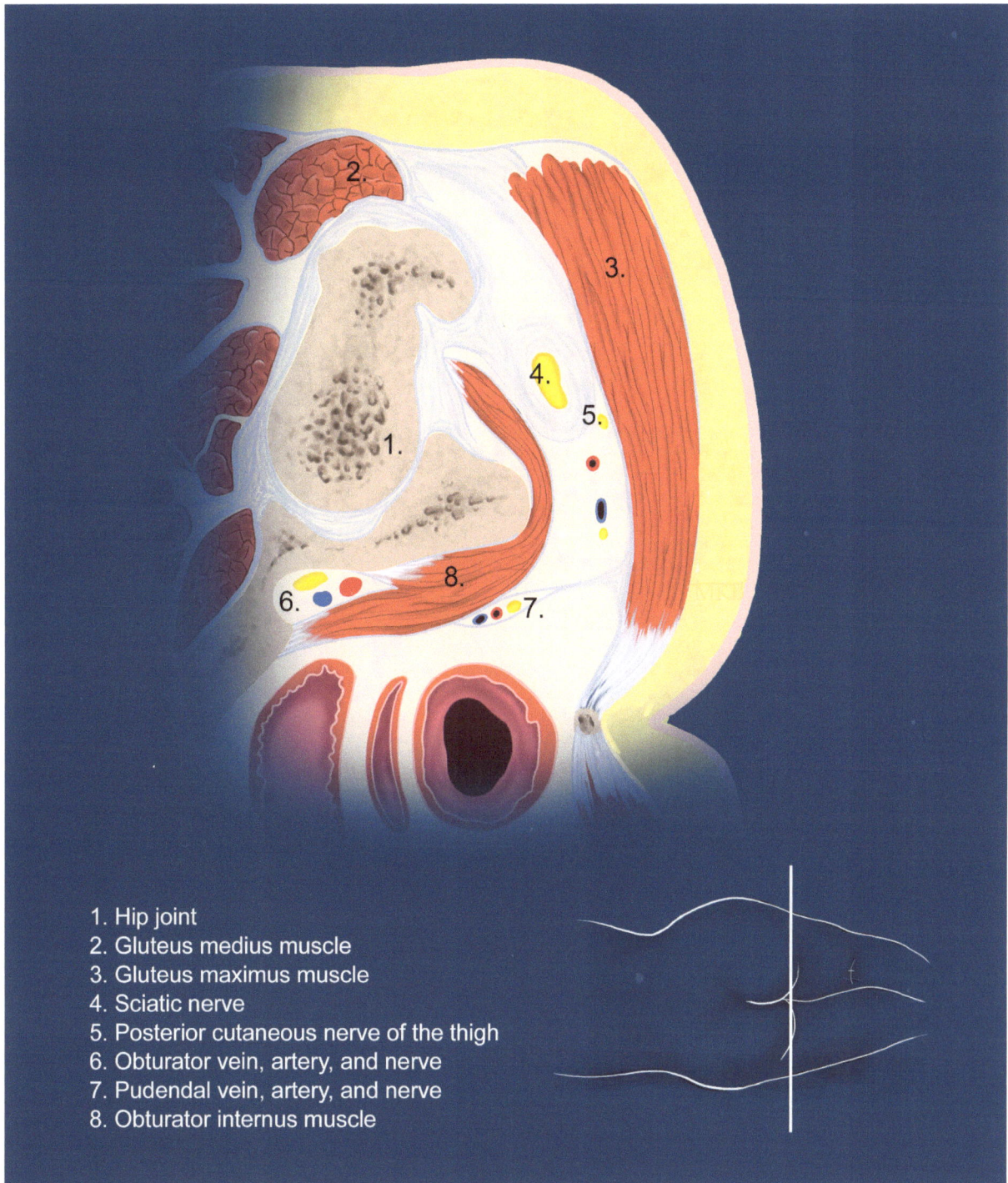

1. Hip joint
2. Gluteus medius muscle
3. Gluteus maximus muscle
4. Sciatic nerve
5. Posterior cutaneous nerve of the thigh
6. Obturator vein, artery, and nerve
7. Pudendal vein, artery, and nerve
8. Obturator internus muscle

*Figure 4-5: Trans-sectional view of the sciatic nerve in the subgluteal area.*

Please note: The posterior cutaneous nerve (5) of the thigh is separate from the sciatic nerve (4) at this level.

# Transection at the Popliteal Level

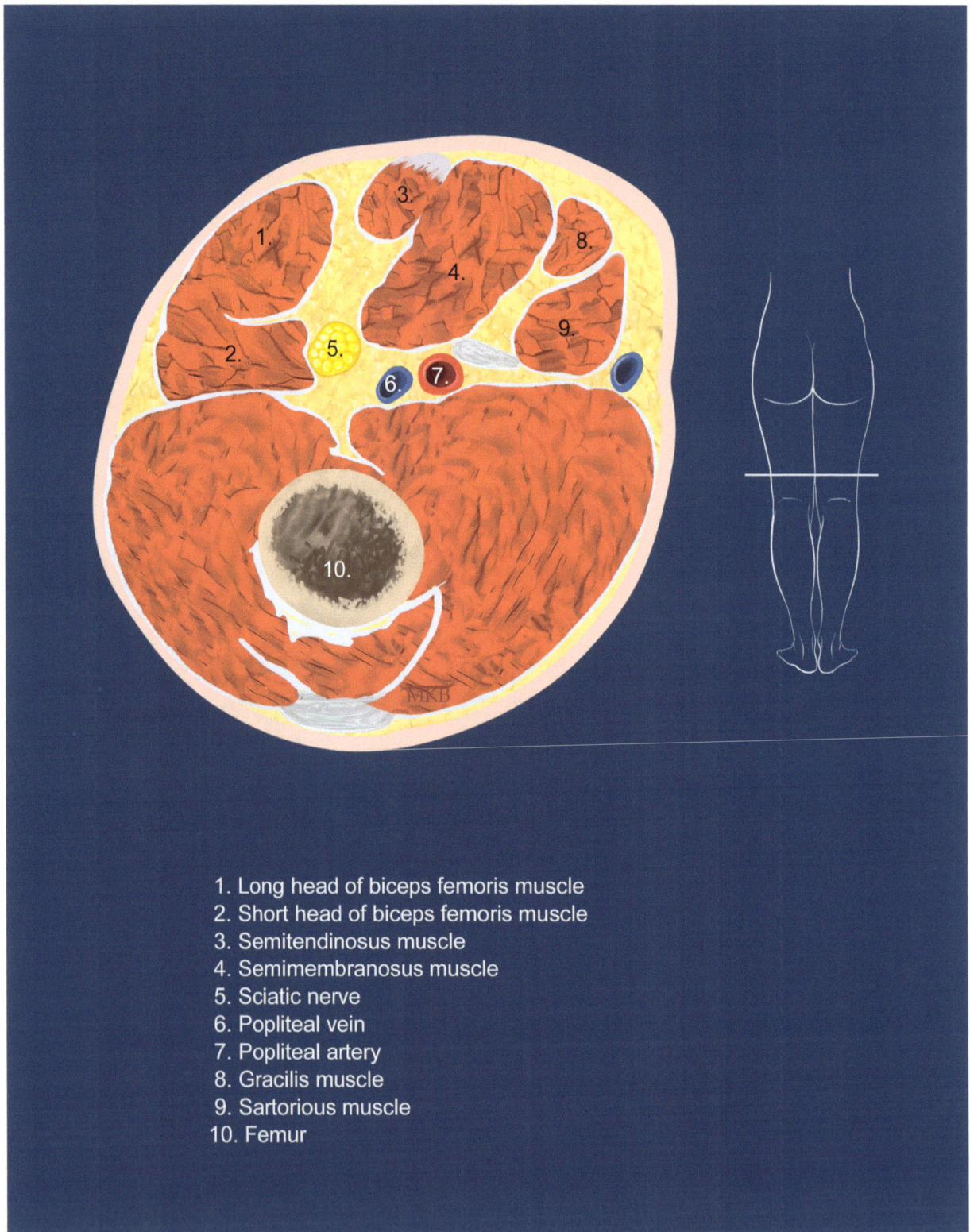

1. Long head of biceps femoris muscle
2. Short head of biceps femoris muscle
3. Semitendinosus muscle
4. Semimembranosus muscle
5. Sciatic nerve
6. Popliteal vein
7. Popliteal artery
8. Gracilis muscle
9. Sartorious muscle
10. Femur

*Figure 4-6: Trans-sectional anatomy of the sciatic nerve in the popliteal fossa.*

# Landmarks for the Subgluteal Sciatic Nerve Block

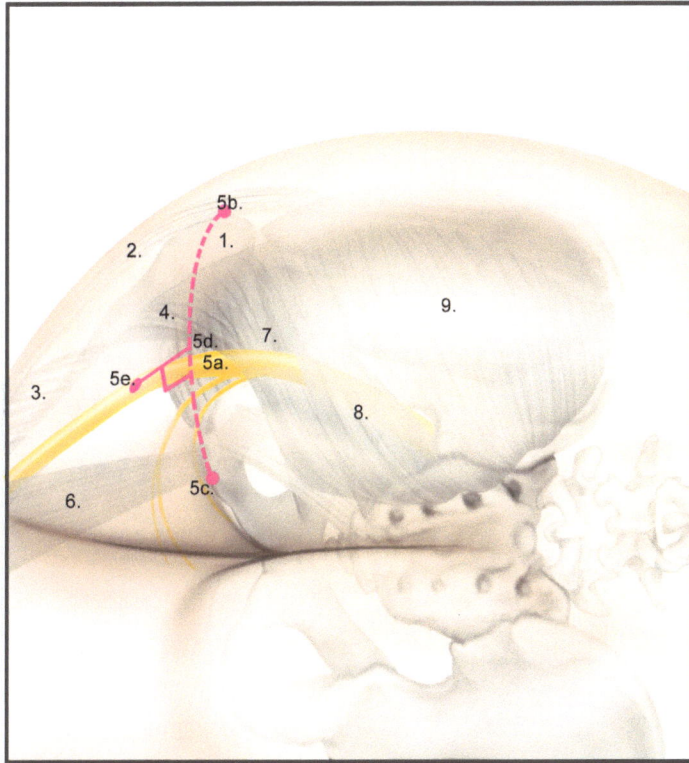

1. Greater trochanter of femur
2. Iliotibial tract
3. Vastus lateralis muscle
4. Gluteus maximus muscle
5a. Sciatic nerve
5b. Line joining greater trochanter of femur with
5c. Ischial tuberosity
5d. Midpoint of line
5e. Needle entry point
6. Biceps femoris muscle
7. Obturator internus muscle
8. Piriformis muscle
9. Gluteus medius muscle

A line (5b) is drawn from the greater trochanter (1) that joins it to the ischial tuberosity (5c). A midpoint of this line (5d) and its perpendicular line (5e) outlines the position of the sciatic nerve. The sciatic nerve seems to be approximately 43% of the distance between the inguinal to the subgluteal creases from the skin.

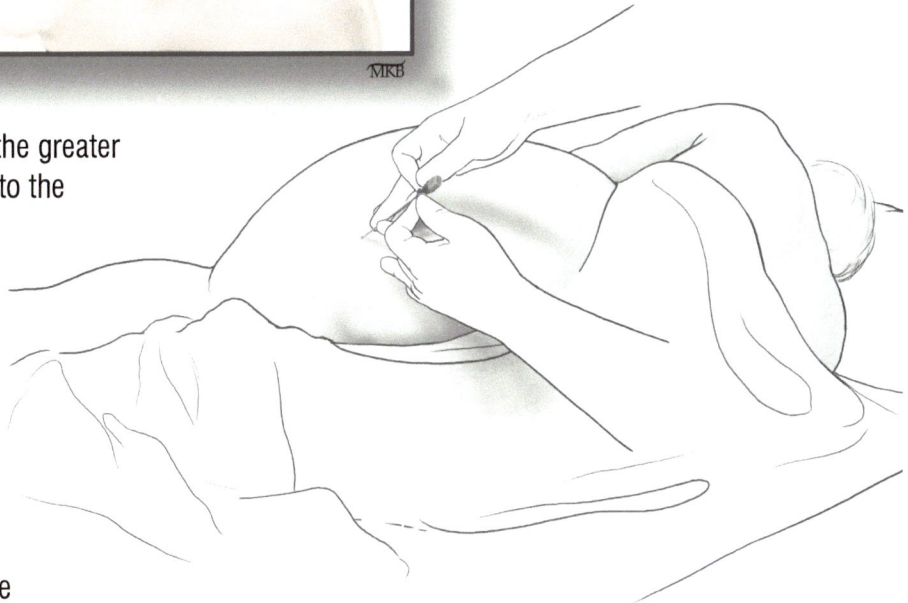

*Figure 4-7: The surface anatomy of the sciatic nerve in the subgluteal area.*

**Please refer to standard textbooks for indications for and techniques of performing any of the blocks referred to in this book.**

*Ref: Crabtree EC, Beck M, Lopp BR, Nosovitch M, Edwards JN, Boezaart AP. A method to estimate the depth of the sciatic nerve during subgluteal block by using thigh diameter as a guide. Reg Anesth Pain Med 2006;31:358-62.*

# Proximal Approaches to the Sciatic Nerve

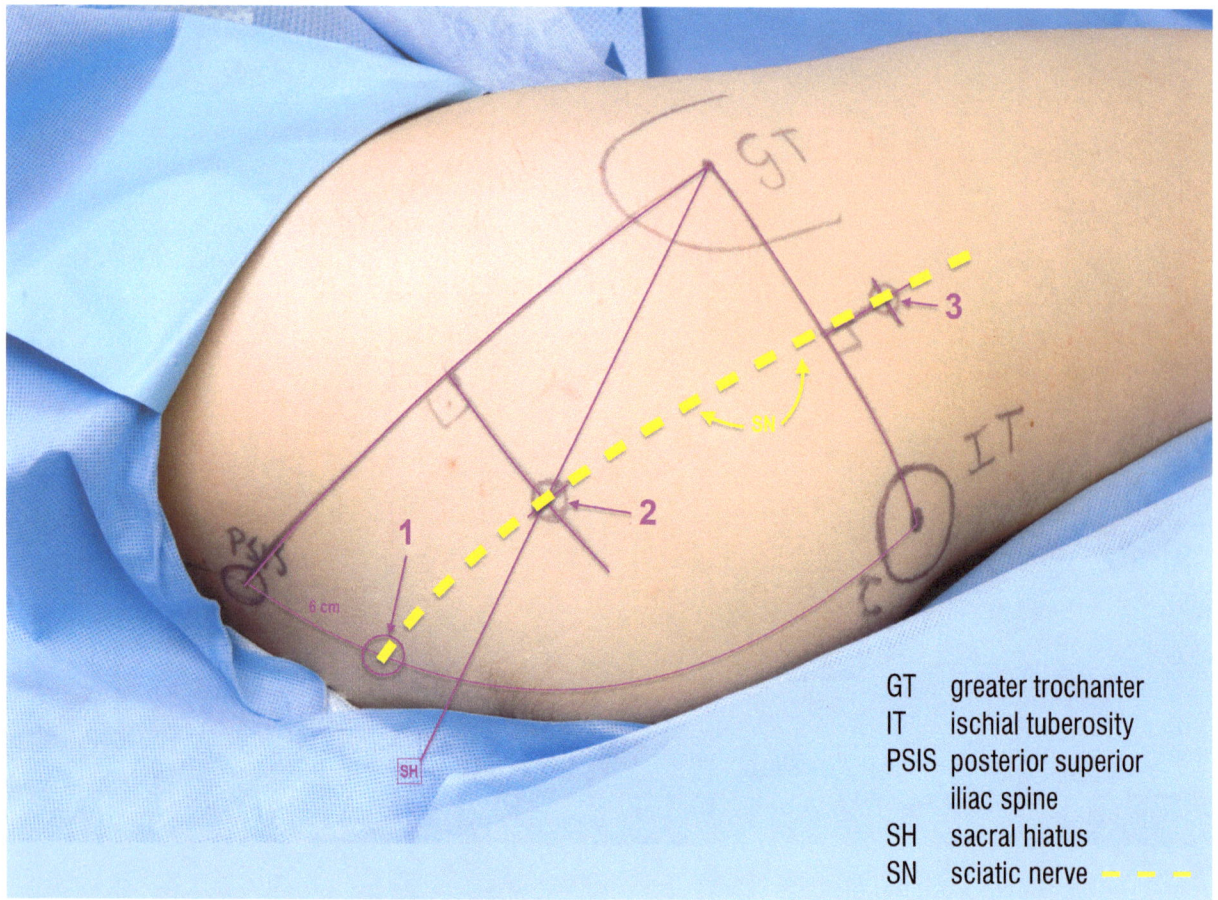

| | |
|---|---|
| GT | greater trochanter |
| IT | ischial tuberosity |
| PSIS | posterior superior iliac spine |
| SH | sacral hiatus |
| SN | sciatic nerve — — — |

*Figure 4-8: Surface anatomy of the sciatic nerve in the parasacral, transgluteal (Labat, Winnie), and subgluteal areas.*

The sciatic nerve can be found at positions 1, 2 & 3 on the photograph:

Position 1: A line is drawn to join the PSIS with the IT, and the sciatic nerve is found 6 cm caudad from the PSIS on this line where it exits the greater sciatic foramen.

Position 2: A line is drawn from the GT to the PSIS, and a perpendicular line is drawn at the midpoint of this line. In the "Labat" transgluteal approach, the sciatic nerve is found 6 cm down this perpendicular line. In the "Winnie" approach, a further line is drawn from the GT to the SH and the sciatic nerve is found transgluteal where this line crosses the perpendicular line, at Position 2.

Position 3: A line is drawn to join the GT with the IT. The sciatic nerve is found in the subgluteal approach on a perpendicular line drawn at the midpoint of this line joining the GR and IT.

**Please refer to standard textbooks for indications for and techniques of performing any of the blocks referred to in this book.**

# Popliteal Approach to the Sciatic Nerve

1. Biceps femoris long head muscle
2. Semitendinosus muscle
3. Popliteal artery
4. Popliteal vein
5. Tibial nerve
6. Common fibular nerve
7. Lateral sural cutaneous nerve
8. Medial sural cutaneous nerve
9. Gastrocnemius muscle
10. Plantaris muscle
11. Semimembranosus muscle
12. Gracilis muscle

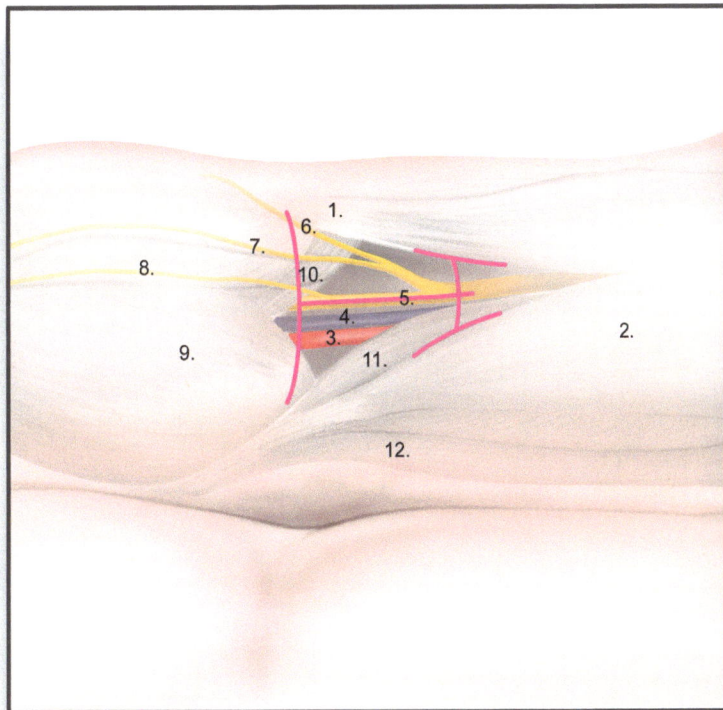

A line (10) is drawn on the popliteal crease line, and two lines are drawn to outline the medial and lateral borders, respectively, of the biceps femoris (1) and semimembranosus and semitendinosus muscles (11). The sciatic nerve is found on a midline (5) that joins the first crease line (10) with a parallel line 7 to 9 cm cephalad that joins the lines outlining the borders of the muscles.

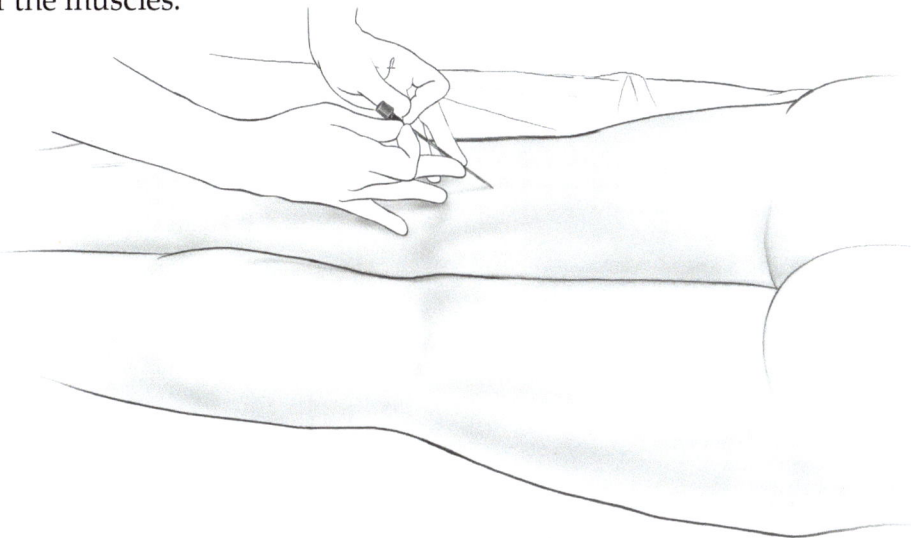

*Figure 4-9: Surface anatomy of the sciatic nerve in the popliteal fossa.*

**Please refer to standard textbooks for indications for and techniques of performing any of the blocks referred to in this book.**

# Microanatomy

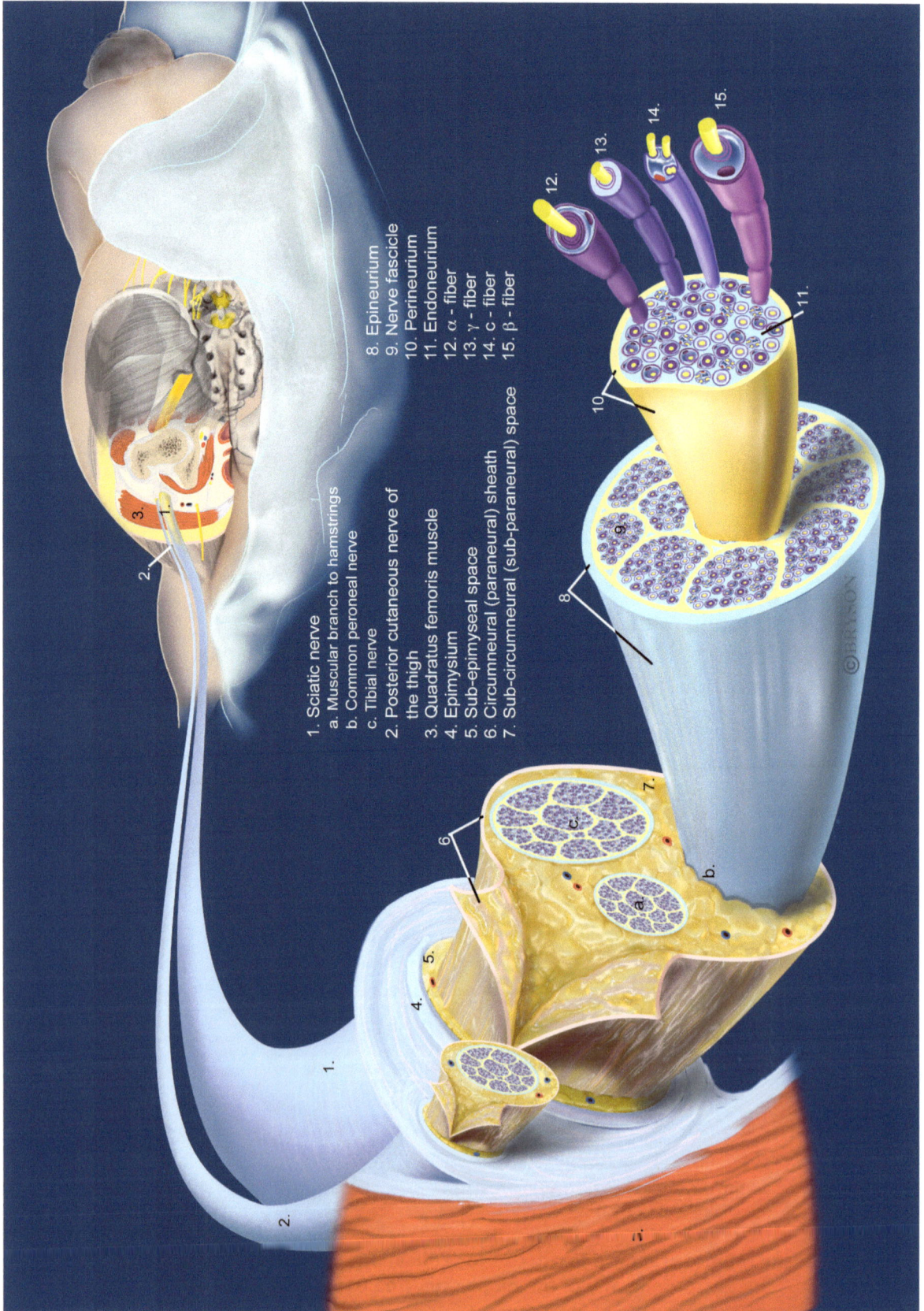

1. Sciatic nerve
   a. Muscular branch to hamstrings
   b. Common peroneal nerve
   c. Tibial nerve
2. Posterior cutaneous nerve of the thigh
3. Quadratus femoris muscle
4. Epimysium
5. Sub-epimyseal space
6. Circumneural (paraneural) sheath
7. Sub-circumneural (sub-paraneural) space
8. Epineurium
9. Nerve fascicle
10. Perineurium
11. Endoneurium
12. α - fiber
13. γ - fiber
14. c - fiber
15. β - fiber

*Figure 4-10: Microstructure of the sciatic nerve.*

Please note:

- The branches of the sciatic nerve are enclosed in a common circumneural sheath (6) (also known as the paraneural sheath).

- There are three branches inside the sciatic nerve: the muscular branch to the hamstring muscles (1a), the common peroneal nerve (1b), and the tibial nerve (1c).

- Outside the circumneural sheath is the sub-epimyseal space (5), which is surrounded by the epimysium (4) – the fascia that surrounds the nerves, muscles, and blood vessels. Injection into this space forms the well-known doughnut sign on an ultrasound-guided nerve block.

- Deep to the circumneural sheath (6); the paraneural sheath) is the sub-circumneural space (7), which is thought to be the ideal space for the needle and catheter placement for a nerve block – the "sweet spot" of the nerve.

- The next layer, which encloses each individual branch, is the epineurium (8), surrounding the fascicles of each branch.

- In turn, each fascicle is surrounded by its own perineurium (10).

- Inside the perineurium are the endoneurium and nerve axons (12-15).

Ref: Boezaart AP. The sweet spot of the nerve: Is the "paraneural sheath" named correctly, and does it matter? Reg Anesth Pain Med 2014;39:557-8.

Ref: Reina MA, Navarro RA, Mateos EMD. Ultrastructure of myelinated and unmyelinated axons. In: Reina MA, Ed. Atlas of Functional Anatomy For Regional Anesthesia And Pain Medicine. New York: Springer, 2015; 3-126.

# The Circumneurium

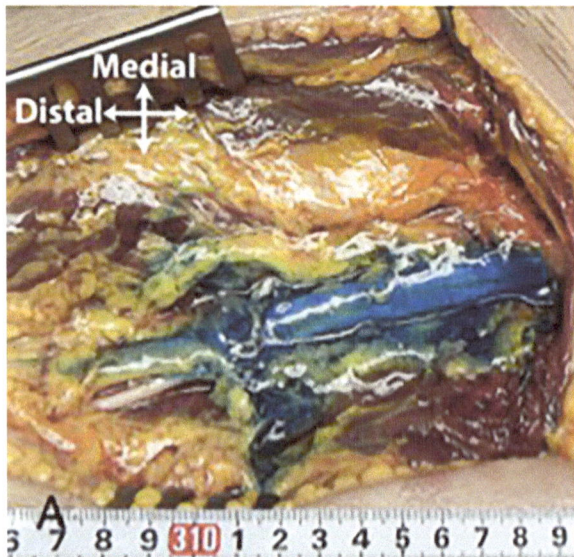

A. The transparent, shiny circumneural (AKA paraneural) sheath is expanded by the injectate around the sciatic nerve and along the tibial nerve. The blue stripe proximal to the bifurcation is the injection site.

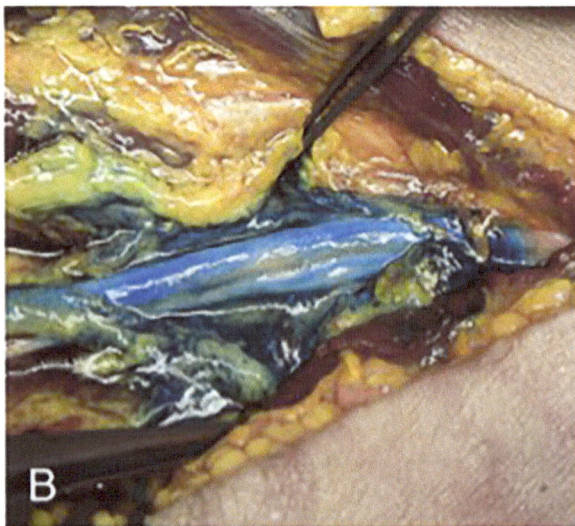

B. The circumneural sheath is cut open and split aside by two pairs of forceps. The sciatic nerve is exposed, and the epineurium is colored by the injectate.

C. The sciatic nerve is opened through a cut in the epineurium to verify that the injection was not intraneural.

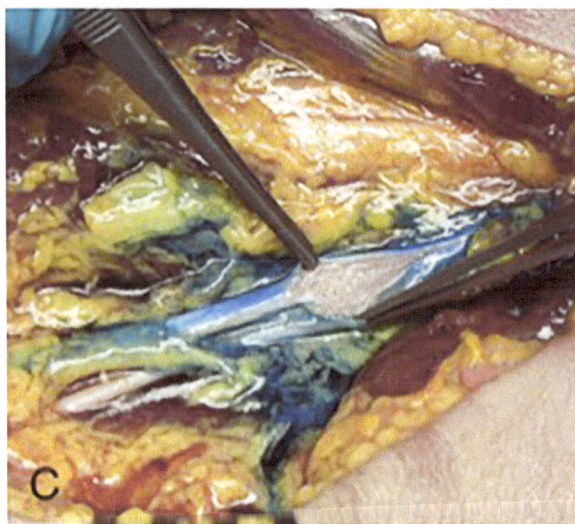

*Reprinted with permission from: Anderson HL, Anderson SL, Tranun-Jensen J. Injecting inside the paraneural sheath or the sciatic nerve: Direct comparison among ultrasound imaging, macroscopic anatomy and histologic analysis. Reg Anesth Pain Med 2012;37:410-14.*

*Figure 4-11: Gross dissection after an ultrasound-guided injection of diluted methylene blue.*

# Interneural Plexus

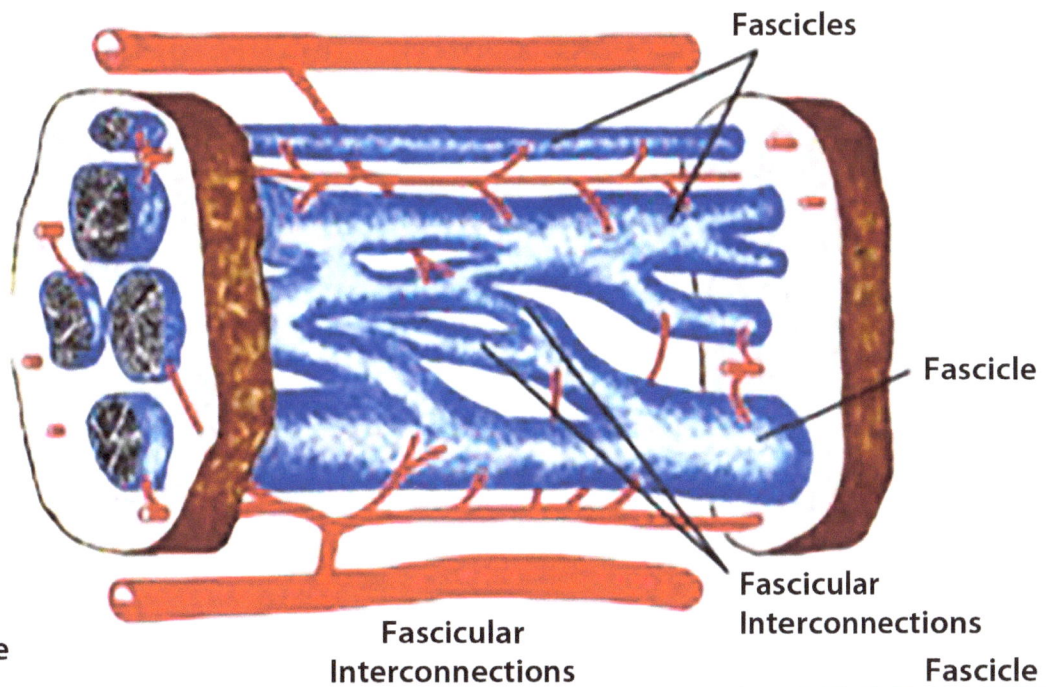

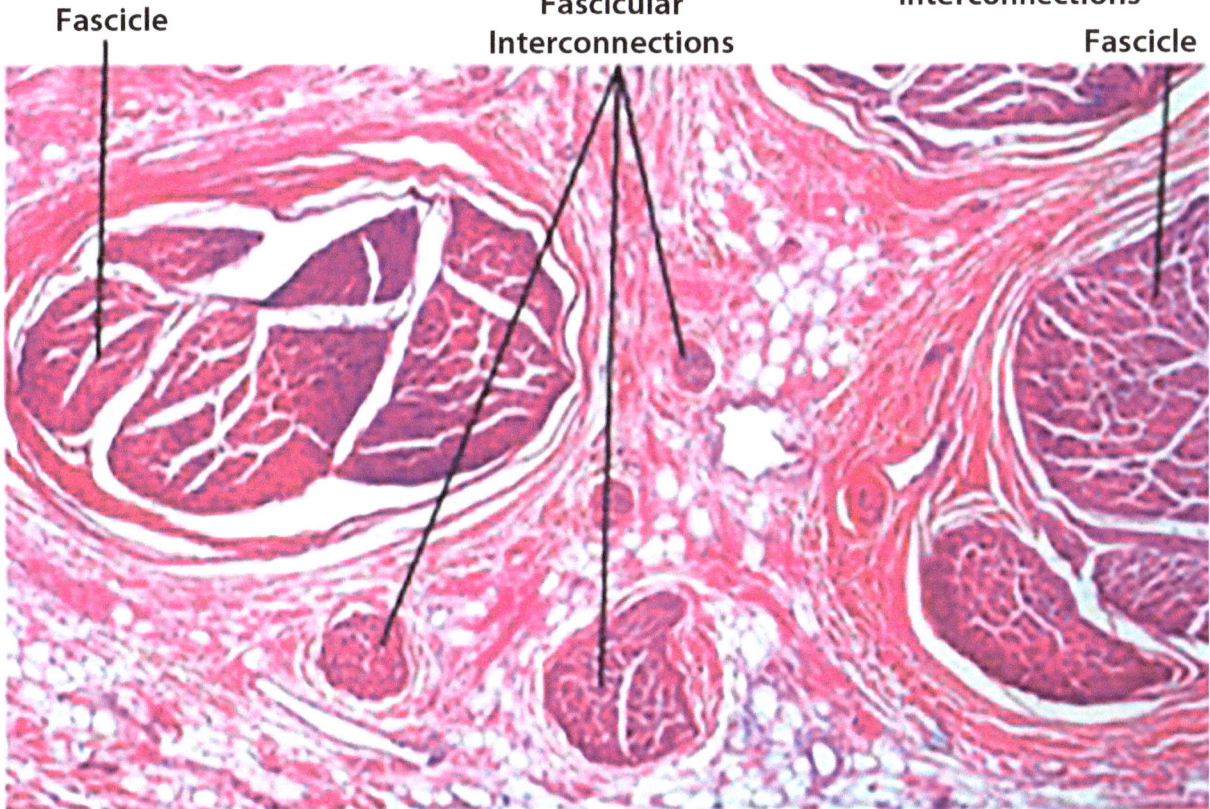

*Figure 4-12: Intraneural plexus.*

This diagram and microscopic photograph shows fascicular interconnections. Nerve fascicles are interconnected inside individual nerves by a complex intraneural plexus.

*Reprinted with permission from: Reina MA, Dominquez MF, Tardieu I. Origin of the fascicles and intraneural plexus. In: Reina MA, Ed. Atlas of Functional Anatomy For Regional Anesthesia And Pain Medicine. New York: 2015, 99-126*

# Sononanatomy
## The Greater Sciatic Notch

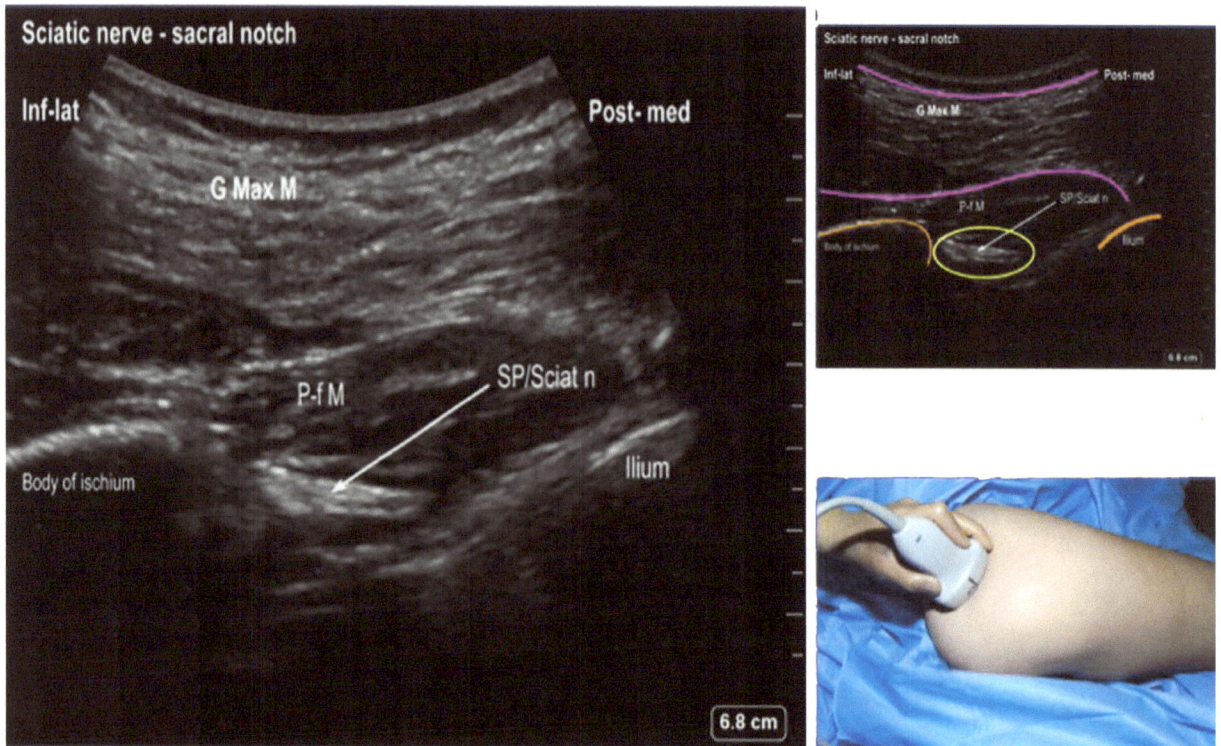

Figure 4-13: Sonoanatomy of the sciatic nerve or sacral plexus in the sciatic notch or sacral paravertebral space.

| | |
|---|---|
| G Max M | gluteus maximus muscle |
| Inf-lat | inferolateral |
| P-f M | piriformis muscle |
| Post-med | postero-medially |
| SP/Sciat | sacral plexus or sciatic nerve |

The distance from the skin in this particular model is 6.8 cm

View Video at RAEducation.com
Acute Pain Medicine - Anatomy -
Sonoanatomy: Parasacral Sciatic Nerve

# The Greater Sciatic Notch

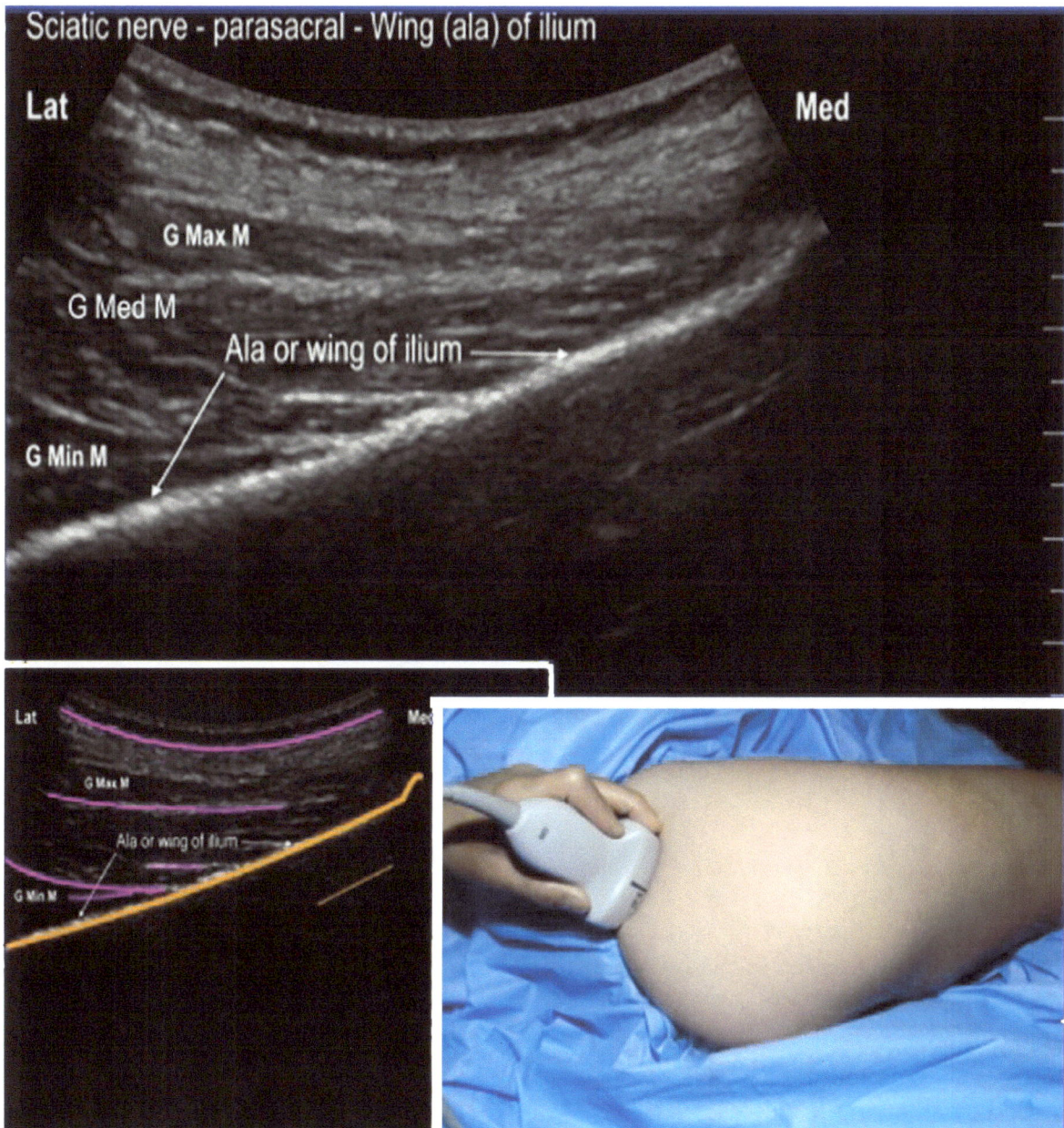

Figure 4-14: Sonoanatomy of the parasacral approach to the sciatic nerve.

| | |
|---|---|
| G Max M | Gluteus maximus muscle |
| G Med M | Gluteus medius muscle |
| G Min M | Gluteus minimus muscle |
| Lat | lateral |
| Med | Medial |

**View Video at RAEducation.com**
**Acute Pain Medicine - Anatomy -**
**Sonoanatomy: Parasacral Sciatic Nerve**

# Subgluteal Sciatic Nerve

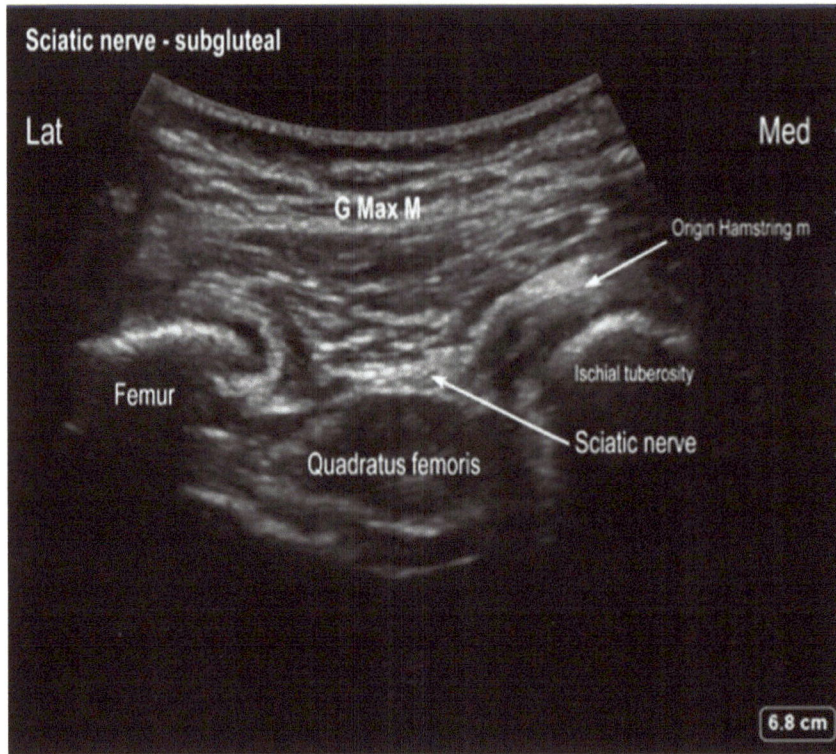

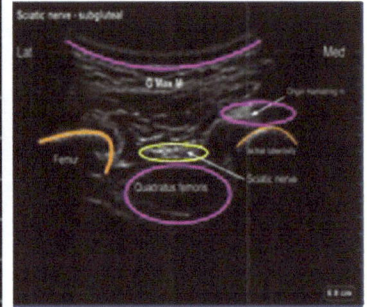

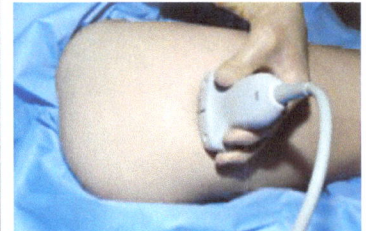

*Figure 4-15: Sonoanatomy of the sciatic nerve in the subgluteal area.*

G Max M      Gluteus maximus muscle
                  (inferior edge)
Lat              Lateral
Med          Medial
Origin of hamstring m muscle

**View Video at RAEducation.com
Acute Pain Medicine - Anatomy -
Sonoanatomy: Subgluteal Sciatic Nerve**

# Mid-femoral Sciatic Nerve

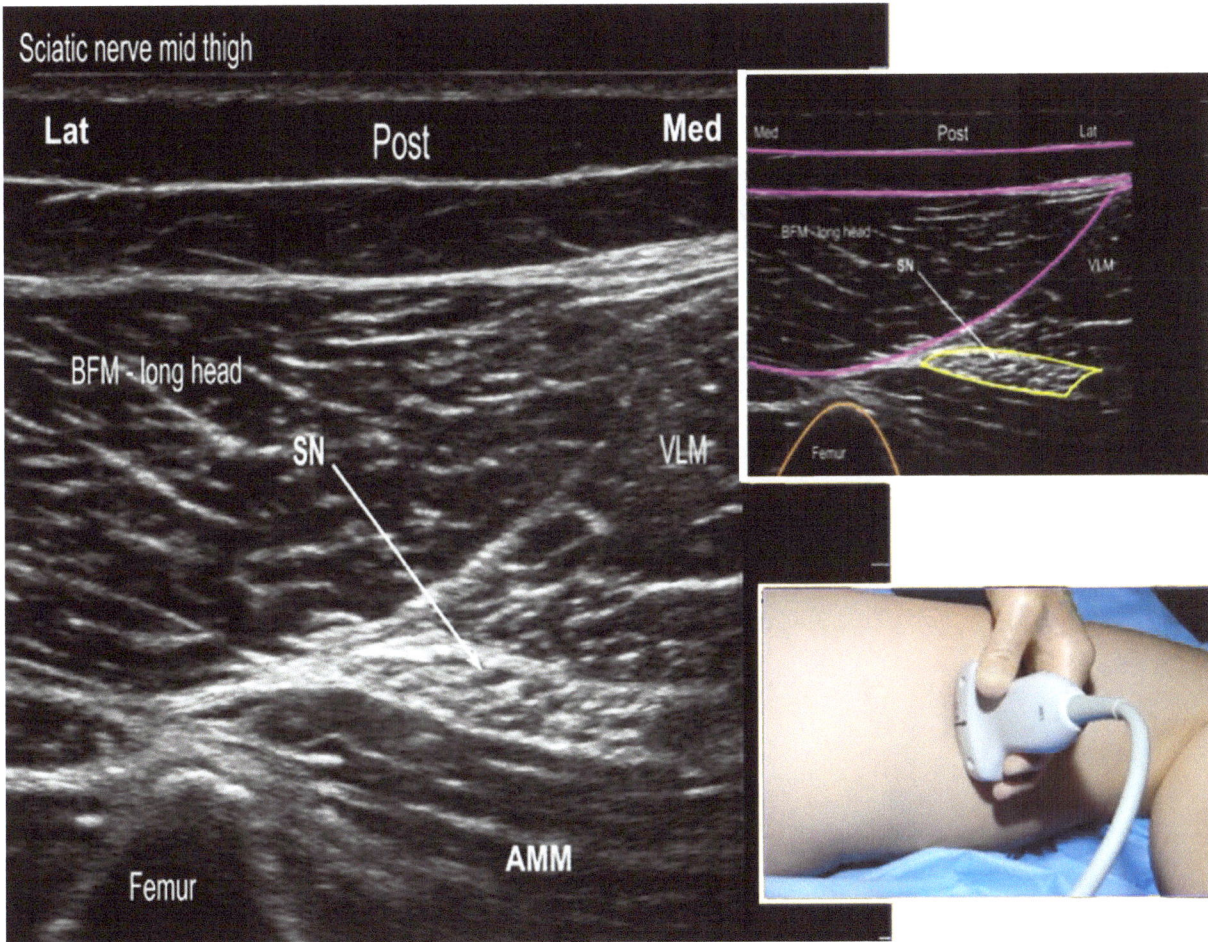

Figure 4-16: Sonoanatomy of the sciatic nerve in the mid-femoral area.

| | |
|---|---|
| AMM | Adductor magnus muscle |
| BFM | Long head of the biceps femoris muscle |
| Lat | Lateral |
| Med | Medial |
| Post | Posterior |
| SN | Sciatic nerve |
| VLM | Vastus lateralis muscle |

# High Popliteal Sciatic Nerve

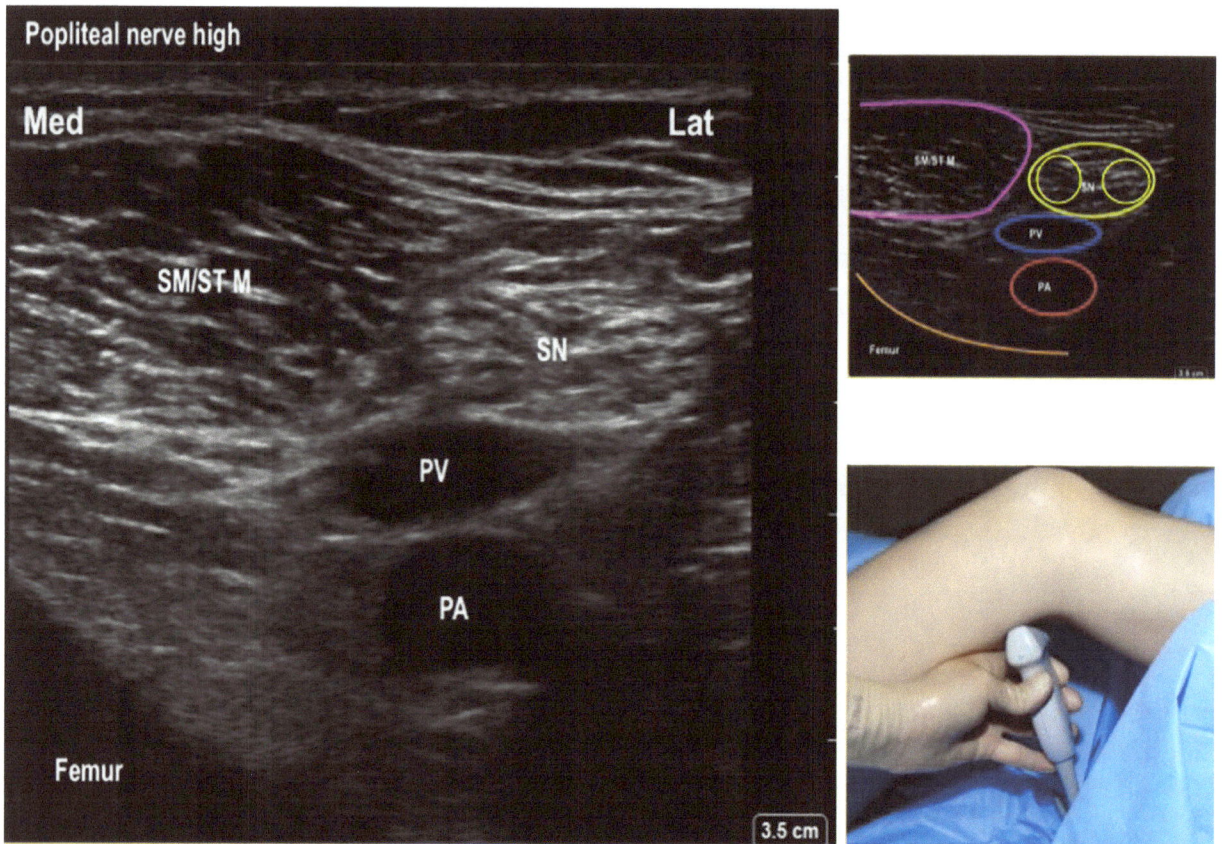

Figure 4-17: Sonoanatomy of the sciatic nerve (popliteal nerve) in the popliteal fossa behind the knee.

Lat          Lateral
Med         Medial
PA           Popliteal artery
PV           Popliteal vein
SM/ST M   Semimembranosus and
               semitendinosus muscles
SN           Sciatic nerve (popliteal part of…)

The distance from the skin is 3.5 cm

View Video at RAEducation.com
Acute Pain Medicine - Anatomy -
Sonoanatomy: Popliteal Sciatic Nerve

# Low Popliteal Sciatic Nerve

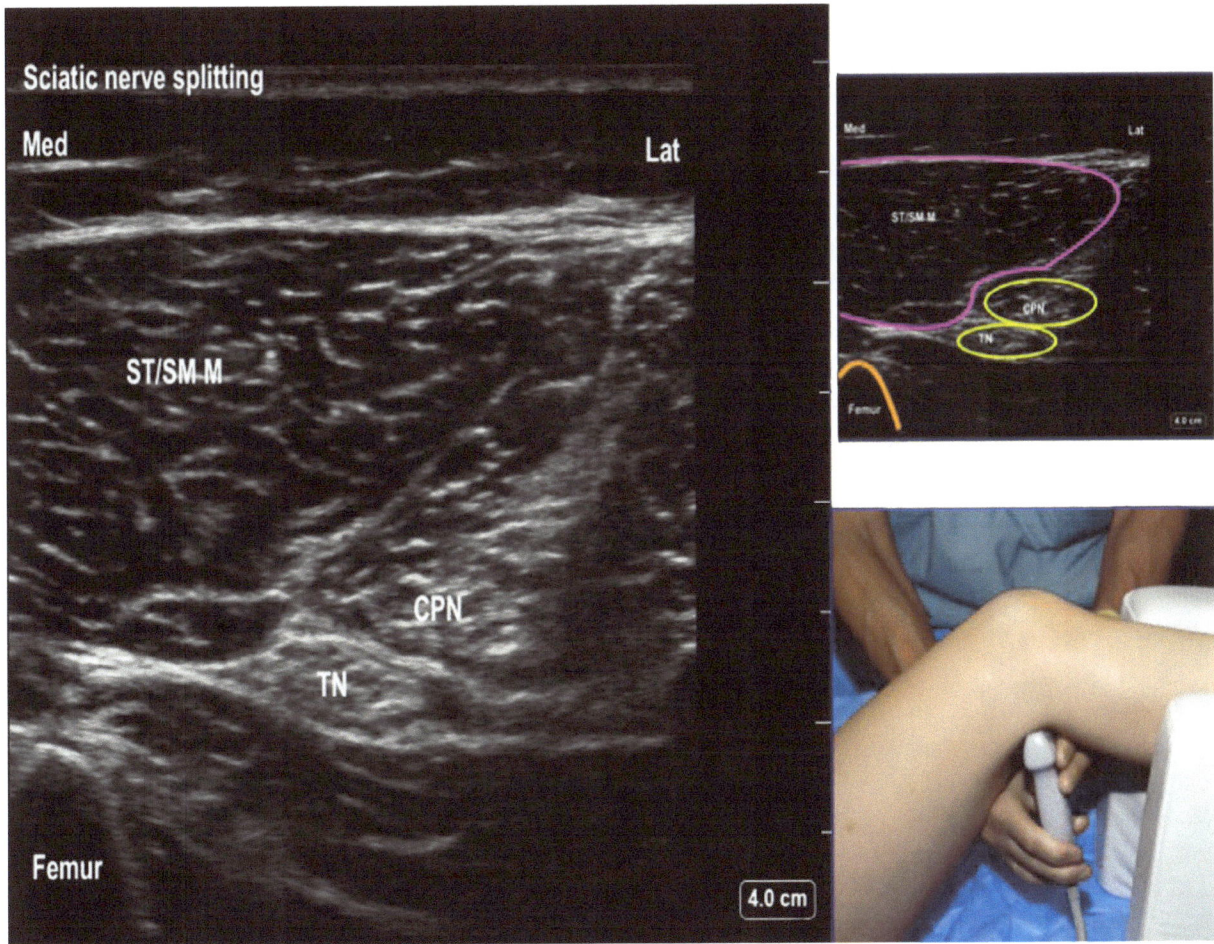

Figure 4-18: Sonoanatomy of the sciatic (popliteal) nerve in the popliteal fossa showing the early splitting of the nerve.

CPN     Common peroneal nerve
           (also called common fibular nerve)
Lat      Lateral
Med    Medial
ST/SM  Semimembranosus and
           semitendinosus muscles
TN      Tibial nerve

4.0 cm is the depth in centimeters from the skin

**View Video at RAEducation.com**
**Acute Pain Medicine - Anatomy -**
**Sonoanatomy: Popliteal Sciatic Nerve**

# Sciatic Nerve in the Popliteal Fossa

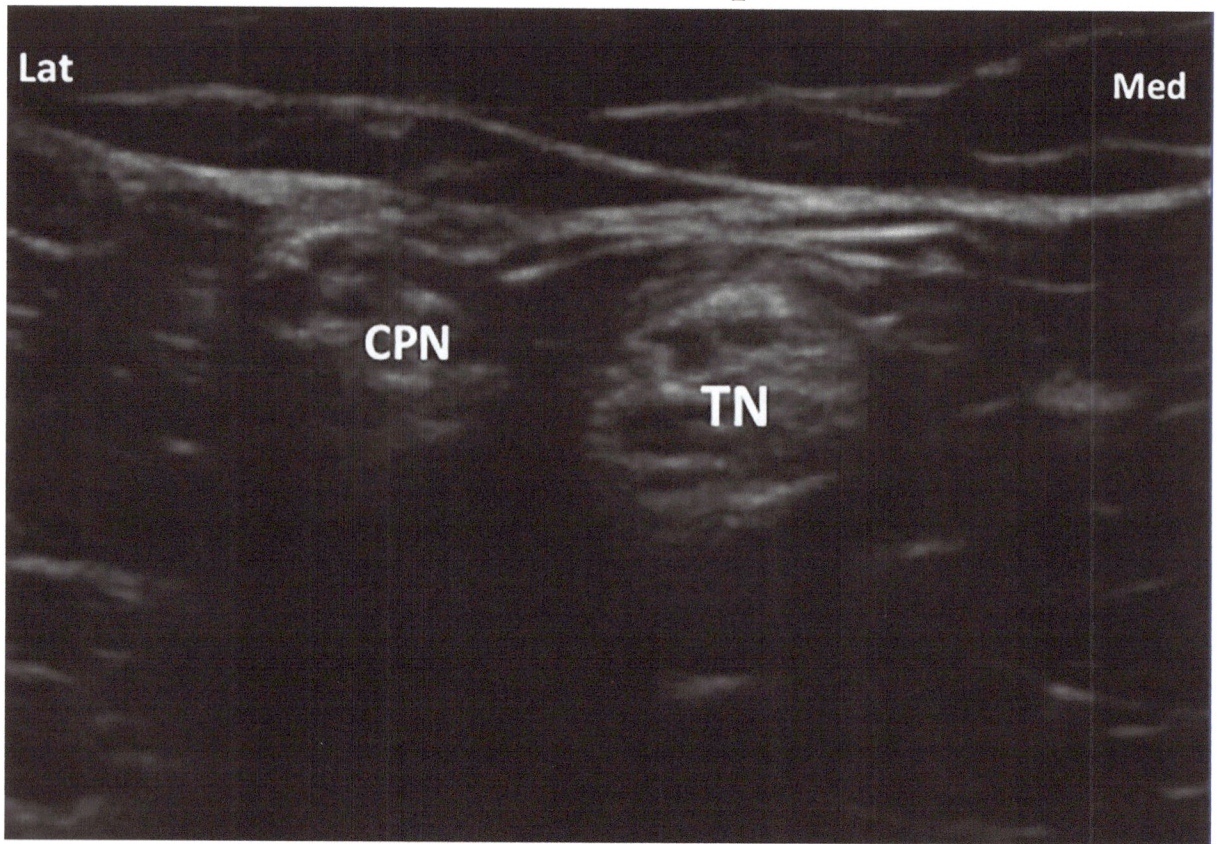

*Figure 4-19: Sonoanatomy of the sciatic nerve (popliteal nerve) in the popliteal fossa after the sciatic nerve has split.*

CPN     Common peroneal nerve
Lat     Lateral
Med     Medial
TN     Tibial nerve

# Close Up of Sciatic Nerve in the Popliteal Fossa??

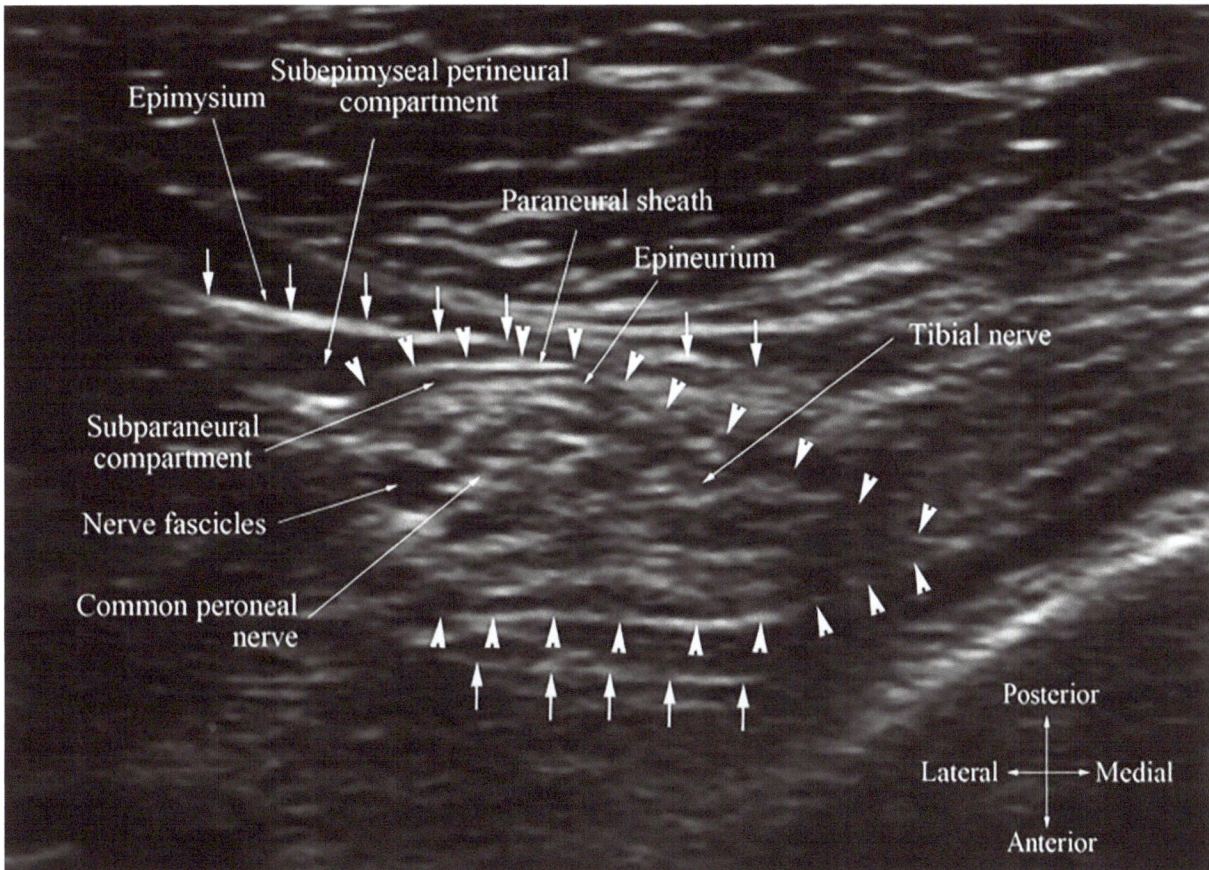

*Figure 4-20: High-definition (and zoomed) transverse sonogram of the sciatic nerve at the level of its bifurcation into the tibial and common peroneal nerve at the popliteal fossa.*

The circumneural sheath (paraneural sheath) (white arrowheads) is interposed between the epimysium (short white arrows) of the surrounding muscles and the outer surface of the sciatic nerve (epineurium), which also appears hyperechoic. The sub-epimyseal and sub-circumneural (sub-paraneural) compartments are seen as hypoechoic areas between the epimysium and the circumneural sheath, and between the circumneural sheath and the epineurium, respectively.

*Reprinted with permission from: Karmakar MK, et al. High-definition ultrasound imaging defines the paraneural sheath and the fascial compartments surrounding the sciatic nerve at the popliteal fossa. Reg Anesth Pain Med 2013;38:447-51.*

# Dermatomes of the Lower Extremity

L1
L2
L3
L4
L5
S1
S2
S3
S4
S5
Co

| Co | coccyx |
| L1-L5 | lumbar roots L2 to L5 |
| S1-S5 | sacral spinal roots S1 to S5 |

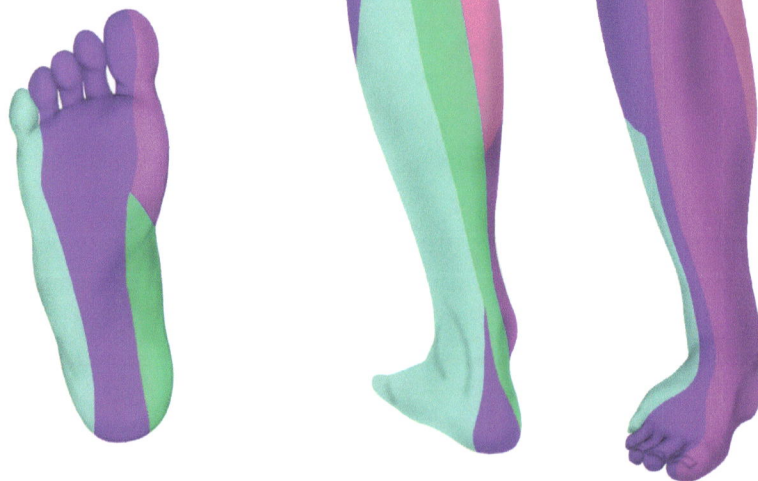

*Figure 4-21: Schematic demarcation of the dermatomes of the lower limb.*

These demarcations are not distinct segments as depicted here because there is significant overlap between adjacent dermatomes.

# Osteotomes of the Lower Extremity

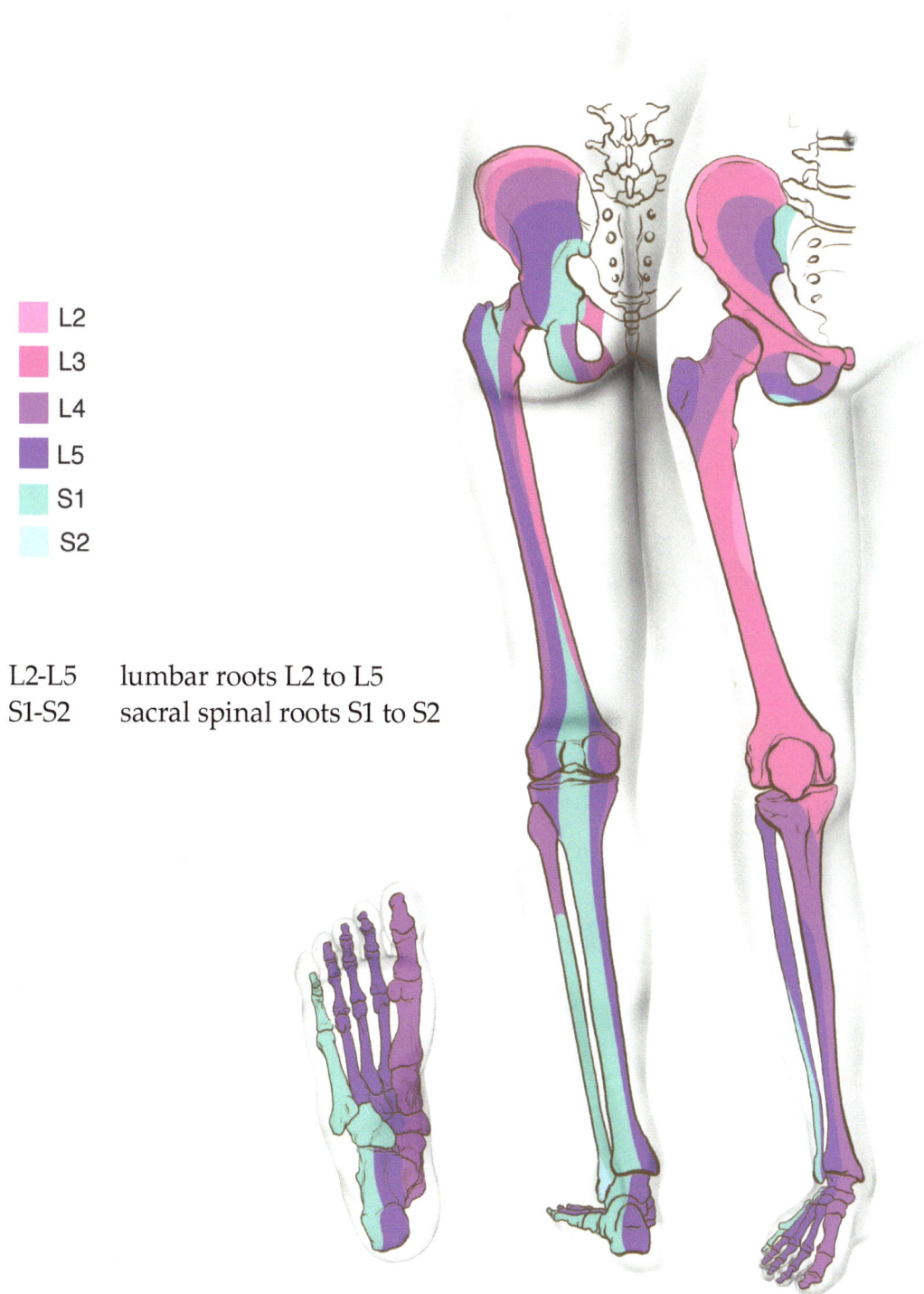

Legend:
- L2
- L3
- L4
- L5
- S1
- S2

L2-L5  lumbar roots L2 to L5
S1-S2  sacral spinal roots S1 to S2

*Figure 4-22: Schematic demarcation of the osteotomes of the lower limb.*

These demarcations are not distinct segments as depicted here because there is significant overlap between adjacent osteotomes.

*Ref: Birnbaum K, Prescher A, Hepler S, Heller KD. The sensory innervation of the hip joint. Surg Radiol Anat 1998;19:371-5.*

# Neurotomes of the Lower Extremity

Posterior femoral cutaneous nerve

Femoral branch of genitofemoral nerve

Genital branch of the genitofemoral nerve

Femoral nerve

Saphenous nerve

Lateral cutaneous nerve of the thigh

Obturator nerve

Common peroneal nerve

Deep peroneal nerve

Superficial peroneal nerve

Sural nerve

Lateral plantar nerve

Calcaneal nerve

Medial plantar nerve

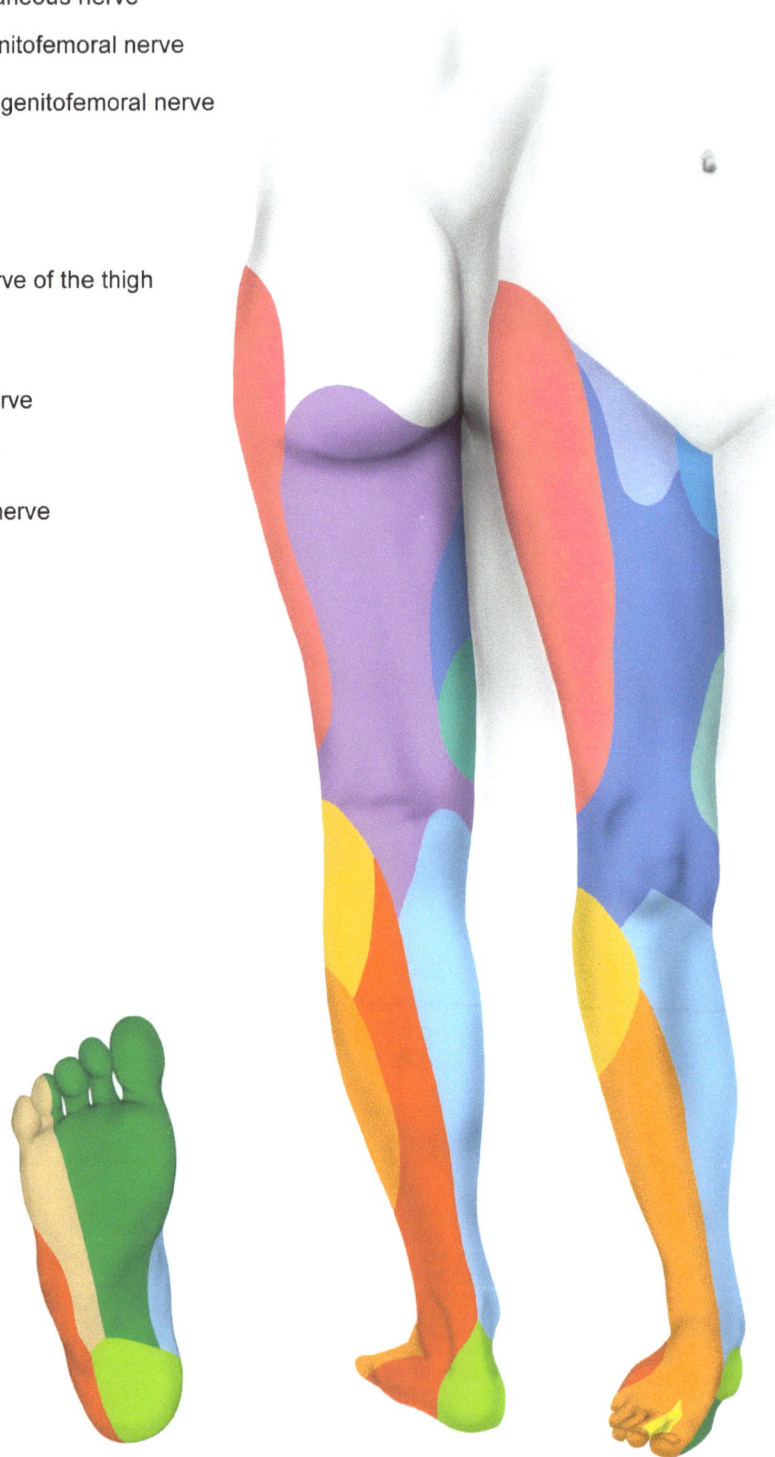

*Figure 4-23: Schematic demarcation of the neurotomes of the upper limb.*

These demarcations are not distinct areas as depicted here because there is significant overlap between adjacent neurotomes.

# Dermatomes of the Sciatic Nerve

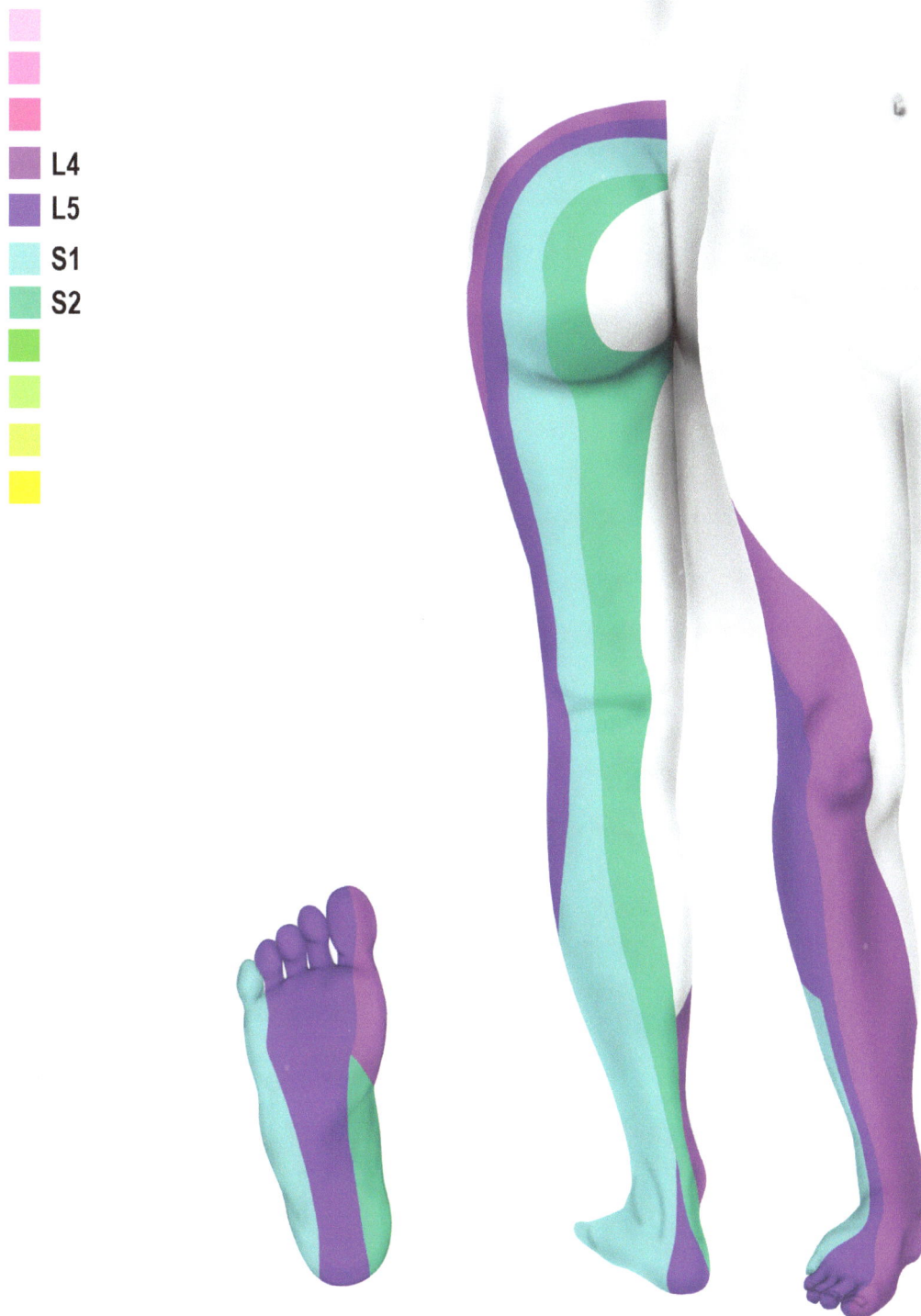

L4
L5
S1
S2

*Figure 4-24: Schematic demarcation of the dermatomes of the lower limb innervated by the sciatic nerve and its branches.*

These demarcations are not distinct areas as depicted here because there is significant overlap between adjacent dermatomes.

# Osteotomes of the Sciatic Nerve

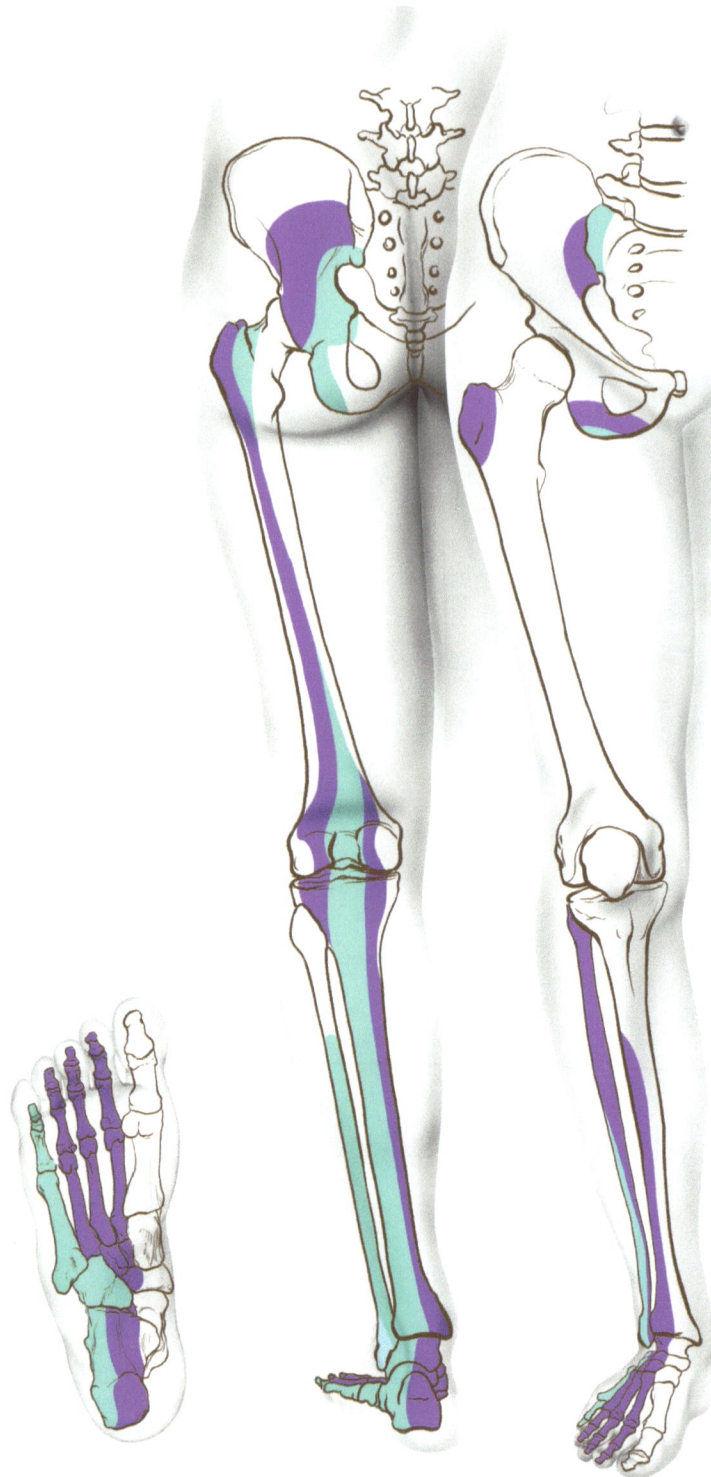

L5

S1

S2

*Figure 4-25: Schematic demarcation of the osteotomes of the lower limb innervated by the sciatic nerve and its branches.*

These demarcations are not distinct areas as depicted here because there is significant overlap between adjacent osteotomes.

# Nuerotomes of the Sciatic Nerve

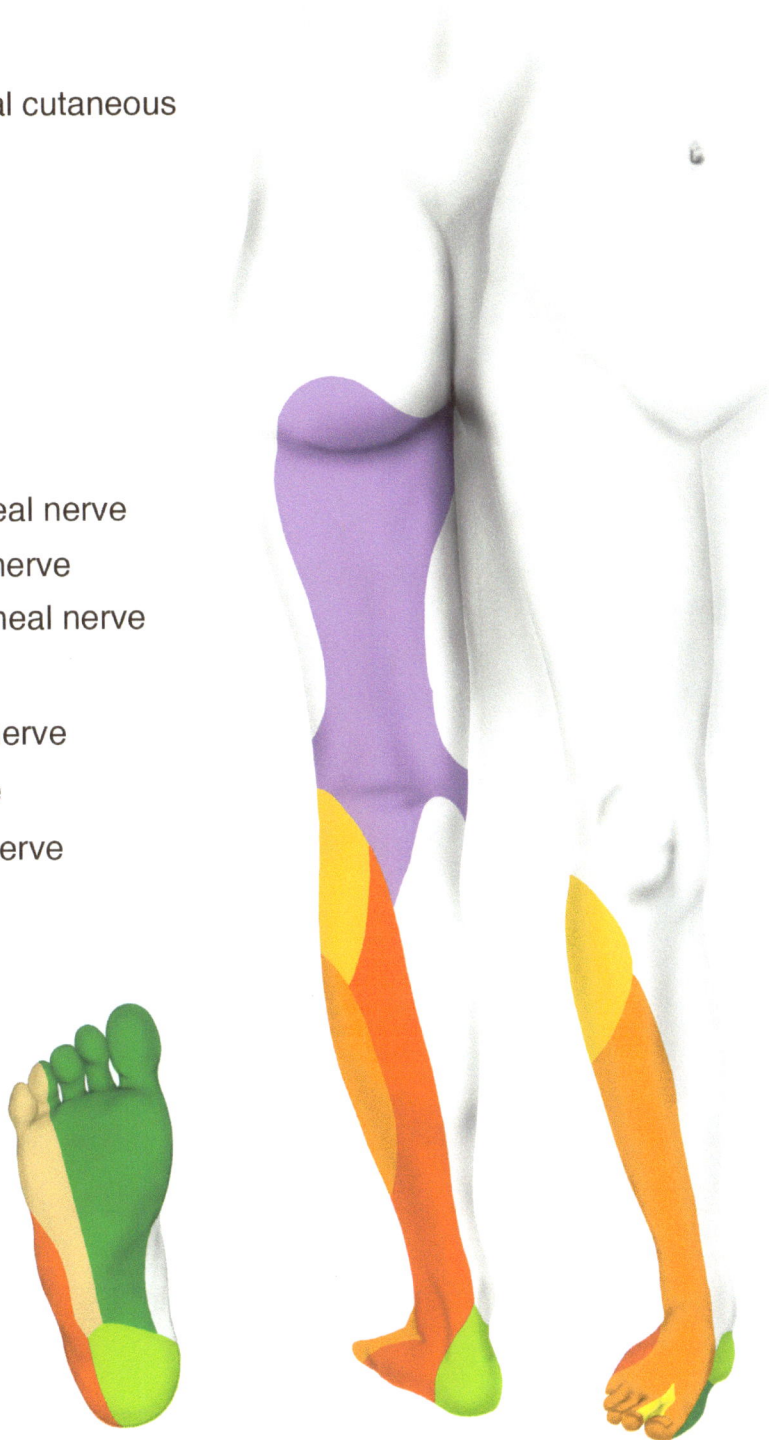

**Posterior femoral cutaneous**

**Common peroneal nerve**
**Deep peroneal nerve**
**Superficial peroneal nerve**
**Sural nerve**
**Lateral plantar nerve**
**Calcaneal nerve**
**Medial plantar nerve**

*Figure 4-26: Schematic demarcation of the neurotomes of the lower limb innervated by the sciatic nerve and its branches.*

These demarcations are not distinct areas as depicted here because there is significant overlap between adjacent dermatomes.

# Chapter 5

# Nerves Around
# The Ankle

*Macroanatomy*
*Sonoanatomy*
*Functional Anatomy*

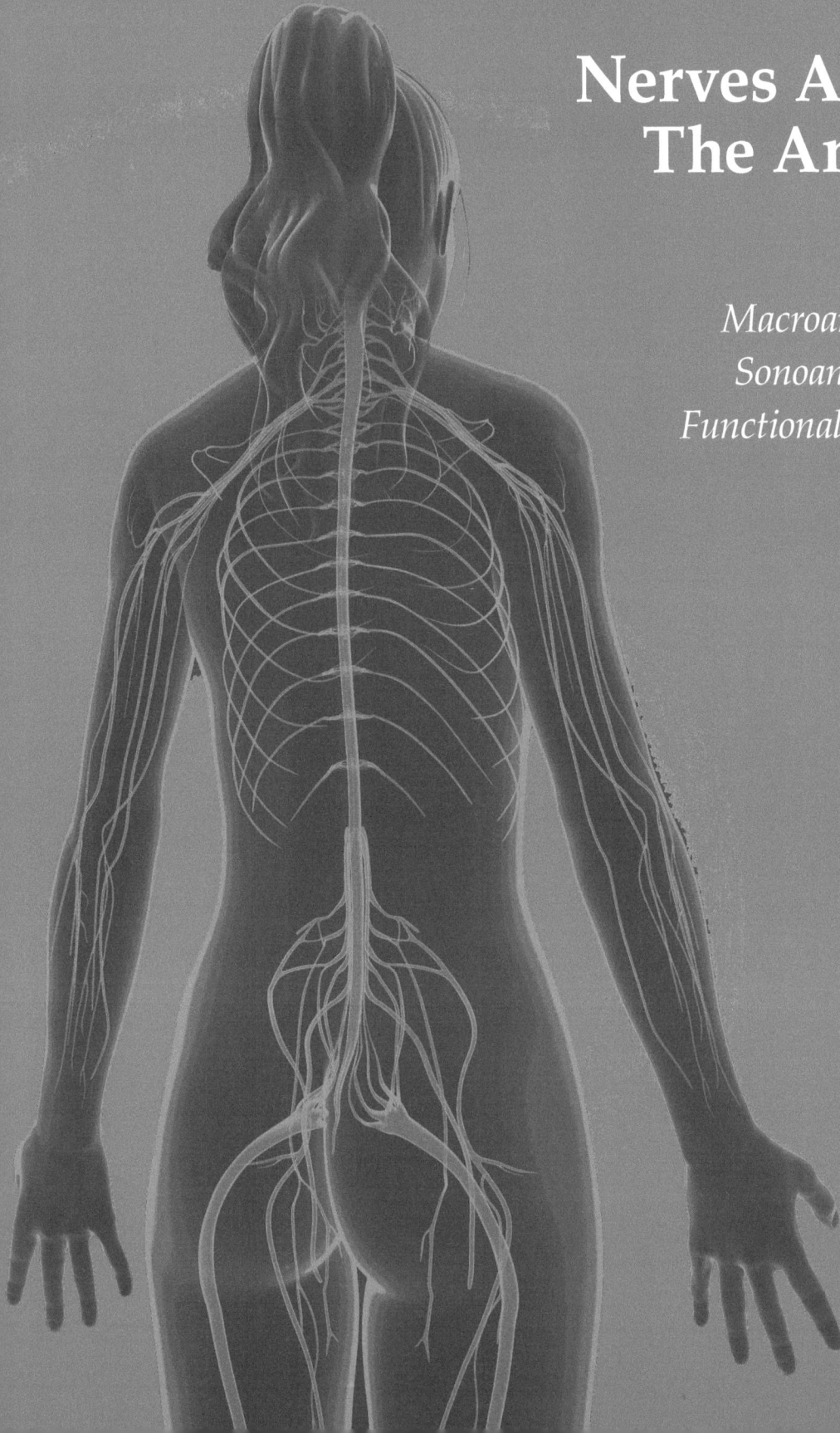

# Macroanatomy
## Transection through the Ankle

1. Superficial peroneal nerve
2. Deep peroneal nerve
3. Saphenous nerve
4. Posterior tibial nerve
5. Sural nerve
6. Achilles tendon
7. Fascia layers
8. Extensor hallucis longus tendon
9. Anterior tibialis tendon

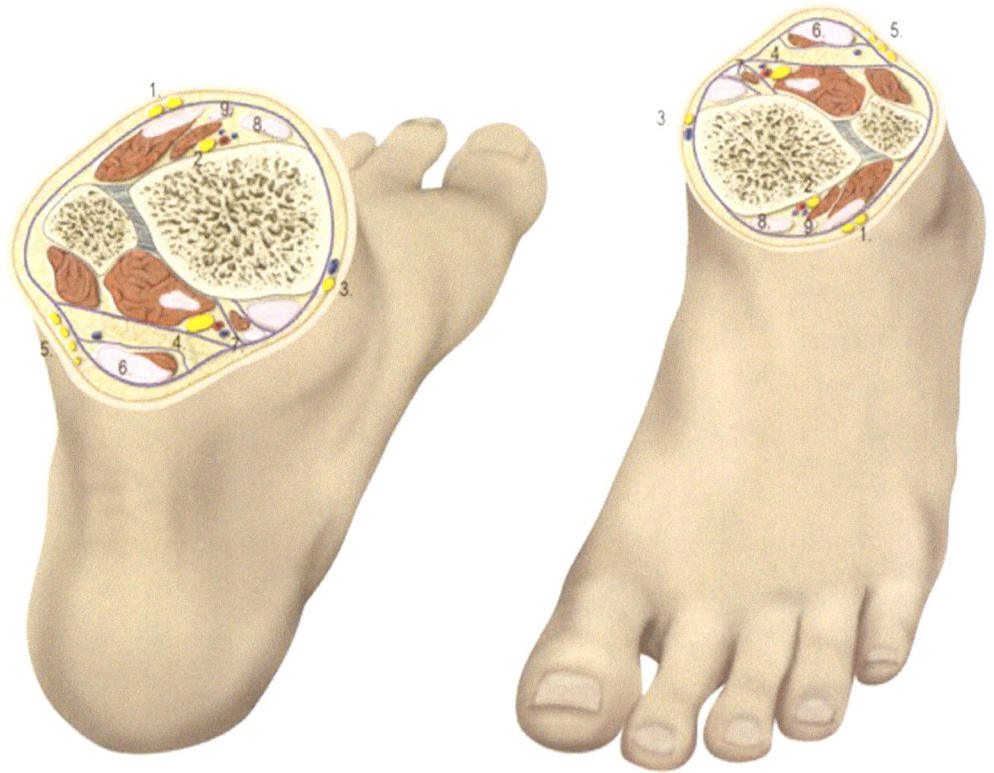

Figure 5-1: Macroanatomy of the nerves at the ankle: transection through ankle.

This illustration identifies the five nerves of the foot in the context of the fascial layers in which they lie.

There are five nerves around the ankle: two deep to the fascia layer and three superficial to it. The two deep nerves are the posterior tibial nerve and the deep peroneal nerve, whereas the three superficial nerves are the superficial peroneal, saphenous, and sural nerves.

Please note: The names of all the superficial nerves start with "s."

Ref: Sarrafian SK. Anatomy of the foot and ankle: Descriptive, topographic, functional. Philadelphia: J.B. Lippincott Company, 1993; 356-90.

# Transection through the Ankle

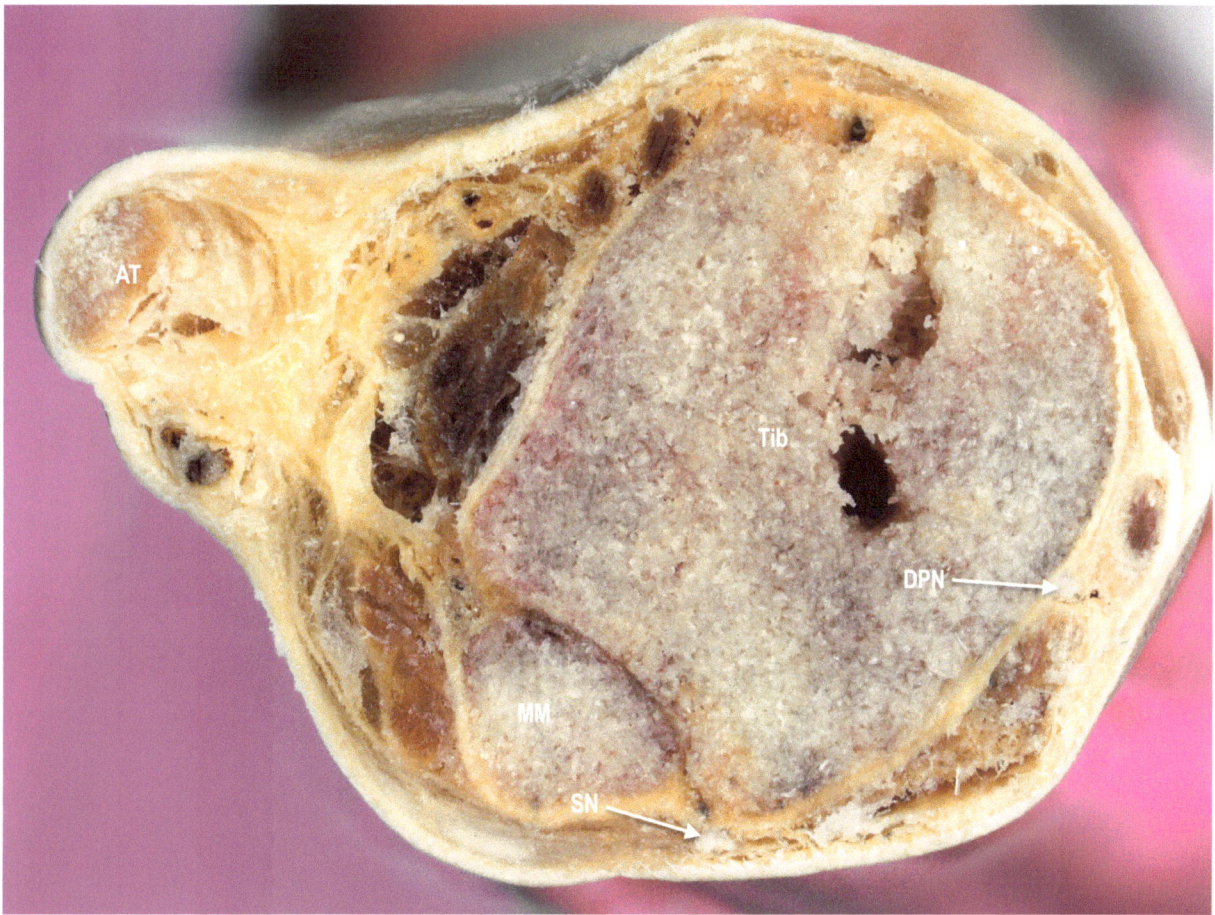

*Figure 5-2: Macroanatomy of the deep peroneal and saphenous nerves.*

AT       Achilles tendon
DPN    Deep peroneal nerve
MM     Medial malleolus
SN      Saphenous nerve
Tib      Tibia

# Dissection of the Posterior Tibial Nerve

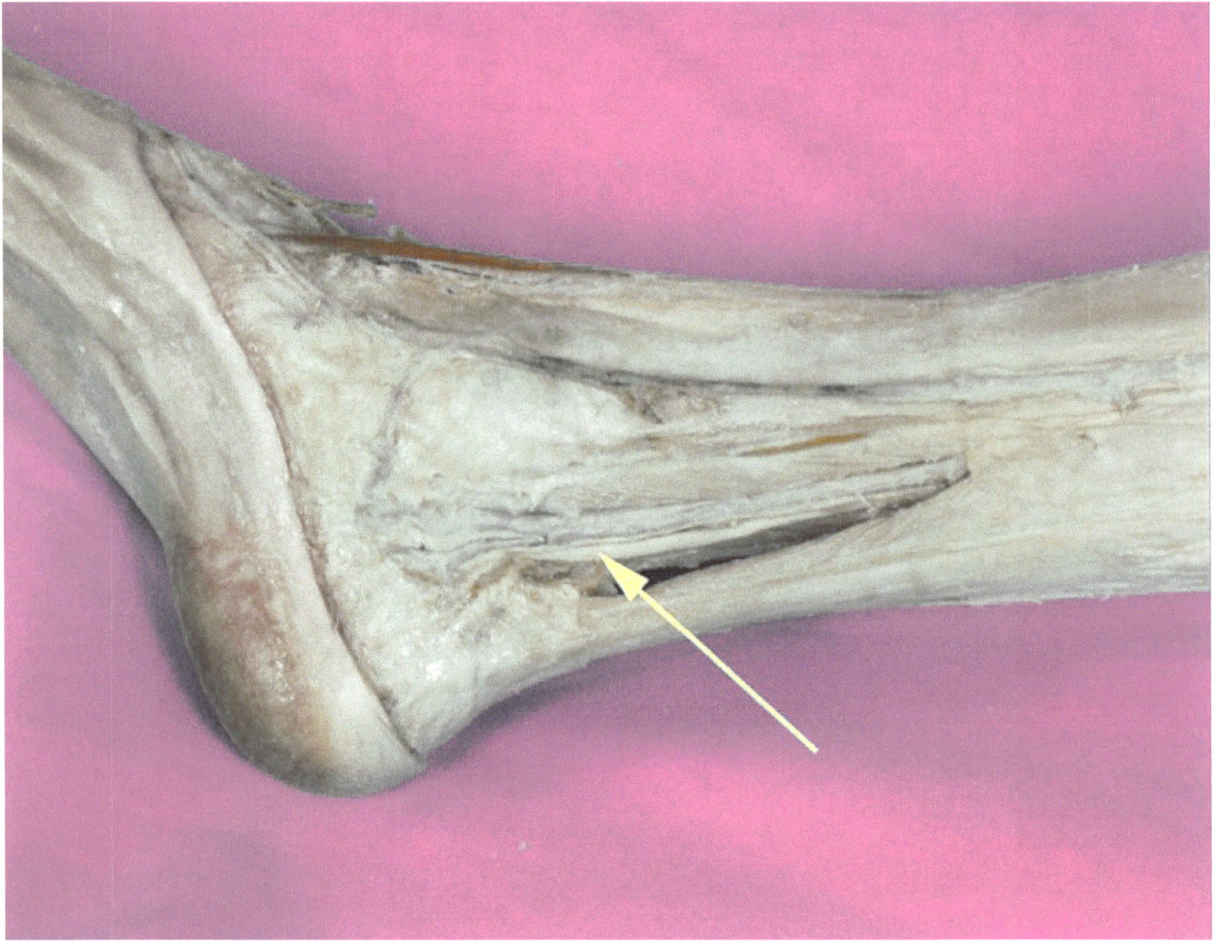

*Figure 5-3: Macroanatomy of the posterior tibial nerve.*

The posterior tibial nerve, indicated by the arrow, is usually posterior to the tibial artery.

# Dissection of the Superficial Peroneal Nerve

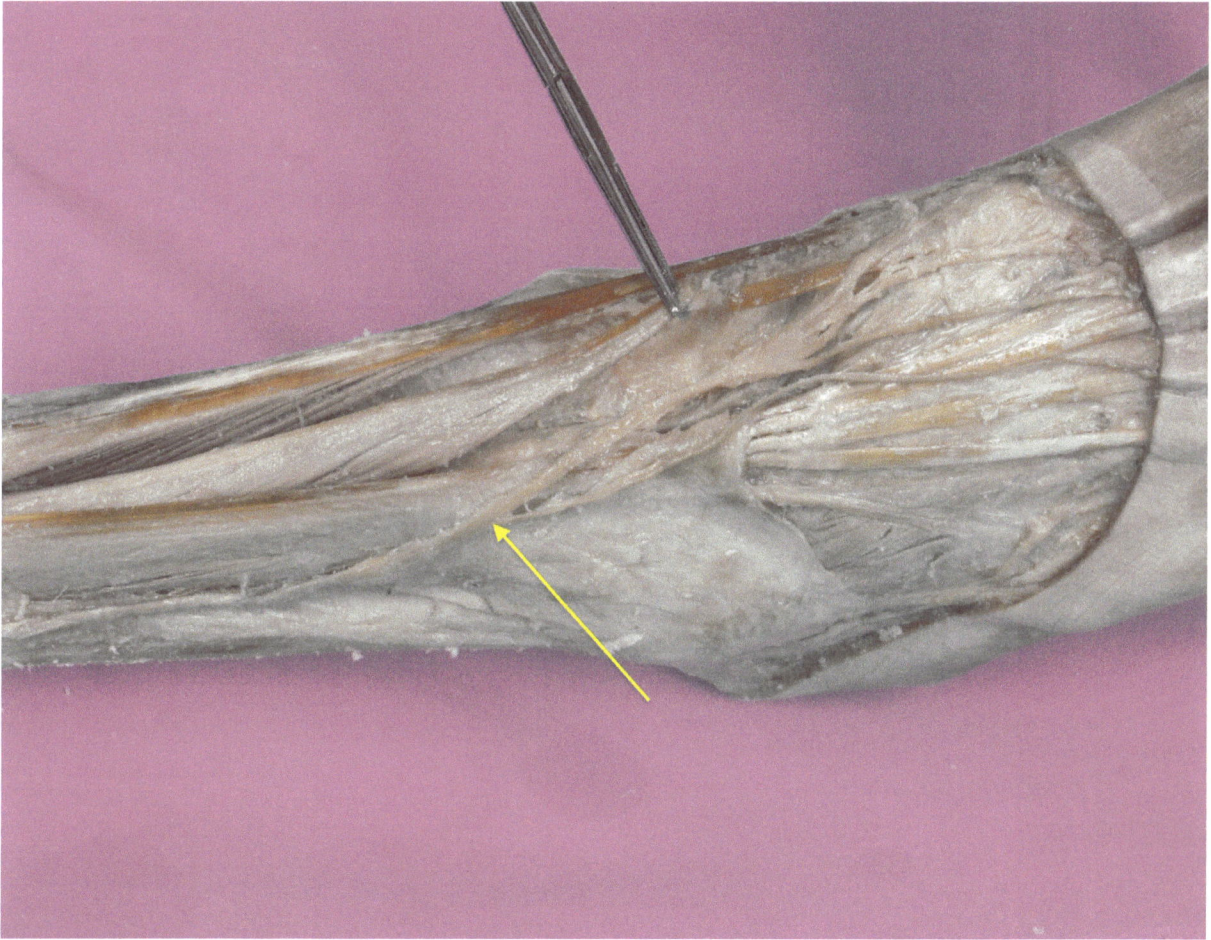

*Figure 5-4: Macroanatomy of the superficial peroneal nerve.*

The superficial peroneal nerve is indicated
by the arrow.

# Dissection of the Sural Nerve

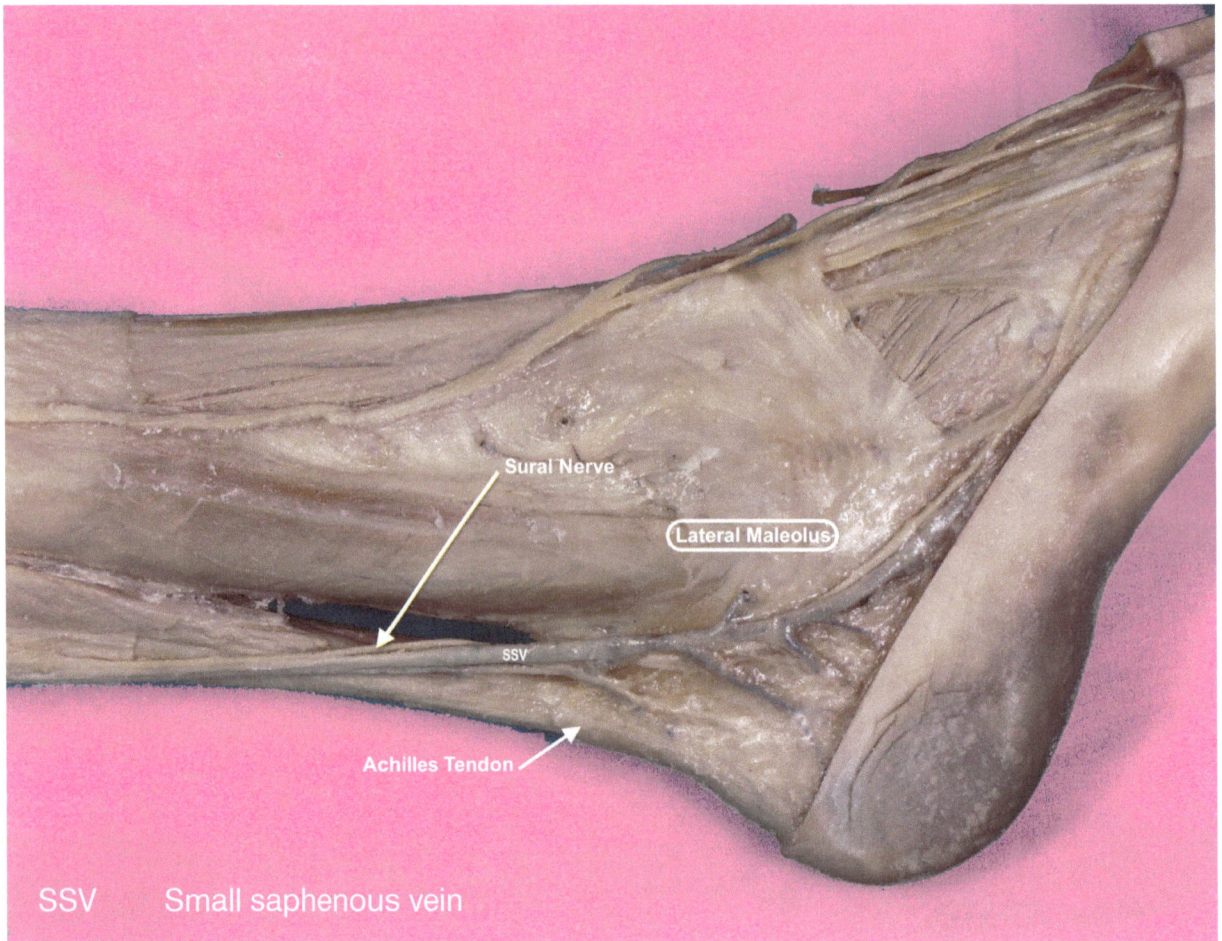

Figure 5-5: Macroanatomy of the sural nerve.

# Surface Landmarks of the Nerves around the Ankle

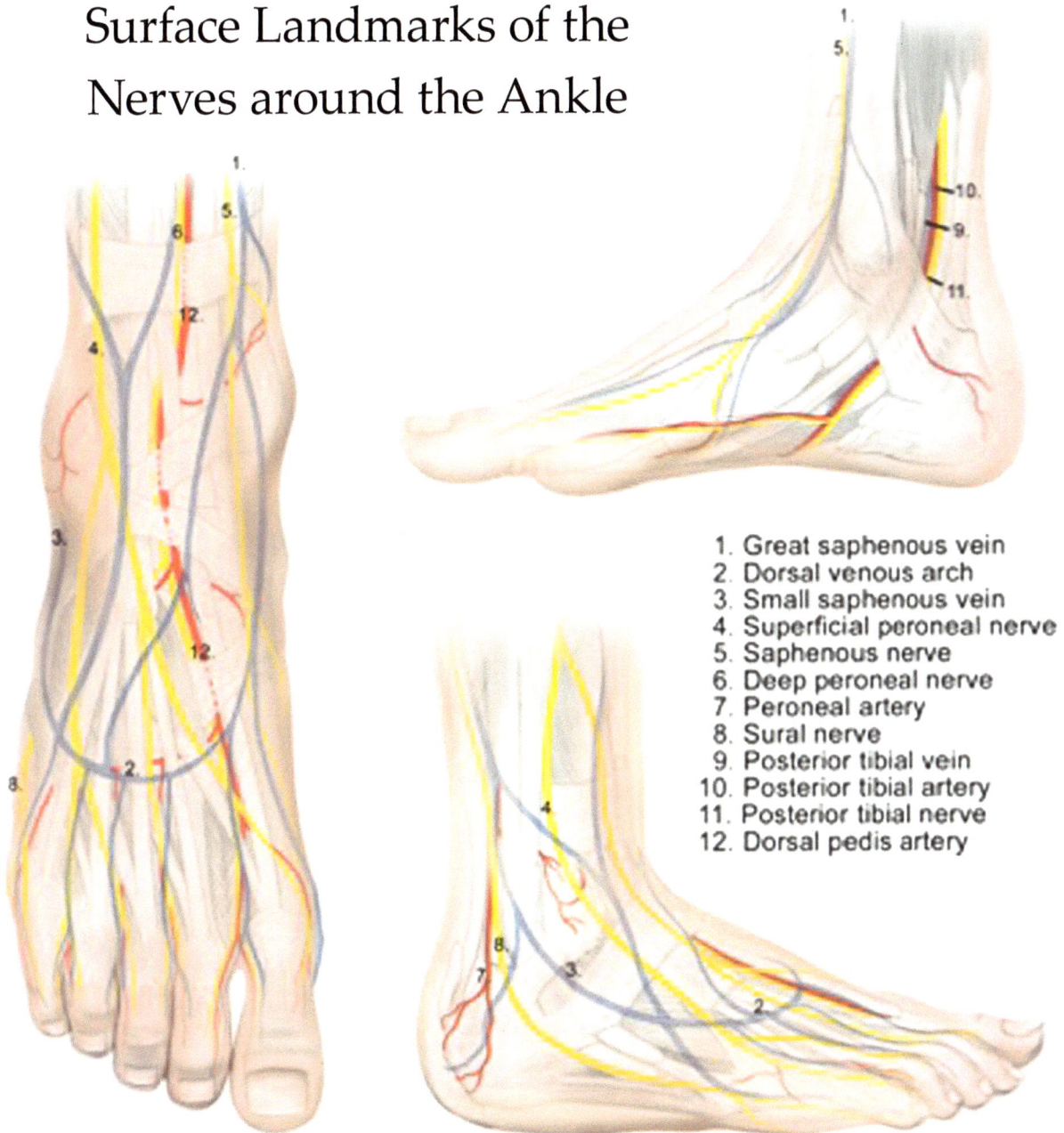

1. Great saphenous vein
2. Dorsal venous arch
3. Small saphenous vein
4. Superficial peroneal nerve
5. Saphenous nerve
6. Deep peroneal nerve
7. Peroneal artery
8. Sural nerve
9. Posterior tibial vein
10. Posterior tibial artery
11. Posterior tibial nerve
12. Dorsal pedis artery

*Figure 5-6: Surface landmarks of the nerves around the ankle.*

- The posterior tibial nerve (11) is two-thirds the distance from the Achilles tendon to the medial malleolus on the lateral side of the ankle, deep to the fascia.
- The deep peroneal nerve (6) is between the tendons of the tibialis anterior and extensor hallucis longus muscles, deep to the fascia.
- The superficial peroneal nerve (4) is situated lateral of the tendon of the extensor digitorum longus muscle, superficial to the fascia.
- The saphenous nerve (5) runs with the great saphenous vein on the anterior aspect of the medial malleolus, superficial to the fascia.
- The sural nerve (8) is situated halfway between the Achilles tendon and lateral malleolus on the lateral side of the ankle.

# Sonoanatomy
## The Deep Peroneal Nerve

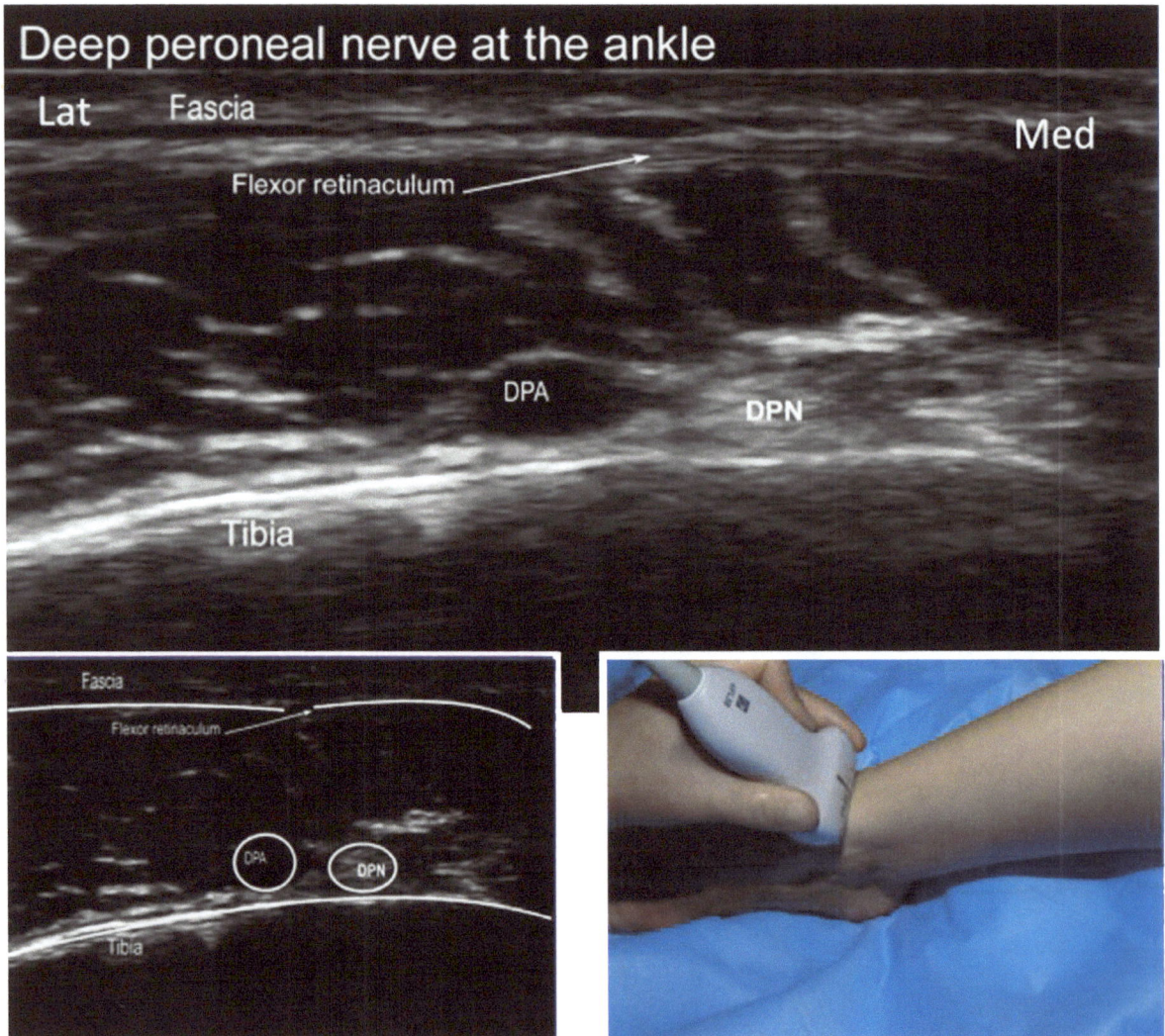

Figure 5-7: Sonoanatomy of the deep peroneal nerve at the ankle.

DPA    Deep peroneal artery
DPN    Deep peroneal nerve

# The Posterior Tibial Nerve

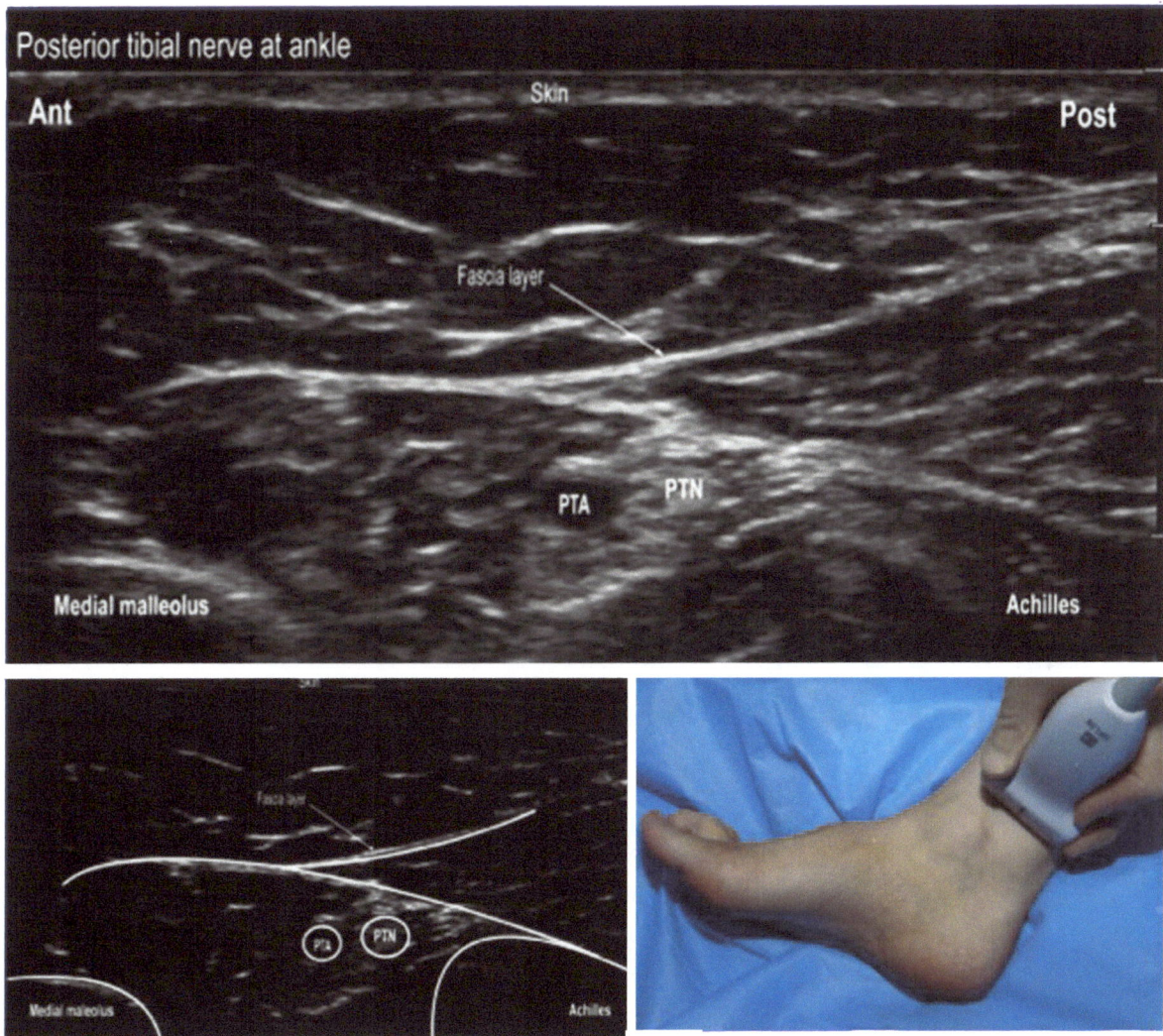

*Figure 5-8: Sonoanatomy of the posterior tibial nerve at the ankle.*

PTA     Posterior tibial artery
PTN     Posterior tibial nerve

**View Video at RAEducation.com**
**Acute Pain Medicine - Anatomy -**
**Sonoanatomy: Posterior Tibial Nerve**

# The Saphenous Nerve

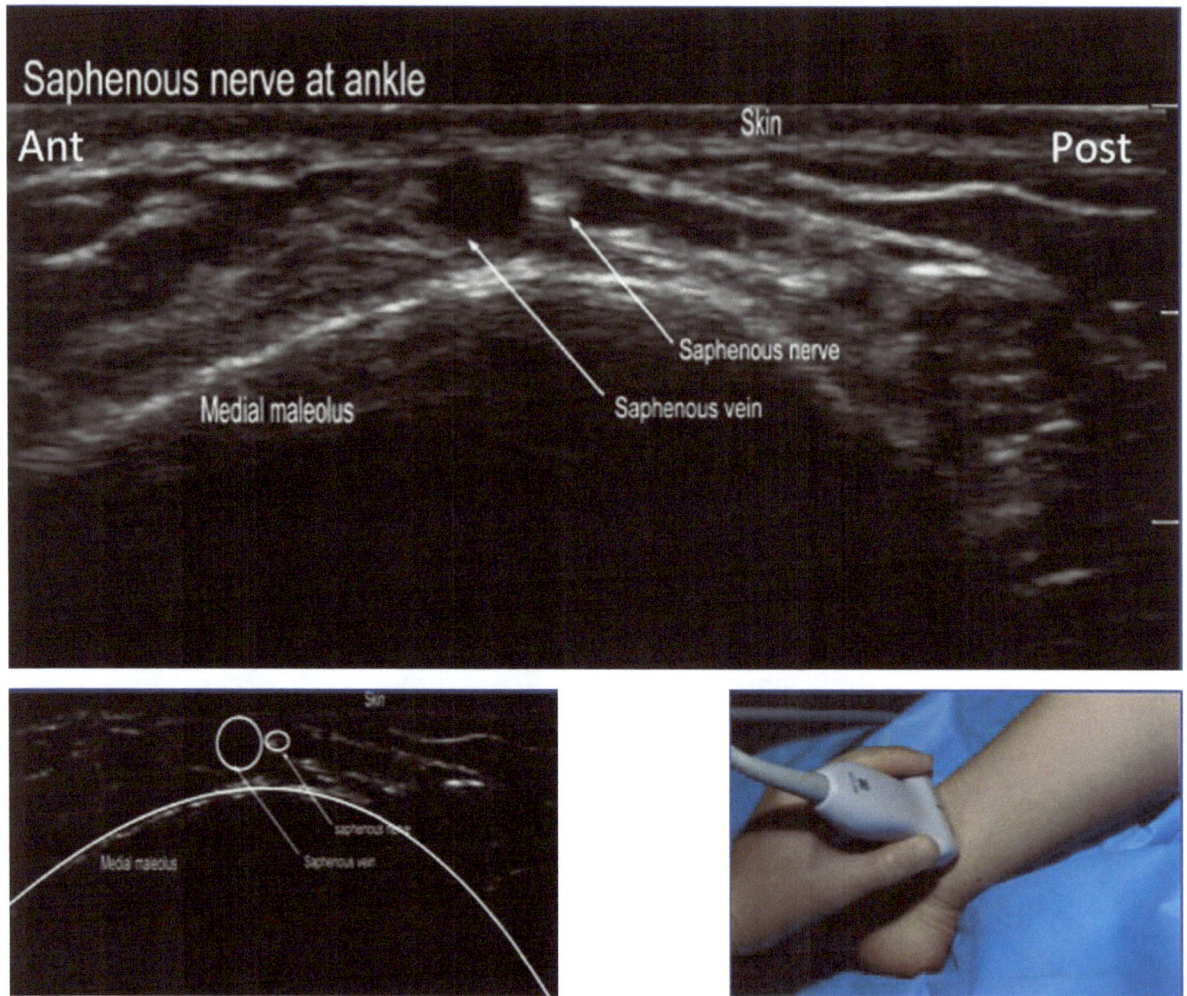

Figure 5-9: Sonoanatomy of the saphenous nerve at the ankle.

# The Sural Nerve

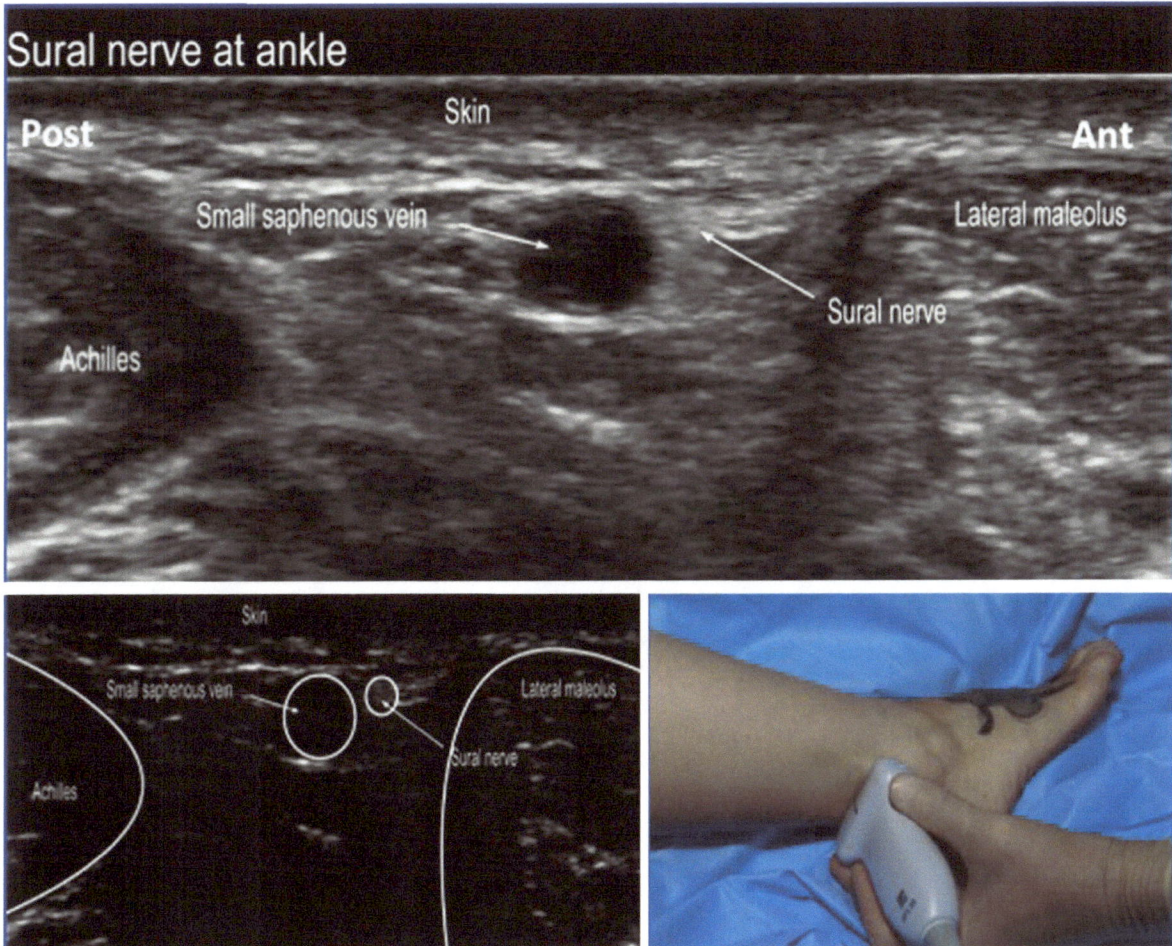

*Figure 5-10: Sonoanatomy of the sural nerve at the ankle.*

Achilles  Achilles tendon

# Functional Anatomy
## Neurotomes of the Foot and Ankle

1. Peroneal cutaneous nerve
2. Saphenous nerve
3. Superficial peroneal nerve
4. Deep peroneal nerve
5. Sural nerve
6. Medial plantar nerve
7. Lateral plantar nerve
8. Lateral calcaneal nerve
9. Medial calcaneal nerve

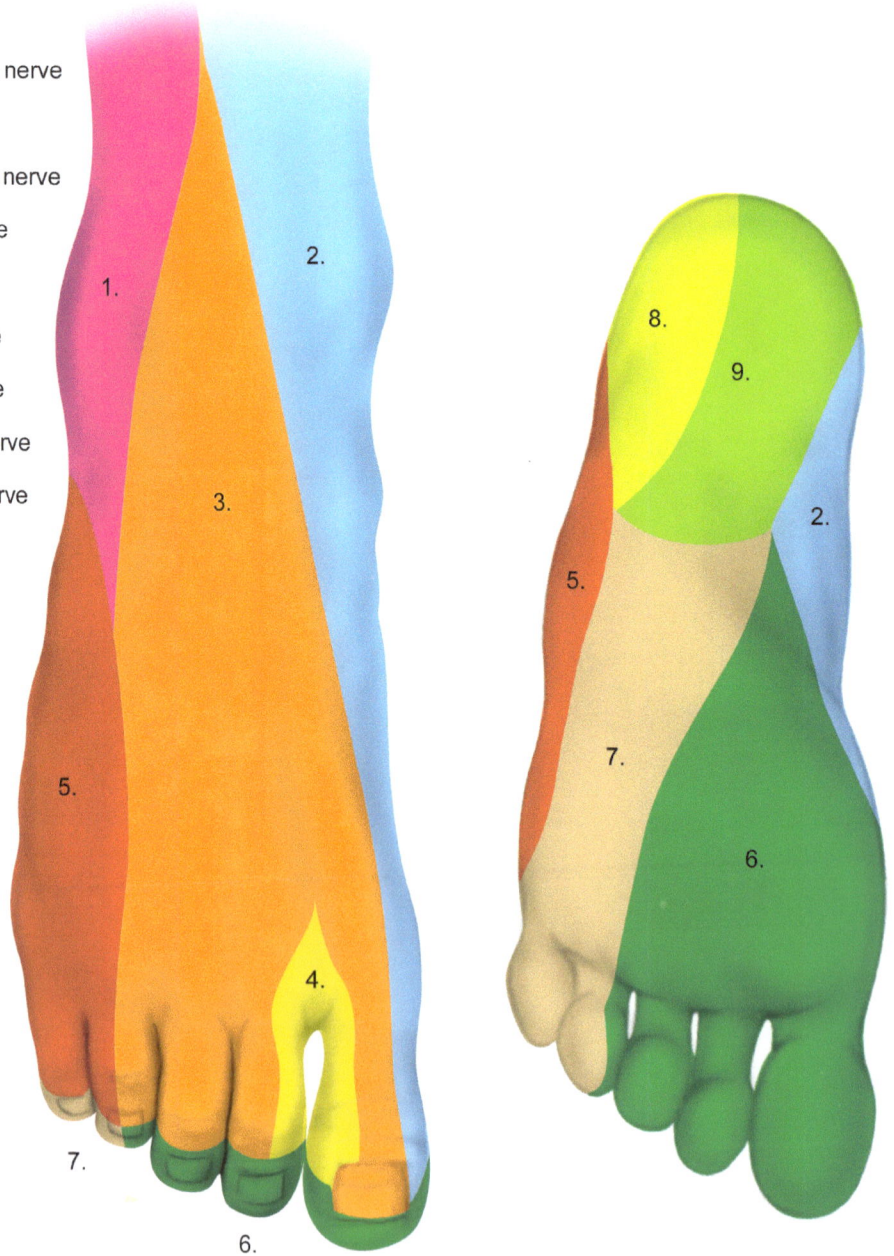

*Figure 5-11: Sensory distribution of the nerves of the foot and ankle.*

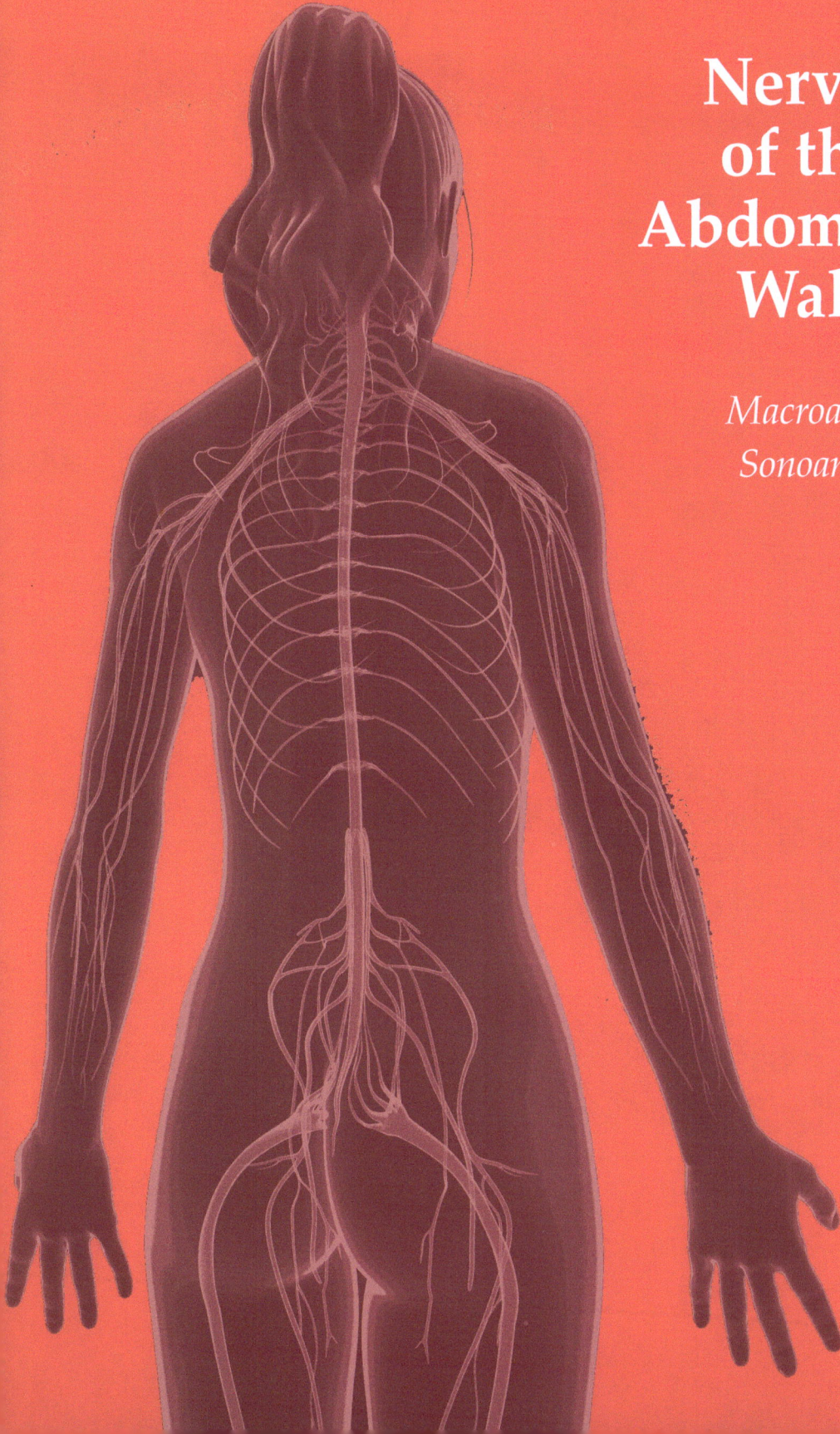

# Chapter 6

# Nerves of the Abdominal Wall

*Macroanatomy*

*Sonoanatomy*

# Macroanatomy
## The Abdominal Wall

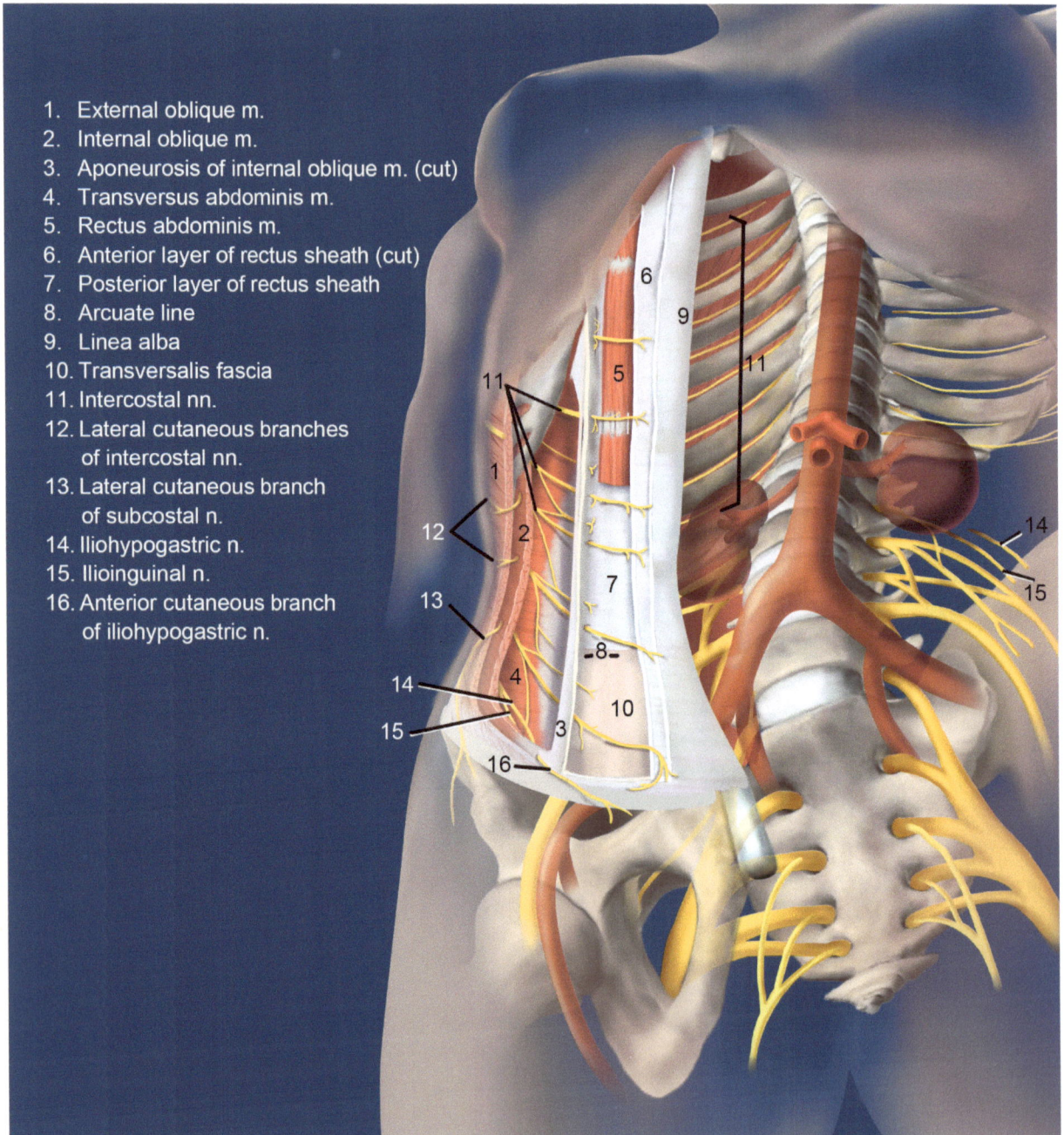

1. External oblique m.
2. Internal oblique m.
3. Aponeurosis of internal oblique m. (cut)
4. Transversus abdominis m.
5. Rectus abdominis m.
6. Anterior layer of rectus sheath (cut)
7. Posterior layer of rectus sheath
8. Arcuate line
9. Linea alba
10. Transversalis fascia
11. Intercostal nn.
12. Lateral cutaneous branches of intercostal nn.
13. Lateral cutaneous branch of subcostal n.
14. Iliohypogastric n.
15. Ilioinguinal n.
16. Anterior cutaneous branch of iliohypogastric n.

*Figure 6-1: Abdominal wall muscles and nerves.*

The transversus abdominis plane (TAP) is between numbers 2 and 4.

# Sonoanatomy
## The Anterior Transversus Abdominus Plane

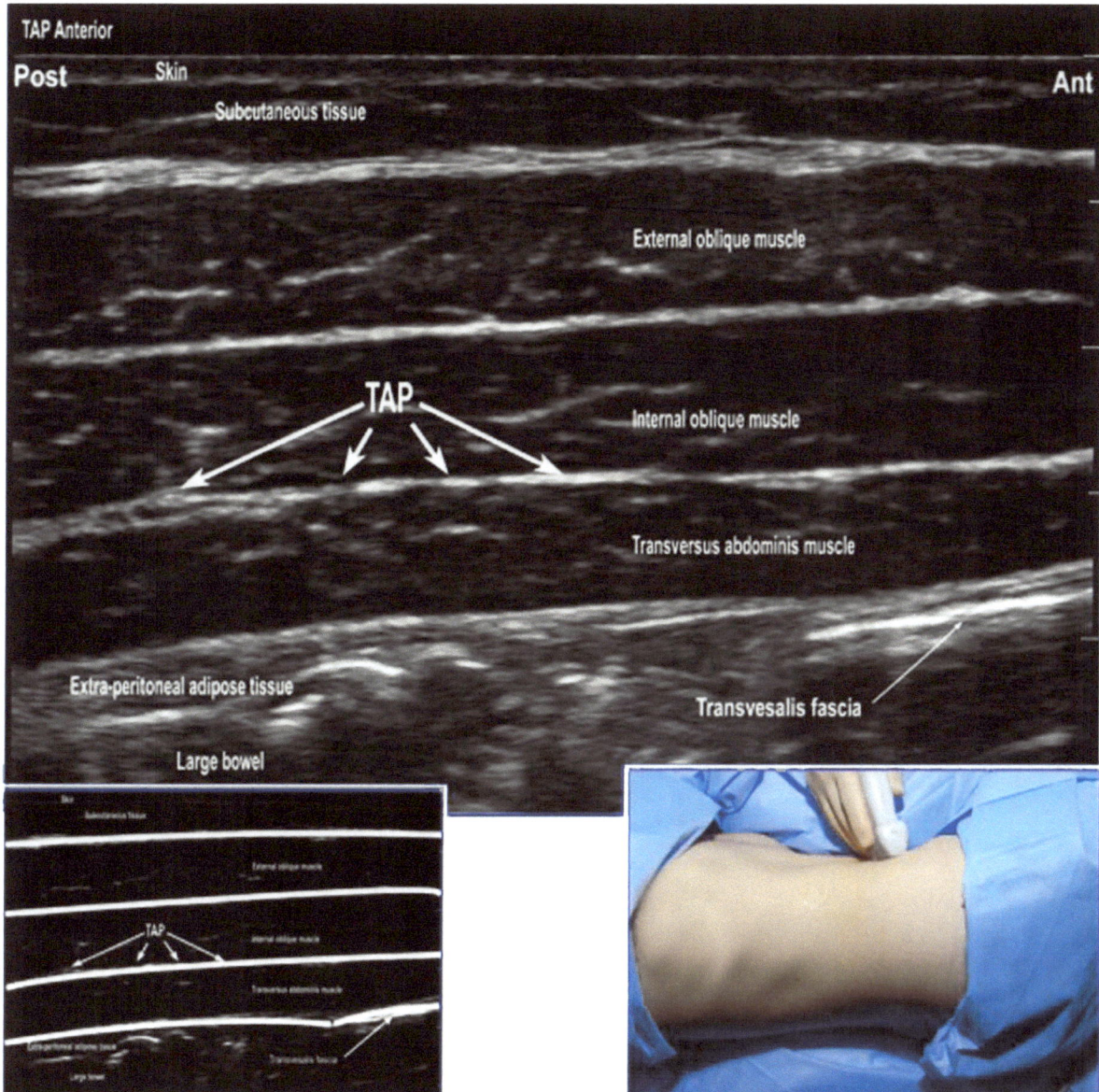

*Figure 6-2: Sonoanatomy of the anterior transversus abdominis plane (TAP).*

Anterior, between the iliac crest and the rib cage, there are three abdominal muscles. From superficial to deep, they are the external oblique, internal oblique, and transversus abdominis muscles. The TAP is the fascia layer between the latter two. An anterior TAP block splits this layer to block the nerves situated here.

**View Video at RAEducation.com**
**Acute Pain Medicine - Anatomy -**
**Sonoanatomy: TAP Space**

# The Posterior Transversus Abdominal Plane

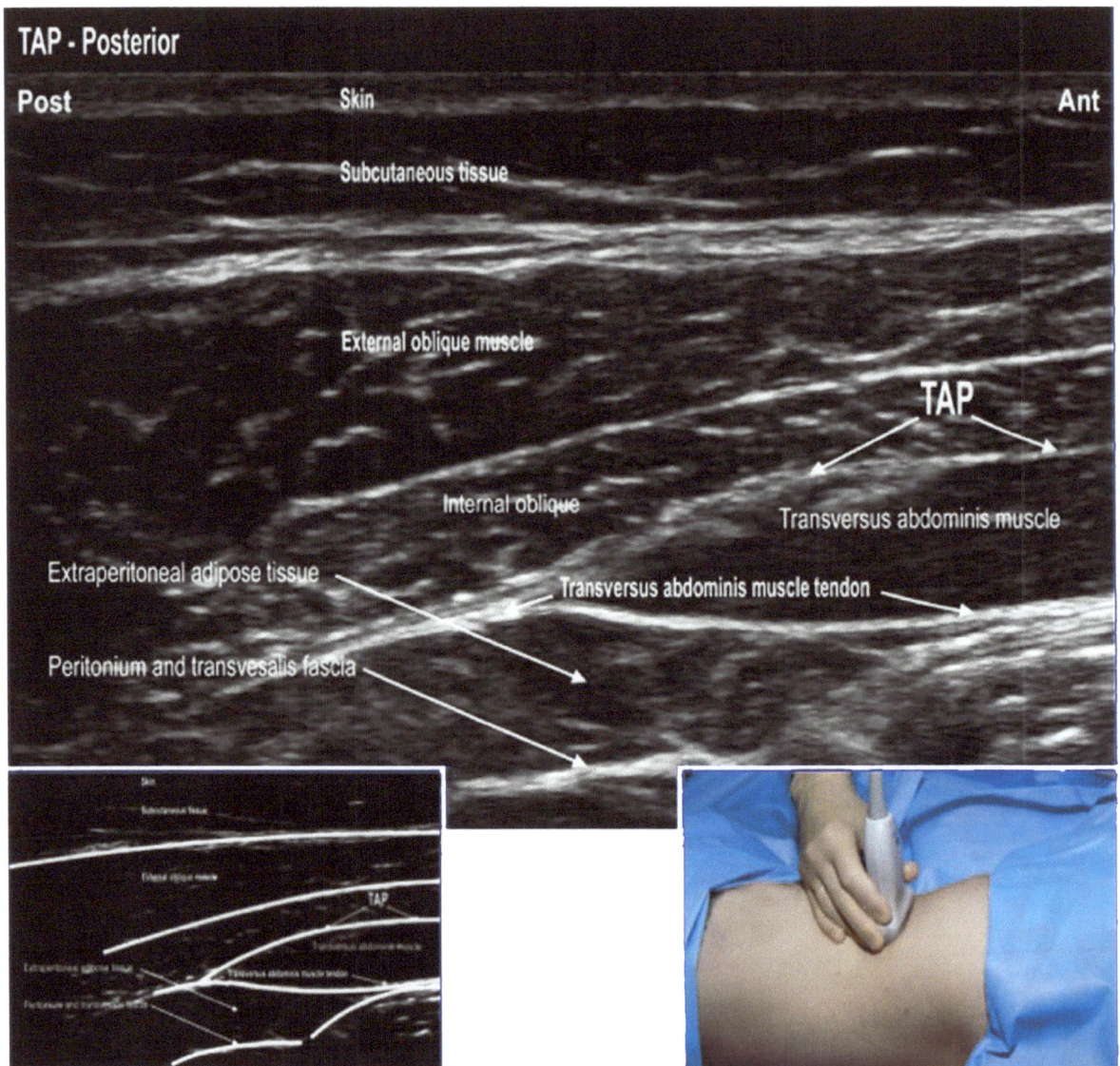

Figure 6-3: Sonoanatomy of the posterior transversus abdominis plane (TAP).

| | |
|---|---|
| Ant | Anterior |
| Post | Posterior |
| TAP | Transversus abdominis plane |

Please note: The transversus abdominis muscle becomes aponeurotic posterior. Note the TAP is again between the internal oblique and transversus abdominis muscles. Also note the extra-peritoneal adipose tissue and the transversalis fascia deep to the transversus abdominis muscle and the bowel deep to these structures.

# The Subcostal Transversus Abdominus Plane

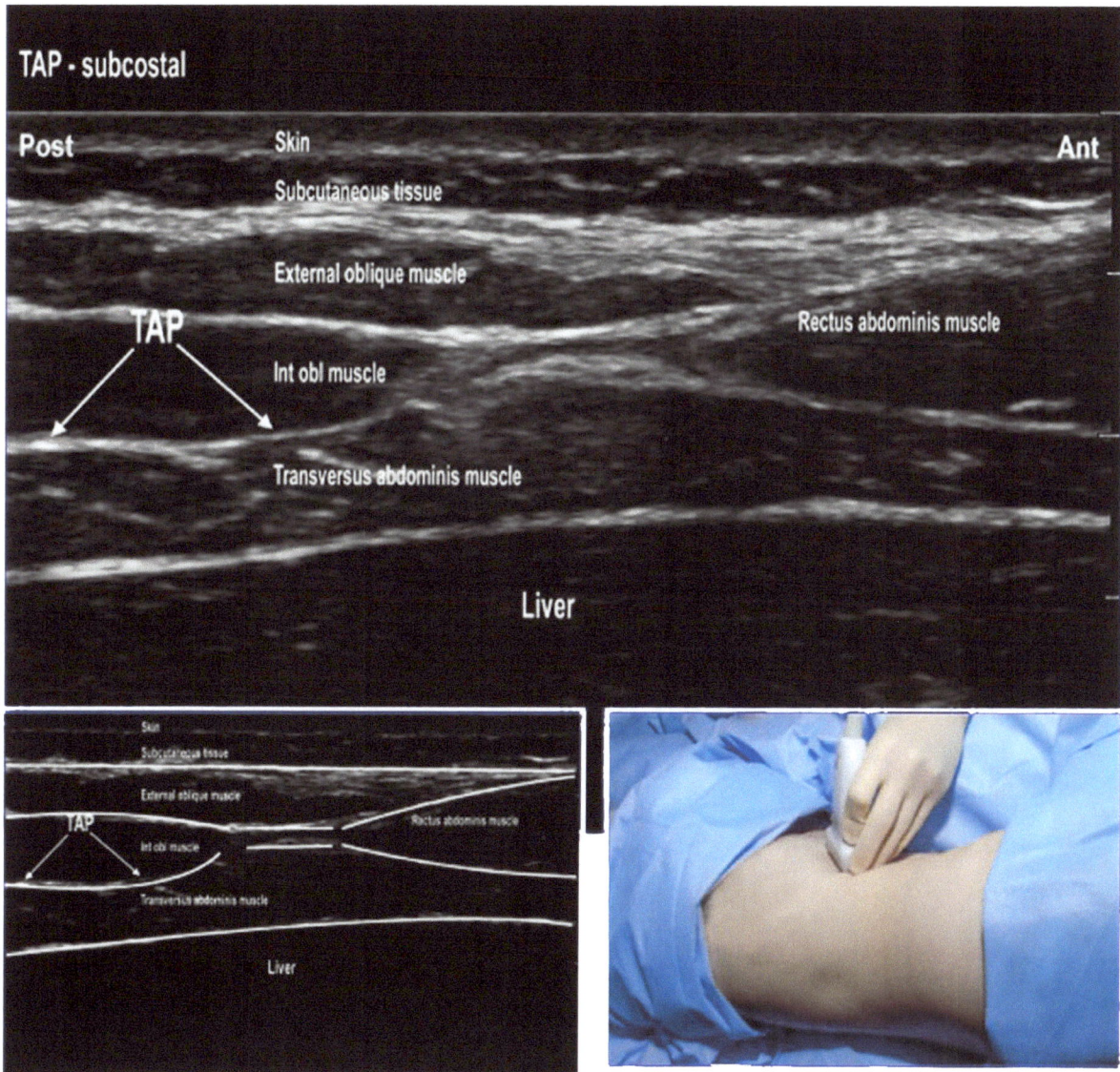

Figure 6-4: Sonoanatomy of the subcostal transversus abdominis plane (TAP).

Ant    Anterior
Post   Posterior
TAP   Transversus abdominis plane

Please note: The tendons of all three abdominal muscles merge to form the anterior and posterior rectus sheath, which hosts the rectus abdominis muscle. Note the presence of the liver deep to the transversus abdominis muscle. Above the arcuate line, the rectus sheath consists of the merged tendons of the abdominal muscles. Below this line, it consists of the transversalis fascia.

# The Ilioinguinal and Iliohypogastric Nerves

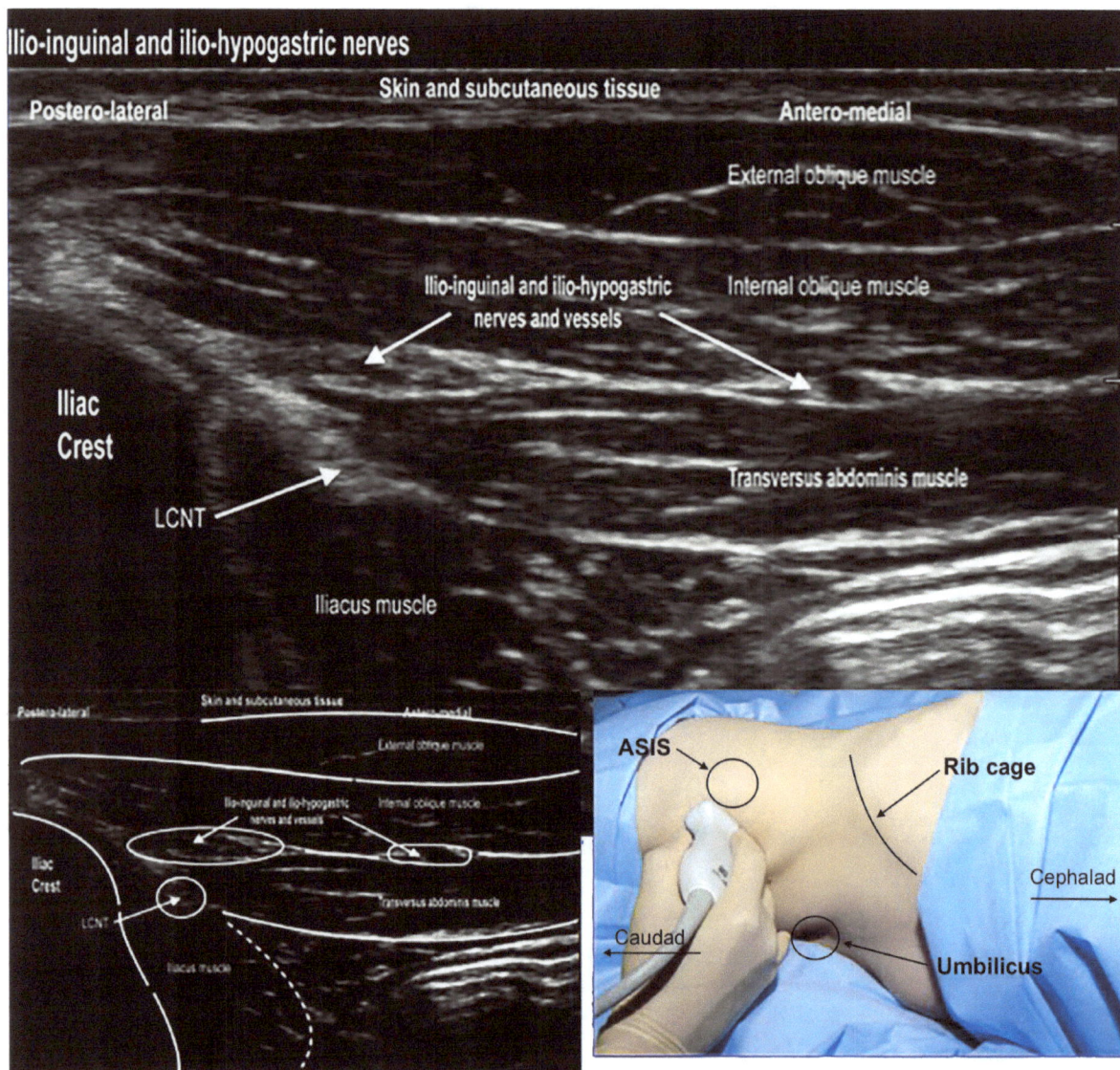

Figure 6-5: Ilioinguinal and iliohypogastric nerves.

LCNT  Lateral cutaneous nerve of the thigh

Please note:  The angle of the ultrasound probe. The abdominal muscles implant on the iliac crest, and the presence of the ilioinguinal and iliohypogastric nerve, arteries, and veins are situated in the fascia layer between the internal oblique and transversus abdominis muscles. The lateral cutaneous nerve of the thigh is on the anterior border of the iliacus muscle, which can be seen anterolateral to the iliac crest.

# Chapter 7

## The Thoracic Paravertebral Space

*Macroanatomy*
*Microanatomy*
*Sonoanatomy*
*Functional Anatomy*

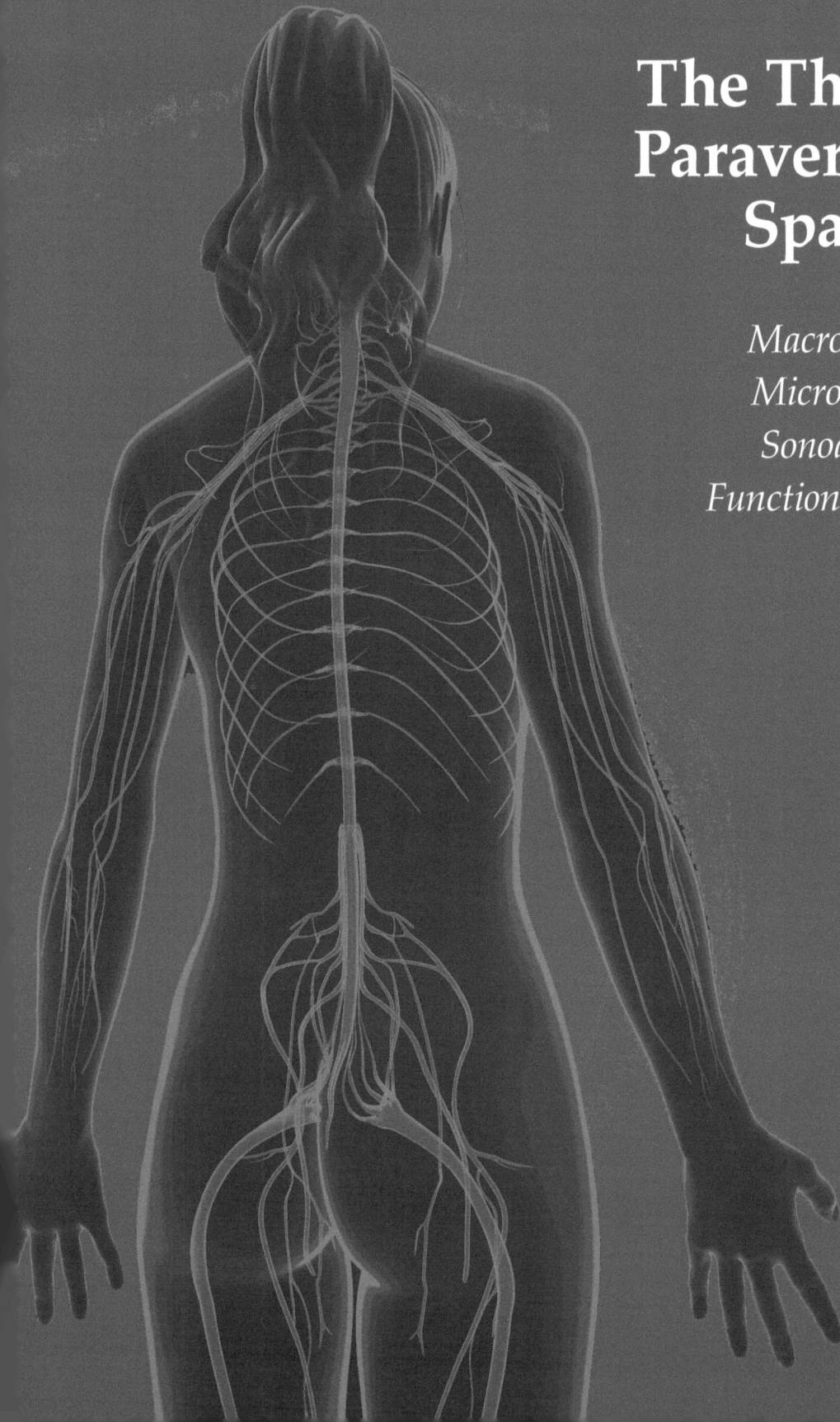

# Macroanatomy
## The Thoracic Paravertebral Space

The blue wedge-shaped area represents the thoracic paravertebral space.

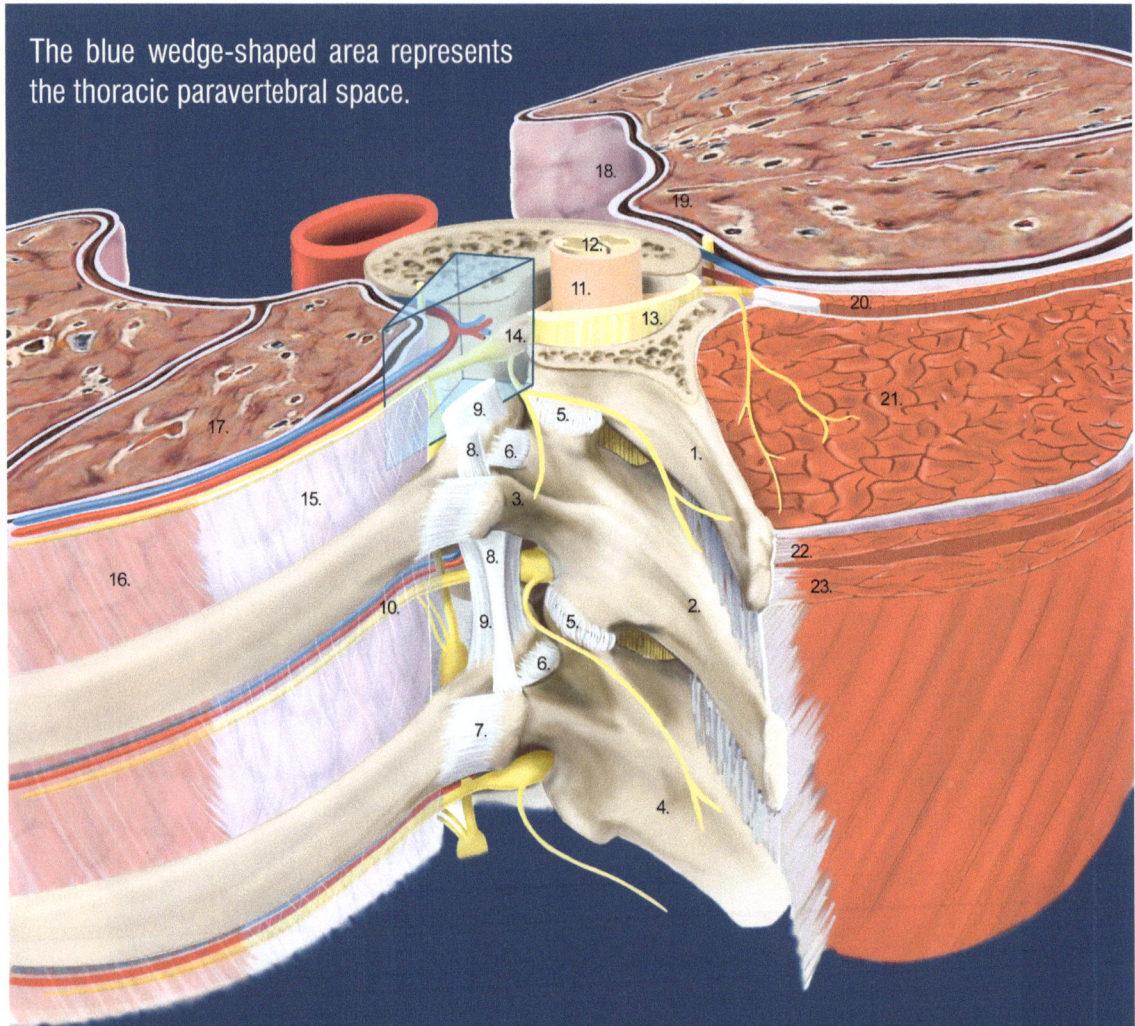

1. Spinous process of T3
2. Spinous process of T4
3. Transverse process of T4
4. Spinous process of T5
5. Zygapophyseal joint capsule
6. Inferior Costotransverse ligament
7. Lateral costotransverse ligament
8. Intertransverse ligament
9. Superior costotransverse ligament
10. Intercostal vein, artery and nerve
11. Dura mater
12. Spinal cord
13. Ligamentum flavum
14. Nerve root
15. Internal intercostal membrane
16. Internal intercostal muscle
17. Left lung
18. Parietal pleura
19. Visceral pleura
20. External intercostal muscle
21. Erector spinae muscle
22. Rhomboid major muscle
23. Trapezius muscle

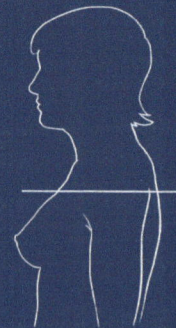

Figure 7-1: *Macroanatomy of the thoracic paravertebral space viewed from the posterior at the level of the 4th thoracic vertebra.*

# The Thoracic Paravertebral Space

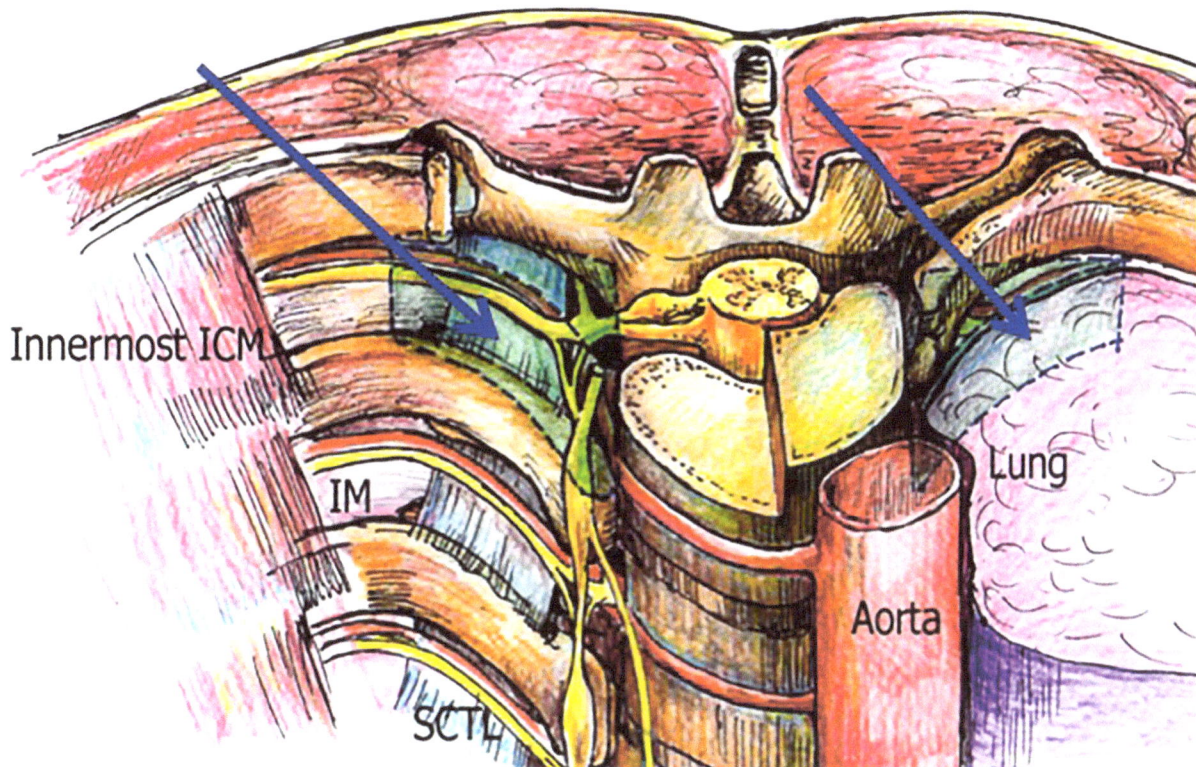

*Figure 7-2: Anterior view of the wedge-shaped space that forms the thoracic paravertebral space.*

→  Thoracic paravertebral
     spaces bilaterally

ICM  Innermost intercostal muscle

IM  Internal intercostal muscle

SCTL  Superior costotransverse ligament

The lung and parietal pleura have been
removed on the right side

*Drawing on this page: Barys V. Ihnatsenka, MD Prior Page Ref: Boezaart AP, Raw RM. Continuous thoracic para-vertebral block for major breast surgery. Reg Anesth Pain Med 2006;31:470-6. • Klein SM, Bergh A, Steele SM , MD, Georgiade GS, Greengrass RA. Thoracic paravertebral block for breast surgery. Anesth Analg 2000;90:1402-5. • Boezaart AP, Lucas SD, Elliott CE. Paravertebral block: cervical, thoracic, lumbar and sacral. Curr Opin Anaesthesiol 2009;22:637-43.*

# The Thoracic Paravertebral Space

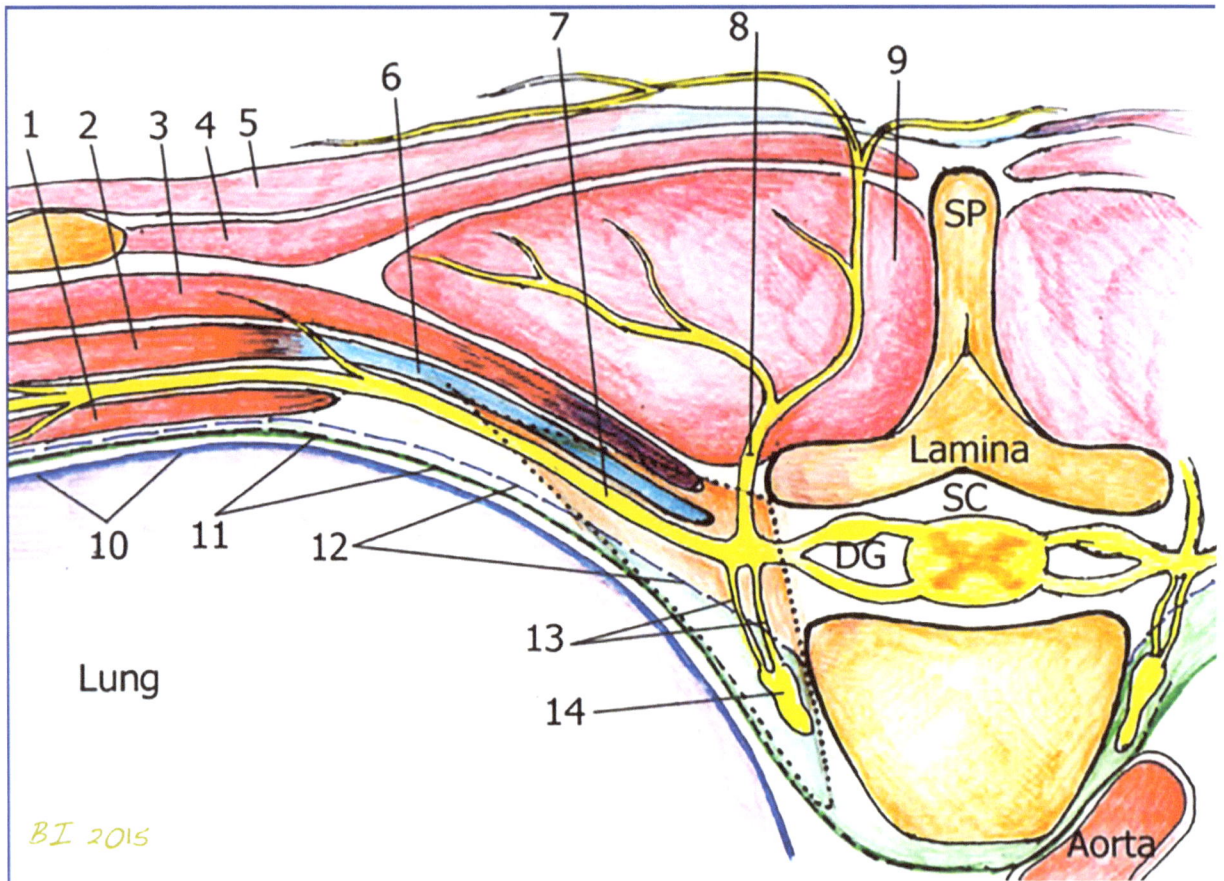

*Figure 7-3: Schematic representation of the wedge-shaped thoracic paravertebral space.*

| | | | |
|---|---|---|---|
| 1 | Innermost intercostal muscle | 8 | Dorsal ramus of thoracic spinal root |
| 2 | Internal intercostal muscle | 9 | Erector spinae muscle |
| 3 | External intercostal muscle, which fuses with the SCTL | 10 | Visceral pleura of the lung |
| 4 | Rhomboid major muscle | 11 | Parietal pleura of the lung |
| 5 | Trapezius muscle | 12 | Endothoracic fascia |
| 6 | Internal intercostal membrane, which covers the external & internal intercostal muscles and fuses with the superior costotransverse ligament | 13 | Gray and white rami communicantes |
| | | 14 | Sympathetic trunk and ganglion |
| | | DG | Dorsal root ganglion |
| | | SC | Spinal cord |
| | | SP | Spinous process of vertebra |
| 7 | Ventral ramus of thoracic spinal root (intercostal nerve) | | |

*Drawing: Barys V. Ihnatsenka, MD*

# Nerves & Ligaments of the Thoracic Paravertebral Space

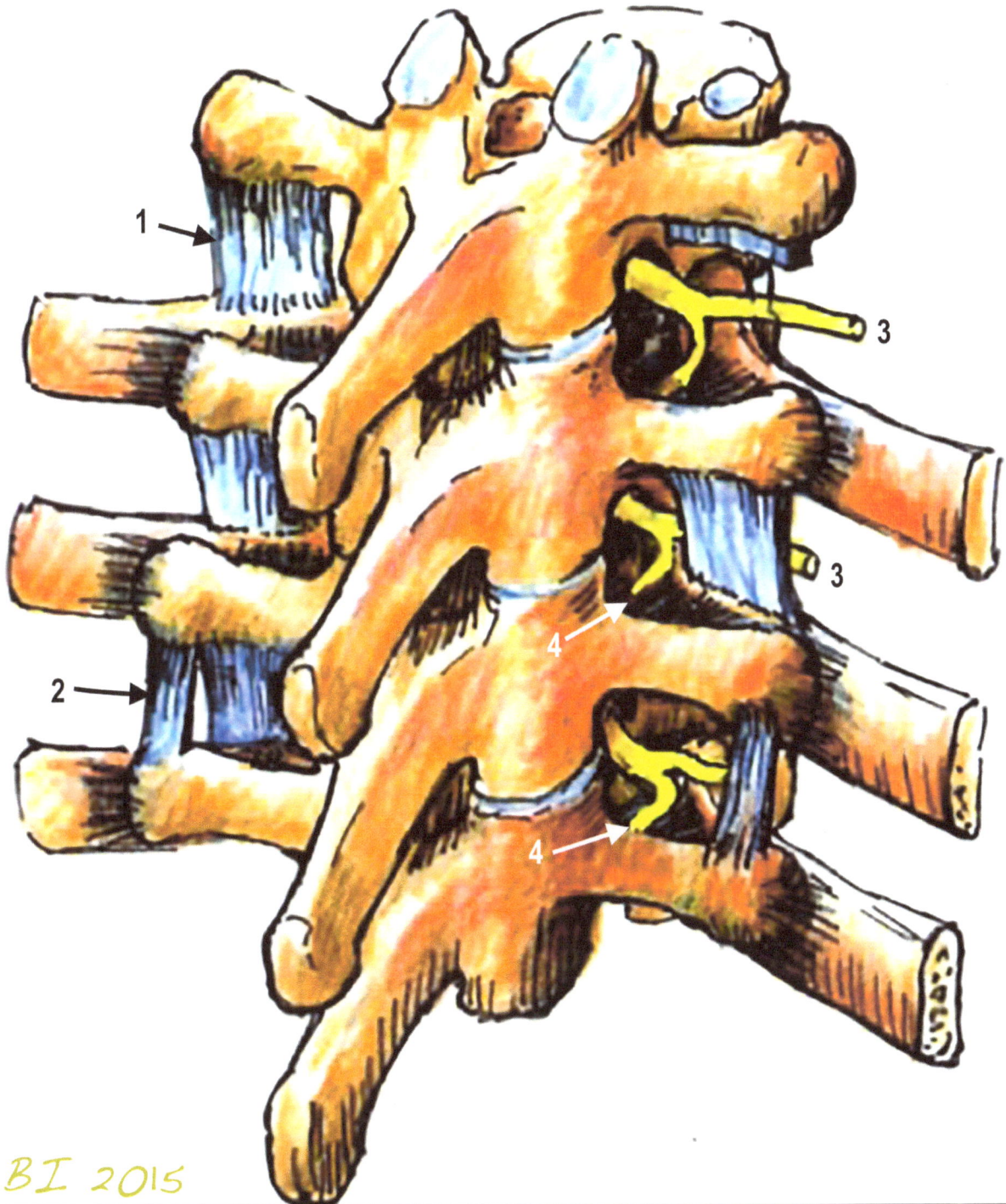

*Figure 7-4: The relationships of the nerves and the ligaments in the thoracic paravertebral space viewed from posterior.*

| | | | |
|---|---|---|---|
| 1 | Superior costo-transverse ligament | 3 | Anterior ramus of spinal nerve |
| 2 | Intertransverse ligament | 4 | Posterior ramus of intercostal nerve |

*Drawing: Barys V. Ihnatsenka, MD*

# The Costotransverse Ligament

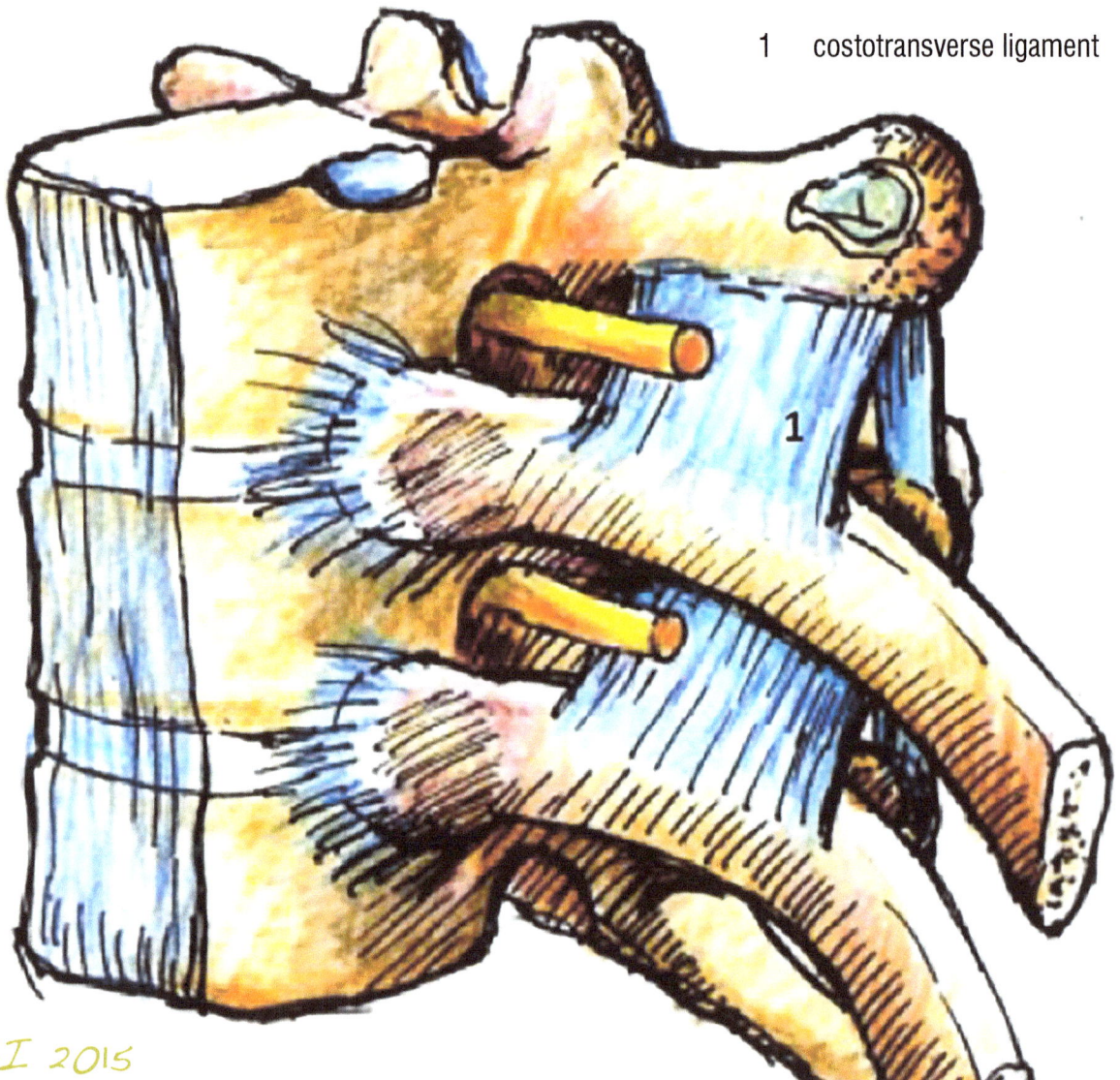

1   costotransverse ligament

BI 2015

Figure 7-5: The relationship of the thoracic spinal root to the superior costotransverse ligament as viewed from anterior.

Drawing: Barys V. Ihnatsenka, MD

# Transverse Process to Skin

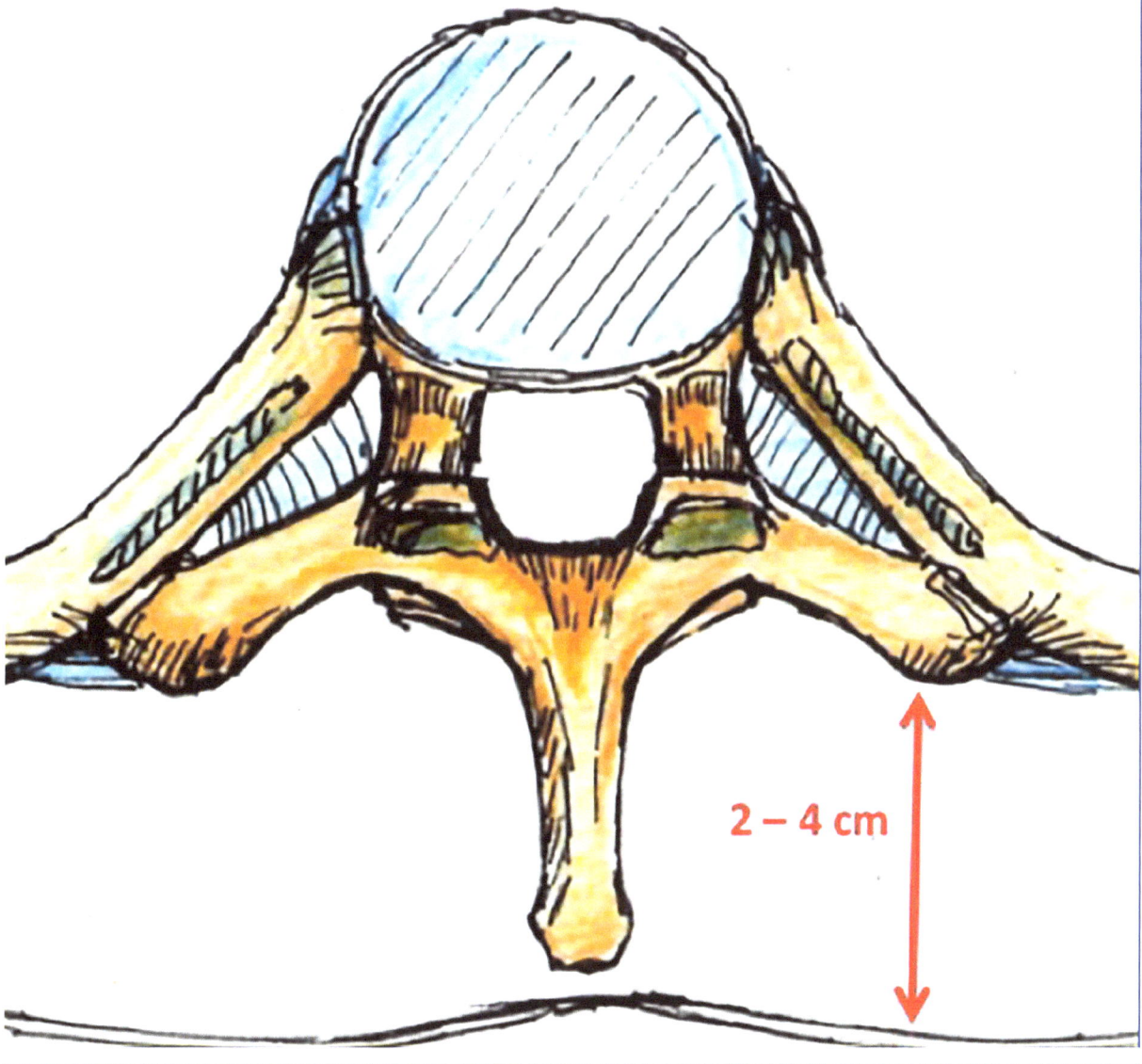

**2 – 4 cm**

*Figure 7-6: Typically, the tip of the transverse process is from 2 to 4 cm from the skin.*

This varies from patient to patient, depending on the body habitus. Note the angle of the transverse process.

*Drawing: Barys V. Ihnatsenka, MD*

# Landmarks of the Thoracic Paravertebral Space

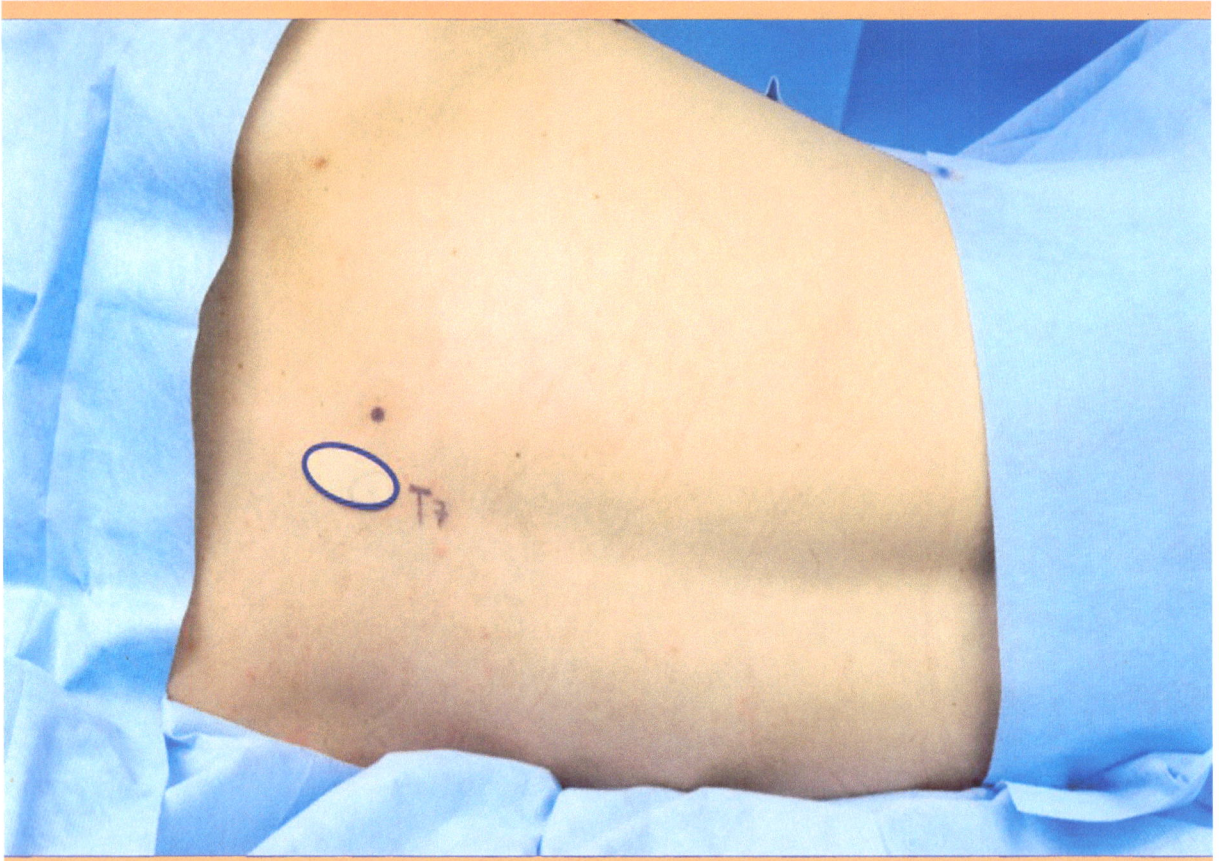

*Figure 7-7: Surface landmarks for the thoracic paravertebral space. Model in left lateral decubitus position. Left is cephalad and right is caudad - posterior view.*

The spinous process of a vertebra, the 7th thoracic vertebra in this case (T7), is identified and marked. It is on the inferior margins of the scapulae. A point 2.5 to 3 cm lateral to the midpoint of the spinous process of T7 marks the position of the transverse process of the 8th thoracic vertebra (T8).

**Please refer to standard textbooks for indications for and techniques of performing any of the blocks referred to in this book.**

# Microanatomy

## Meningeal Layers around Spinal Nerve Roots

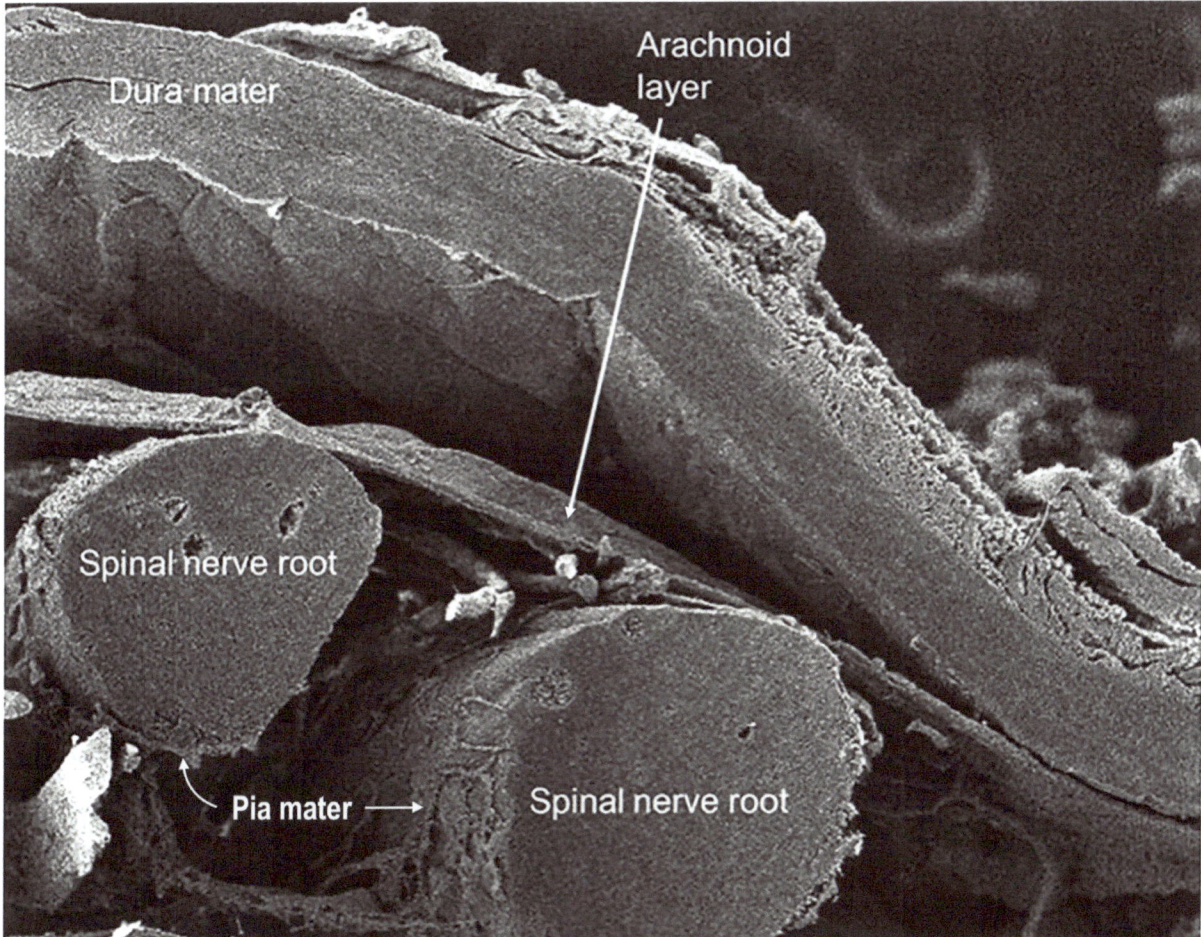

*Figure 7-8: Ultrastructure of the meninges (dura, arachnoid, and pia maters) surrounding nerve root. Scanning electron microscopy – magnification ×40.*

Please note: The subdural–extra-arachnoid space between the dura and arachnoid maters.

*Reprinted with permission from: Collier CB, Reina MA. Unintentional subdural and intradural placement of epidural catheters. In: Reina MA, Ed. Atlas of Functional Anatomy For Regional Anesthesia And Pain Medicine. New York: Springer Science and Business Media, 2015; 439. Ref: Boezaart AP, Kadieva VS. Inadvertent extra-arachnoid [subdural] injection of a local anaesthetic agent during epidural anaesthesia. S Afr Med J 1992;81:325-6.*

# The Meningies around the Spinal Roots

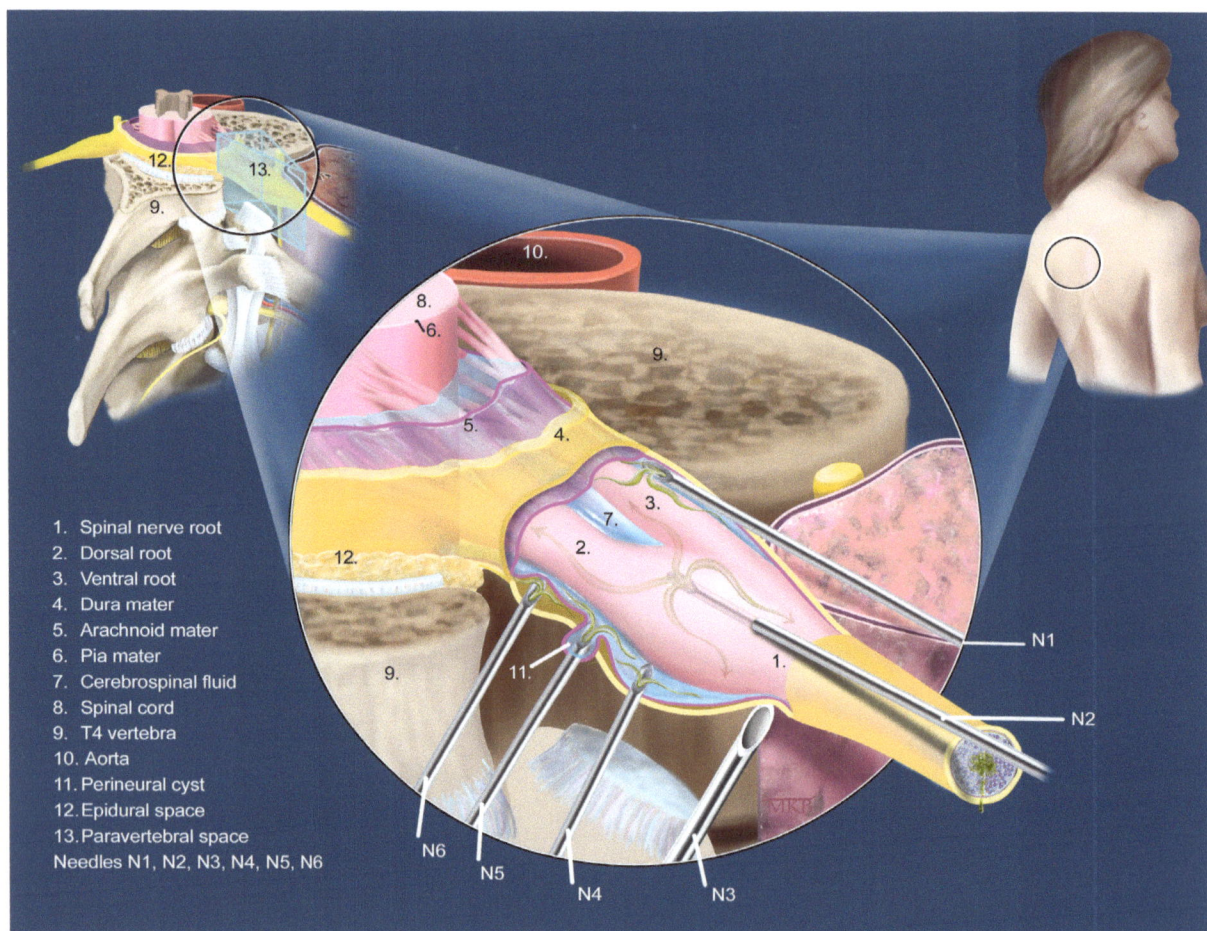

1. Spinal nerve root
2. Dorsal root
3. Ventral root
4. Dura mater
5. Arachnoid mater
6. Pia mater
7. Cerebrospinal fluid
8. Spinal cord
9. T4 vertebra
10. Aorta
11. Perineural cyst
12. Epidural space
13. Paravertebral space
Needles N1, N2, N3, N4, N5, N6

*Figure 7-9: Schematic representation of the thoracic paravertebral space and the meninges surrounding the spinal root.*

## Specification and Placement of Needles in Meningeal Spaces
Note: Implications can be devastating. (See page 192)

Needle 1 (N1): Subarachnoid placement of a relatively thin needle during a trans-foraminal injection (usually steroids).

Needle 2 (N2): Intraparenchymal placement of a relatively thin needle during a nerve root block (e.g., interscalene block at the cervical level) or an intercostal nerve block.

Needle 3 (N3): Extradural needle or Tuohy needle during a paravertebral block.

Needle 4 (N4): Subarachnoid placement of a relatively thin needle during a paravertebral block.

Needle 5 (N5): Needle placement into a perineural cyst during a paravertebral block.

Needle 6 (N6): Subdural (extra-arachnoid) needle placement during a paravertebral block.

# Types of Arachnoid Villi

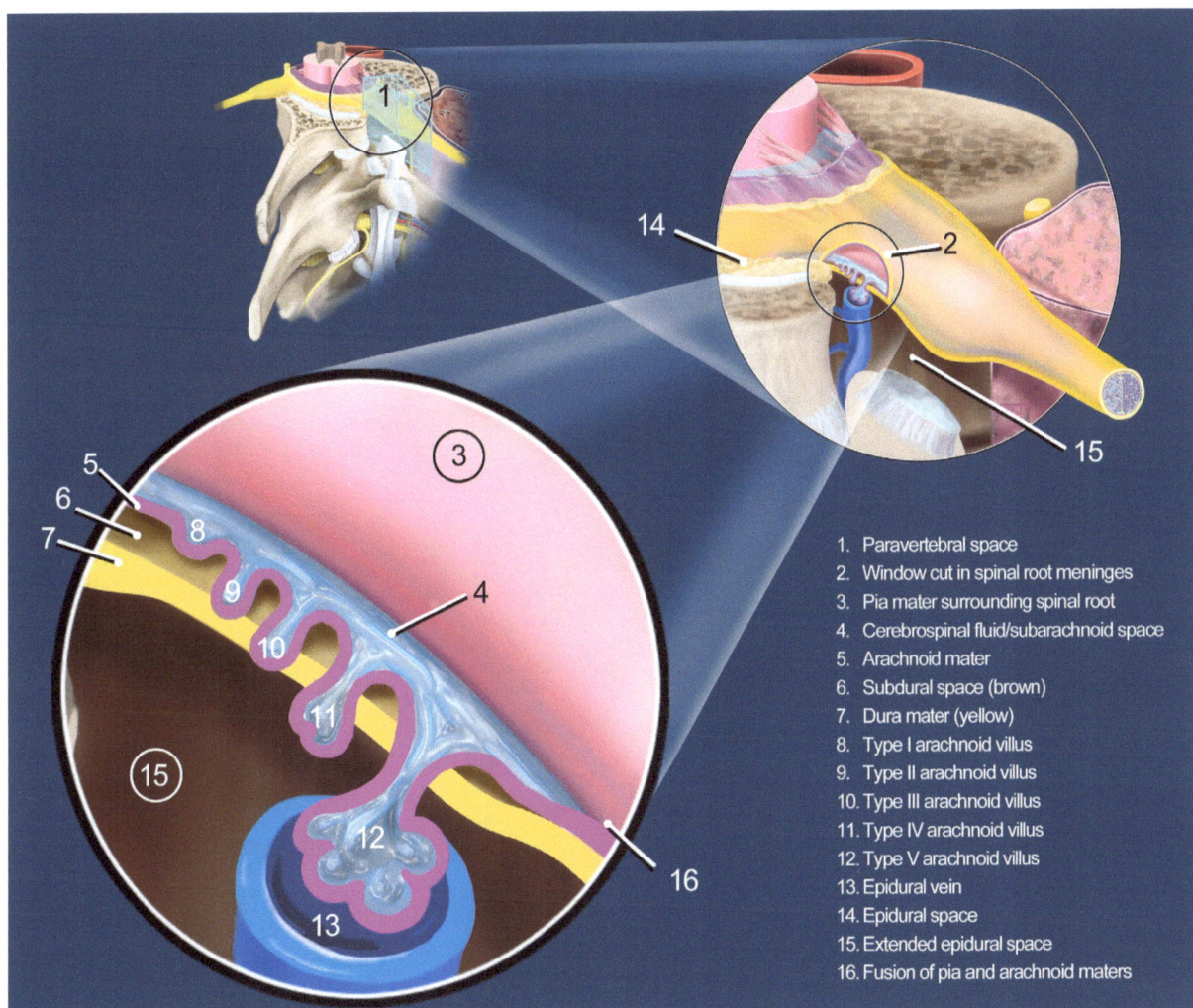

1. Paravertebral space
2. Window cut in spinal root meninges
3. Pia mater surrounding spinal root
4. Cerebrospinal fluid/subarachnoid space
5. Arachnoid mater
6. Subdural space (brown)
7. Dura mater (yellow)
8. Type I arachnoid villus
9. Type II arachnoid villus
10. Type III arachnoid villus
11. Type IV arachnoid villus
12. Type V arachnoid villus
13. Epidural vein
14. Epidural space
15. Extended epidural space
16. Fusion of pia and arachnoid maters

*Figure 7-10: Arachnoid villi.*

Type I: Simple arachnoid proliferations, consisting of several layers of arachnoid epithelial cells, are found along the root arachnoid. They are consistently found where the pia and arachnoid come together to obliterate the subarachnoid space. These proliferations come in many shapes and sizes and may protrude into adjacent subdural spaces.

Type II: Arachnoid villi partially protruding into the dural sheath without breaching the dural continuity, at the same time reducing the thickness of the dura at the site.

Type III: Villi that completely breach the dura but do not protrude beyond it.

Type IV: Villi protruding out of the dura lying in the epidural space.

Type V: Villi protruding beyond the dura in proximity to epidural veins and partially protruding into the veins, as commonly observed in the sagittal sinus.

Note: Types I through III are commonly found, especially in the young, whereas Types IV and V are less frequent, but their numbers increase with advancing age.

# Paravertebral Arachnoid Cyst

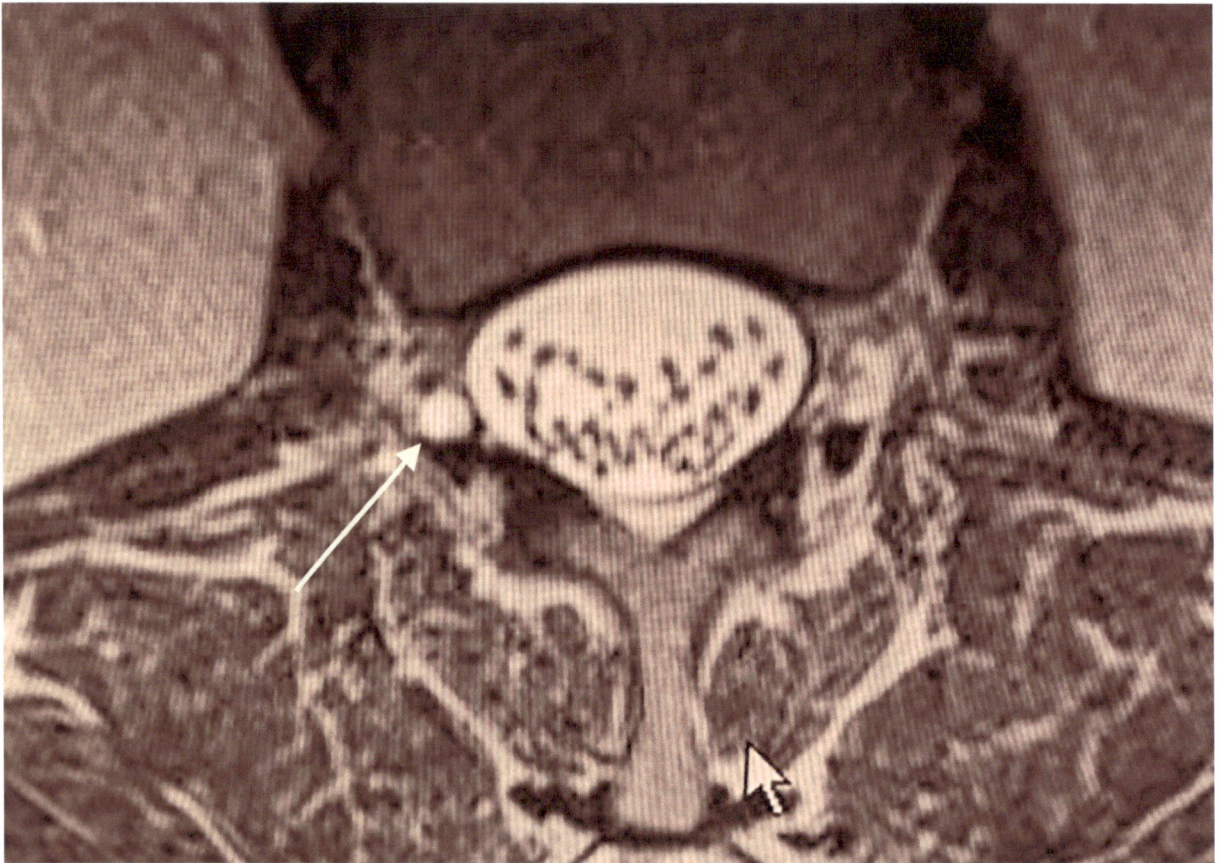

*Figure 7-11: Magnetic resonance image (MRI) of a paravertebral arachnoid cyst.*

Arrow points to a paravertebral arachnoid cyst. (Tarlov cyst)

*Ref: Nabors M, Pait TG, Byrd EB. Updated assessment and current classification of spinal meningeal cysts. J Neurosurg 1988;68:366-77. • Holt S, Yates PO. Cervical nerve root "cysts." Brain 1964;87:481-90.*

# Sonoanatomy
## Meningeal Layers around Spinal Nerve Roots

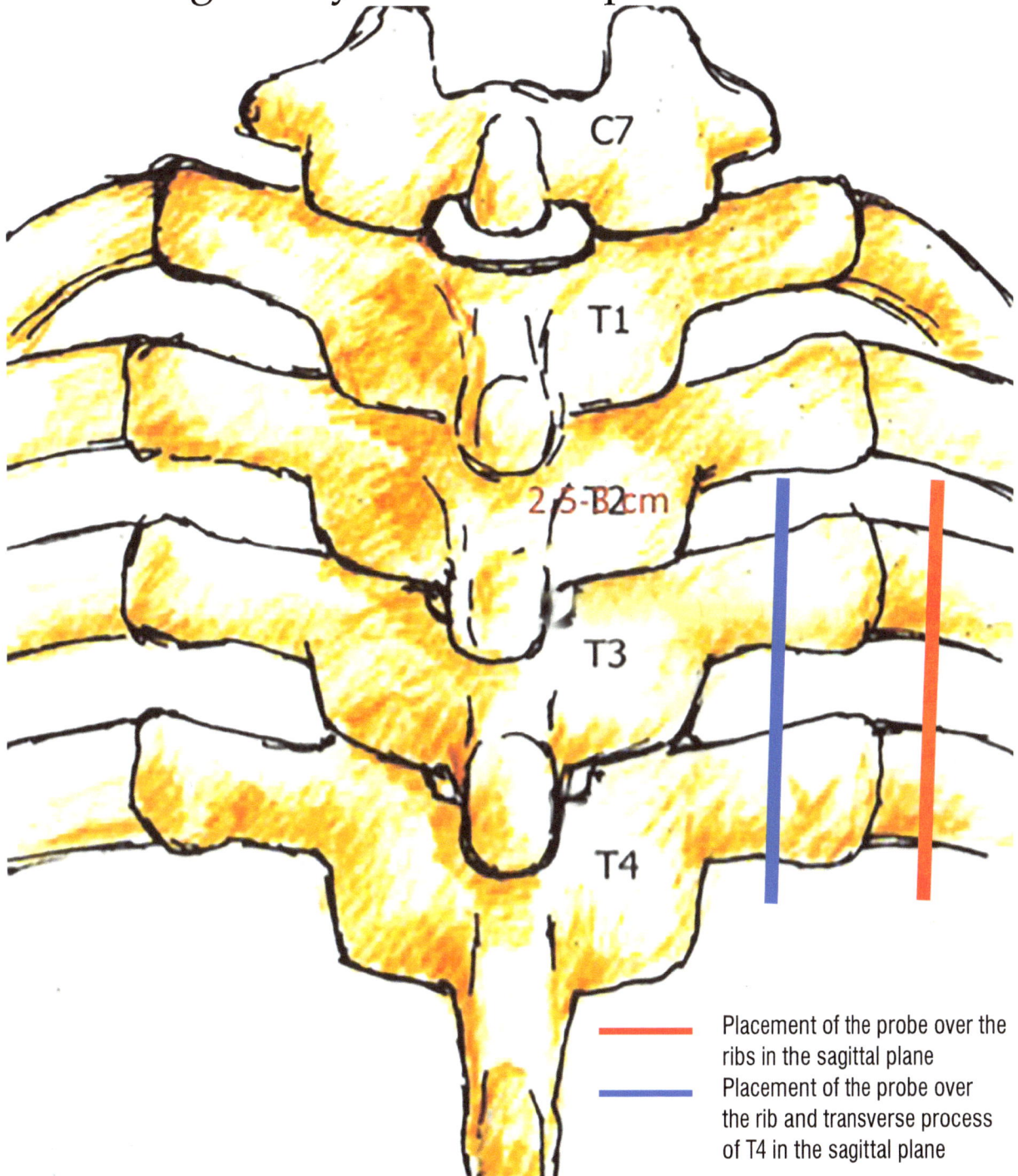

C7

T1

2.5-3 cm

T3

T4

- — Placement of the probe over the ribs in the sagittal plane
- — Placement of the probe over the rib and transverse process of T4 in the sagittal plane

*Figure 7-12: Orientation of the ultrasound transducer probe from the ribs to the rib below and the transverse process superior.*

*Drawing: Barys V. Ihnatsenka, MD*

# Intercostal Placement of Probe
## (Red Line -Fig 12)

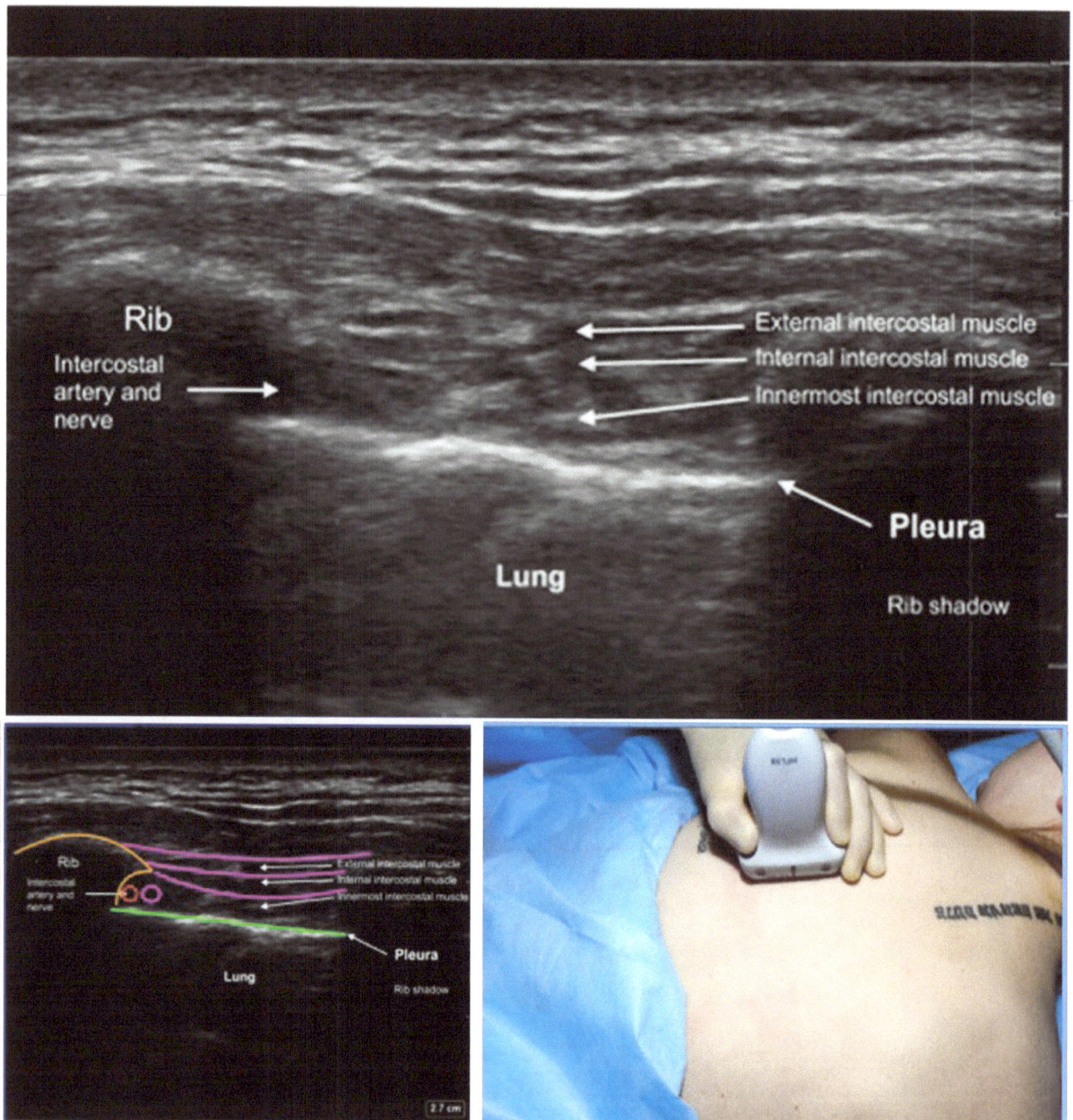

Figure 7-13: Sonoanatomy of the thoracic paravertebral space. Intercostal.

The right side of the image is cephalad and the left side is caudad.

View Video at RAEducation.com
Acute Pain Medicine - Anatomy -
Sonoanatomy: Thoracic Paravertebral Space

# Placement of Probe Over Transverse Process
## (Blue Line -Fig 12)

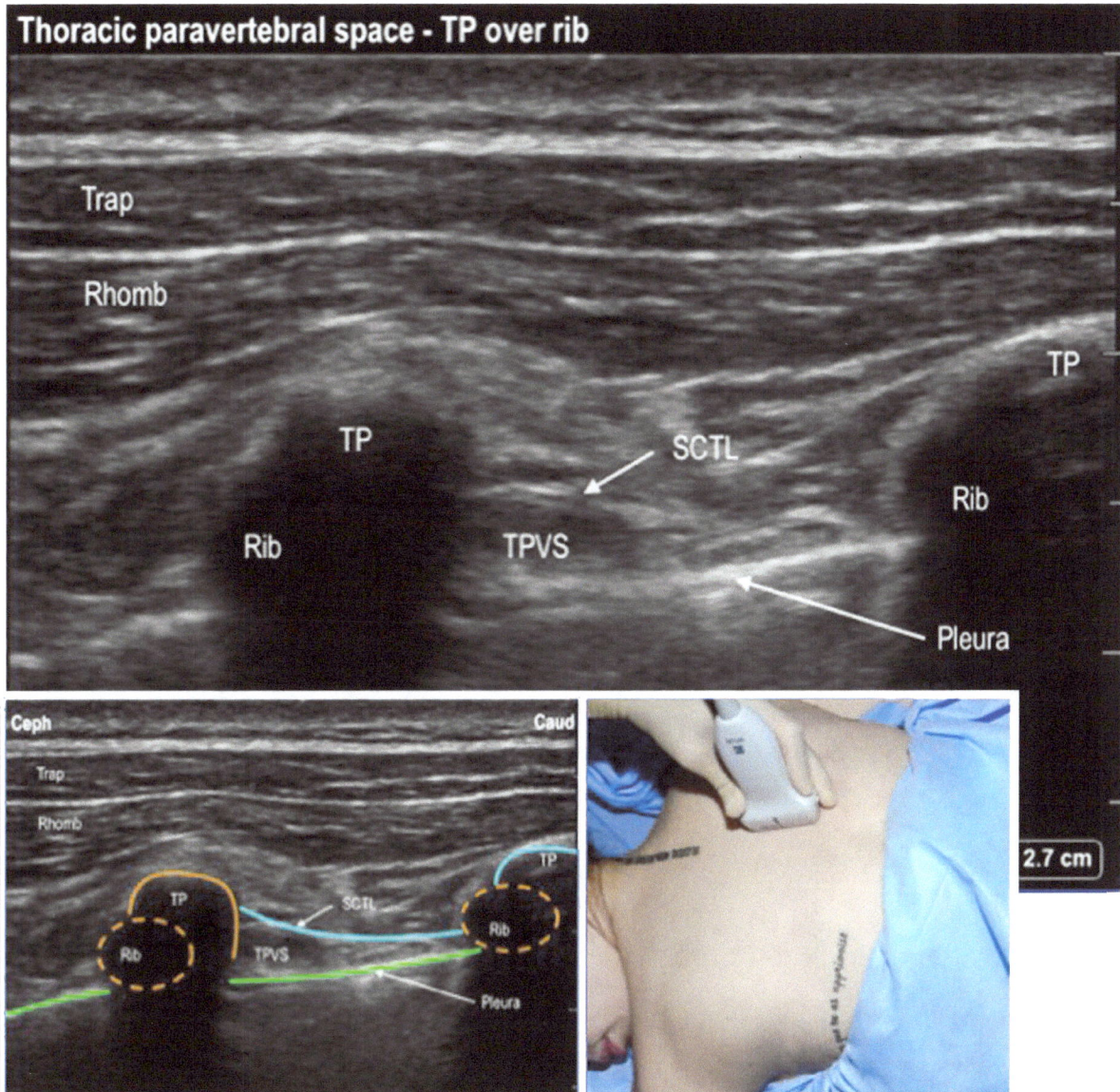

*Figure 7-14: Sonoanatomy of the thoracic paravertebral space in the sagittal plane showing the superior transverse process and the rib below.*

The probe is held slightly oblique here. The left side of the image is cephalad.

2.7 cm — Distance from skin in centimeters

| | |
|---|---|
| Rhomb | Rhomboid muscle |
| SCTL | Superior costotransverse ligament |
| TP | Transverse process of the 4th thoracic vertebra |
| TPVS | Thoracic paravertebral space |
| Trap | Trapezius muscle |

# Oblique View of Paravertebral Space

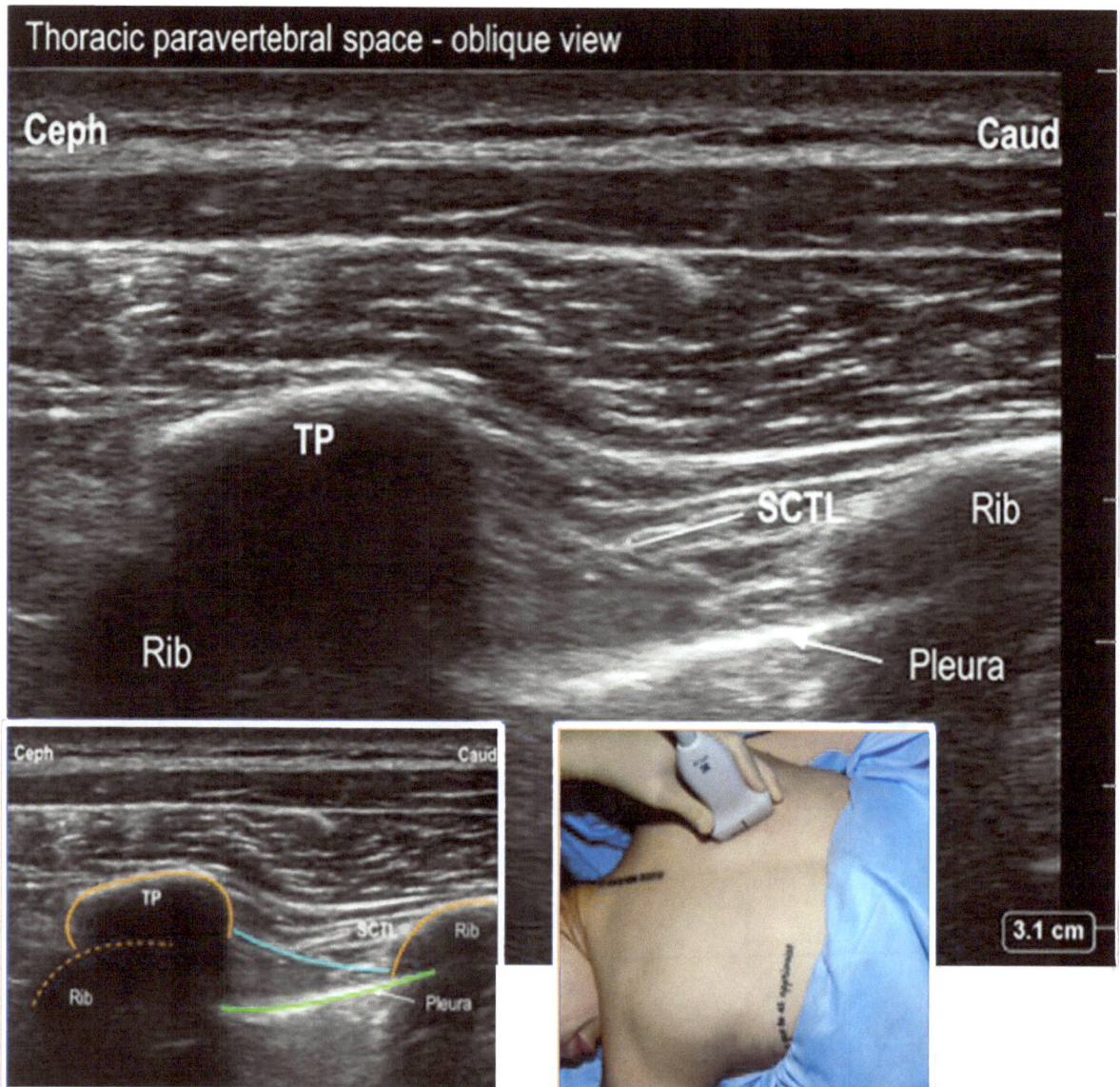

Figure 7-15: Sonoanatomy of the thoracic paravertebral space in the sagittal plane.

The probe is held more oblique than in the previous figure (Fig. 7-14).

| | |
|---|---|
| Ceph | Cephalad |
| Caud | Caudad |
| PV Space | Thoracic paravertebral space |
| SCTL | Superior costotransverse ligament |
| TP T4 | Transverse process of the 4th thoracic vertebra |

# Moving Probe from Lateral (Blue Line) to Medial (Red Line)

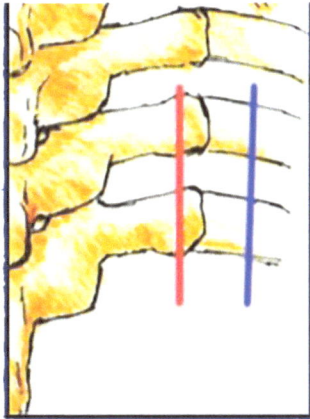

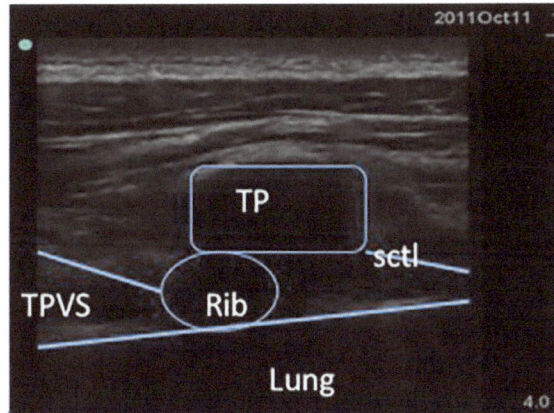

**As the probe moves from lateral to medial, the round rib outline is replaced by a squarer TP outline at a shallower depth. Rib is completely overshadowed by TP. Lung outline becomes deeper.**

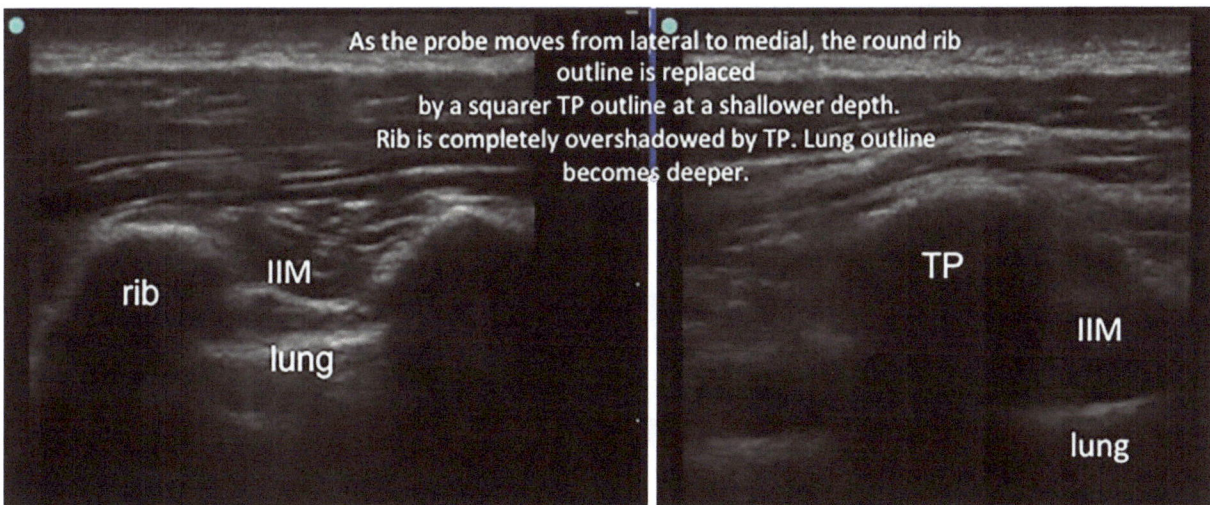

*Figure 7-16: Sonoanatomy of the thoracic paravertebral space with the probe in the vertical sagittal place.*

The ultrasound probe is on the blue line in the drawing on the top left and in the left-hand ultrasound image and moved to the red line in the right-hand ultrasound image.

| | |
|---|---|
| 4.0 | Depth in centimeters from skin |
| IMM | Internal intercostal membrane |
| sctl | Superior costotransverse ligament |
| TP | Transverse process |
| TPVS | Thoracic paravertebral space |

*Drawing: Barys V. Ihnatsenka, MD*

# Axial View of Transverse Process and Rib (Red Line)

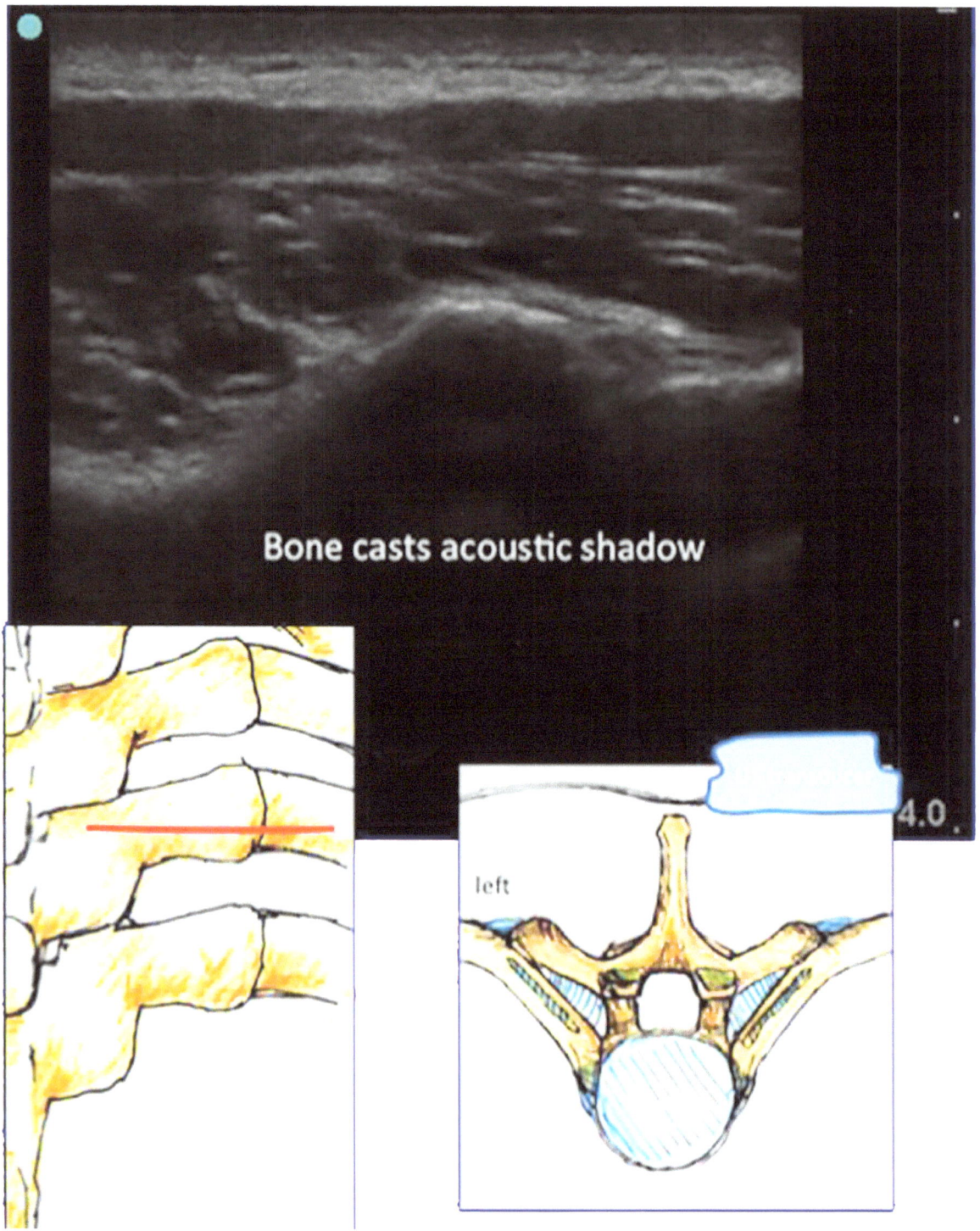

Bone casts acoustic shadow

left

4.0

*Figure 7-17: Sonoanatomy of the thoracic paravertebral space in the axial view.*

The top figure depicts the ultrasound image and the acoustic shadow cast by the transverse process and the rib seen when the ultrasound transducer is placed on the red line shown in the bottom left picture.

*Drawing: Barys V. Ihnatsenka, MD*

# Axial View of the Paravertebral Space

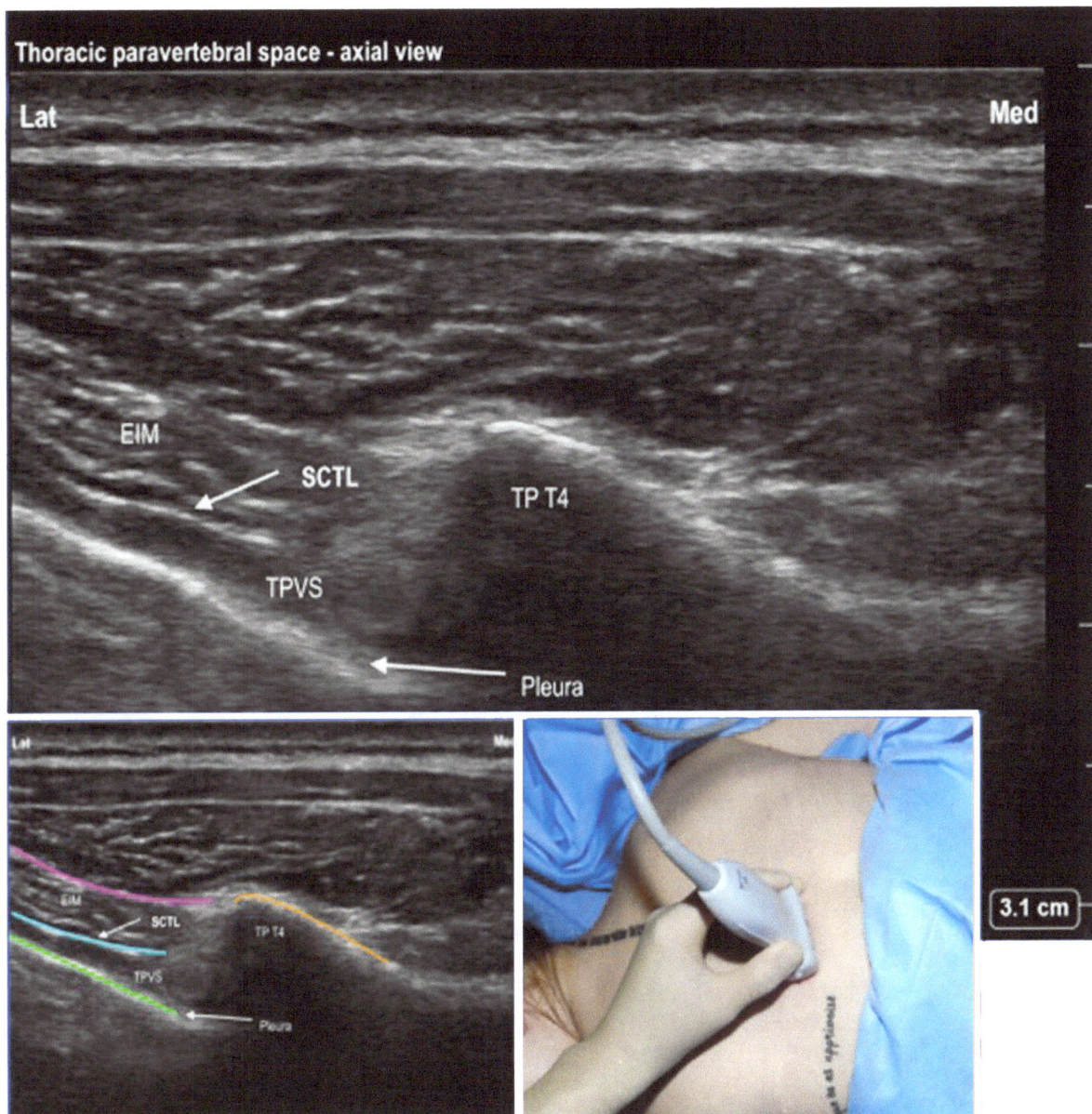

Figure 7-18: Sonoanatomy of the thoracic paravertebral space in the axial paravertebral view.

The probe is placed over the transverse process and just below the rib.

EIM      External intercostal membrane
Lat      Lateral
Med      Medial
SCTL      Superior costotransverse ligament
TPVS      Thoracic paravertebral space
TP T4      Transverse process of the 4th thoracic vertebra

3.1      Distance from the skin
NOTE: The EIM and IMM (Internal intercostal membrane) are both present but cannot be distinguished with ultrasound (see Fig. 7-16)

**View Video at RAEducation.com**
**Acute Pain Medicine - Anatomy -**
**Sonoanatomy: Thoracic Paravertebral Space**

# Moving Probe from Red to Blue Line

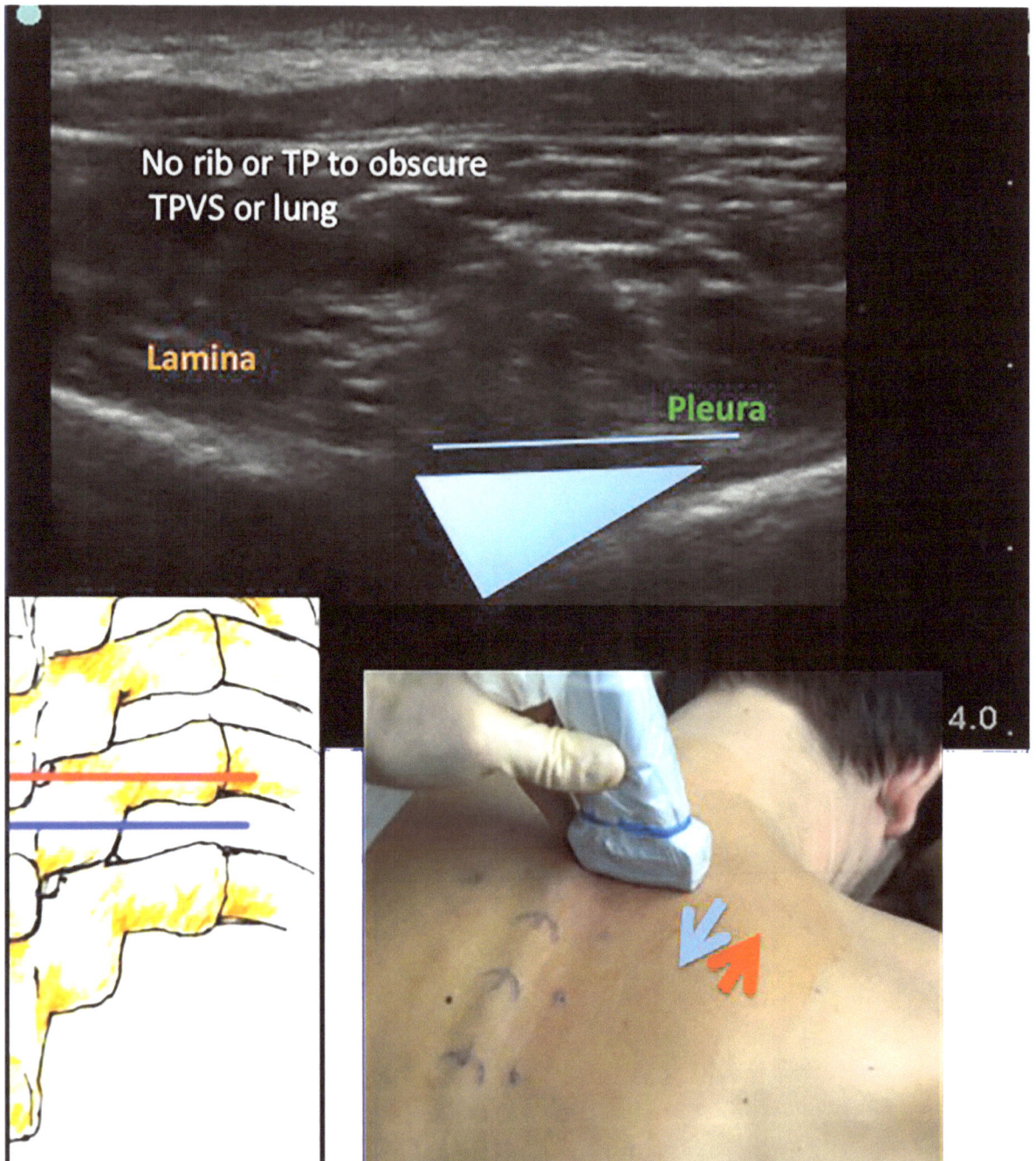

No rib or TP to obscure
TPVS or lung

Lamina

Pleura

4.0

*Figure 7-19: Sonoanatomy of the thoracic paravertebral space in the axial view.*

The ultrasound probe is moved from the red line position to that of the blue line. The thoracic paravertebral space is indicated by the blue triangle.

TP — Transverse process
TPVS — Thoracic paravertebral space

*Drawing: Barys V. Ihnatsenka, MD*

# Axial View of Thoracic Paravertebral Space

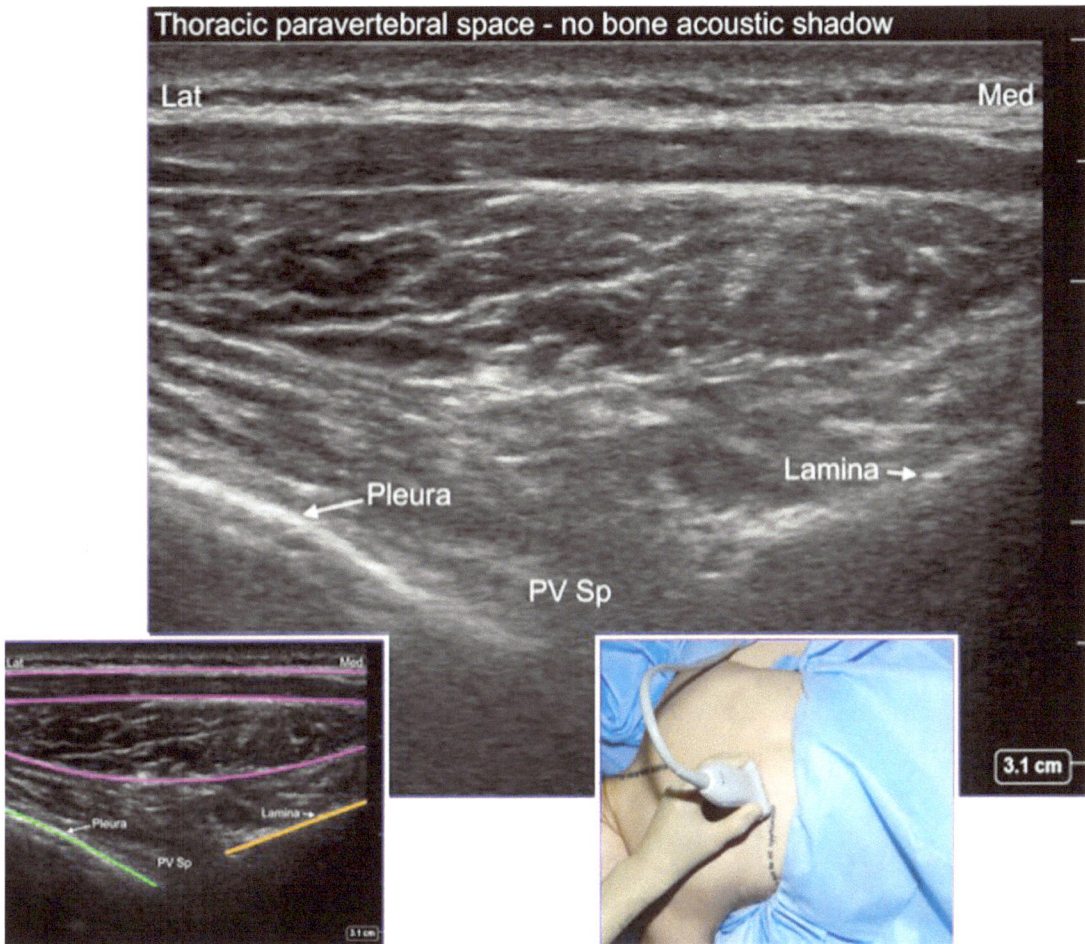

Figure 7-20: Sonoanatomy of the thoracic paravertebral space in the axial view.

The acoustic shadow cast by the transverse process and rib disappears as the probe is moved caudad and the paravertebral space comes into view.

Lat — Lateral
Med — Medial
PV Sp — Thoracic paravertebral space
3.1 cm — Depth in centimeters from skin

# Distances of Skin to Lung at Different Positions

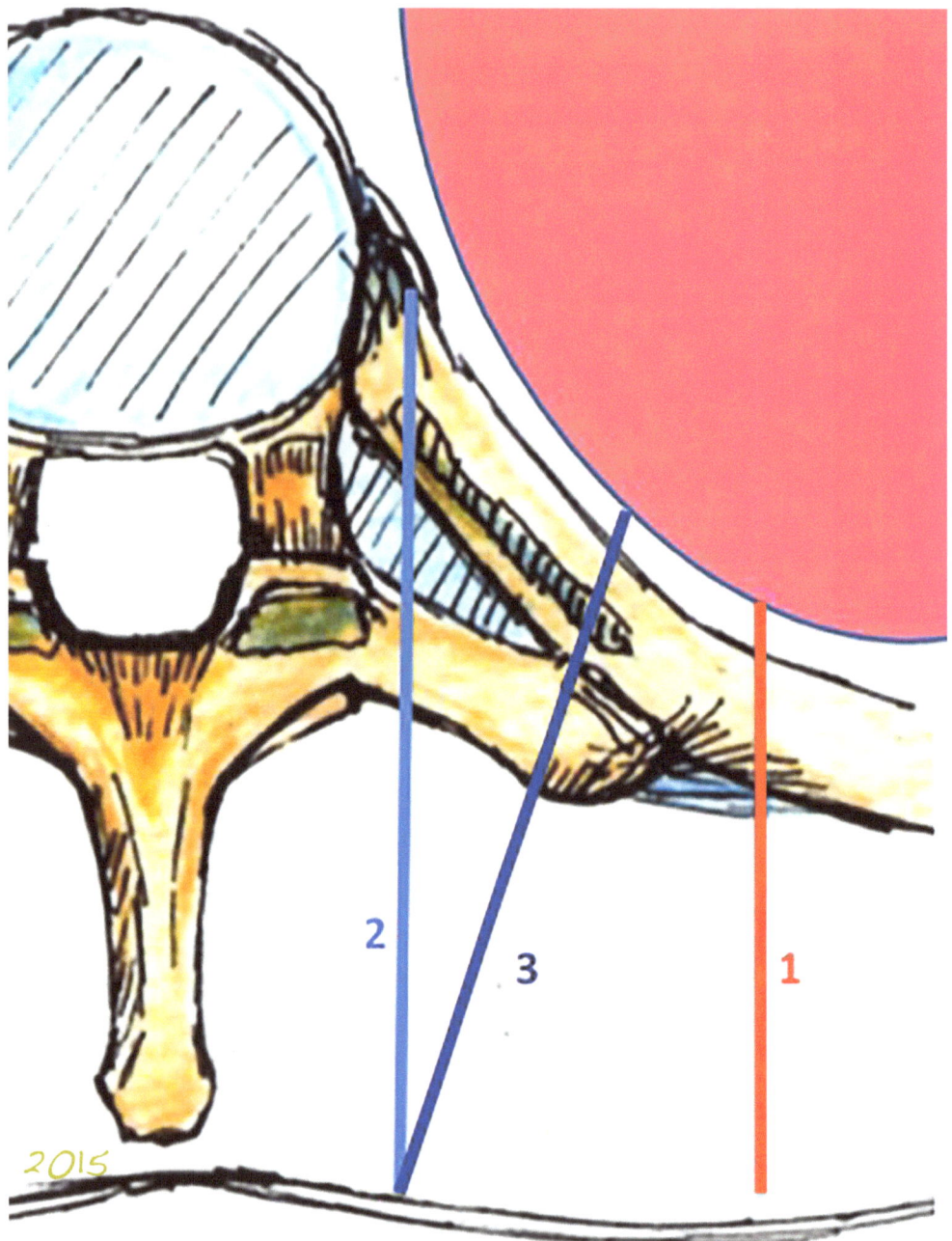

Figure 7-21: Lung visualization with the ultrasound beam at thoracic paravertebral area.

1    the lung is well visualized typically about 4 to 6 cm lateral of the spinous process of the vertebra

2    the lung is not visible because the ultrasound beam is directed between the lung and the vertebral body

3    tilting the beam laterally brings the lung into view again

*Drawing: Barys V. Ihnatsenka, MD*

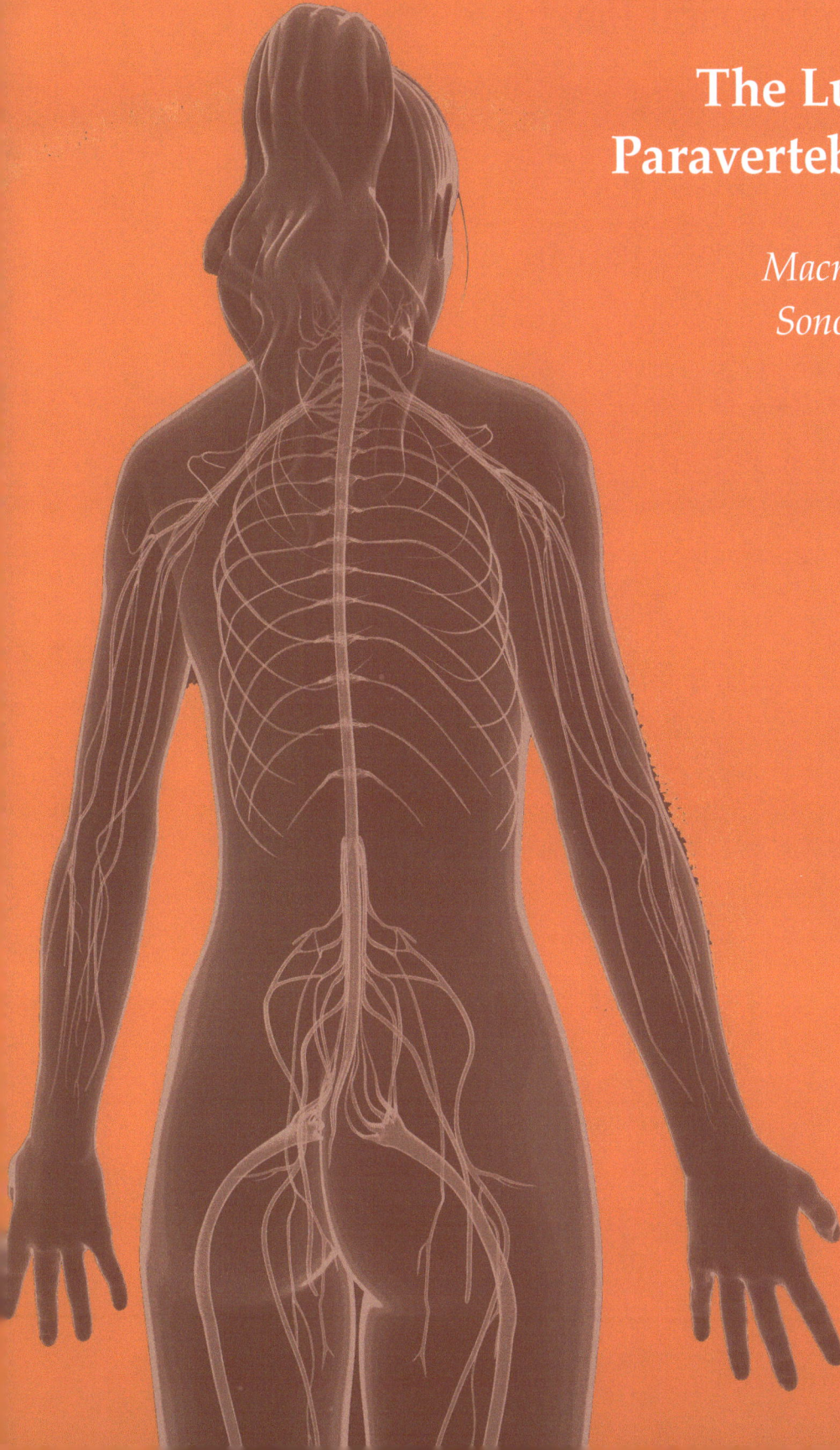

# Chapter 8

## The Lumbar Paravertebral Space

*Macroanatomy*
*Sonoanatomy*

# Macroanatomy

## The Lumbosacral Plexus

### Nerves

1. Subcostal nerve (T12)
2. Iliohypogastric nerve (L1)
3. Ilioinguinal nerve (L1)
4. Lateral femoral cutaneous nerve (L2,3)
5. Femoral branch of genitofemoral nerve (L1,2)
6. Genital branch of genitofemoral nerve (L1,2)
7. Femoral nerve (L2,3,4)
8. Sciatic nerve
   a. Common peroneal nerve (L4,5,S1,2)
   b. Tibial nerve (L4,5,S1,2,3)
9. Posterior femoral cutaneous nerve (S1,2,3)
10. Nerve to Sartorius muscle (L2,3,4)
11. Saphenous branch of the Femoral nerve
12. Obturator nerve (L2,3,4)
13. Pudendal nerve (S1,2,3)
14. Sympathetic trunk
15. Lumbosacral trunk

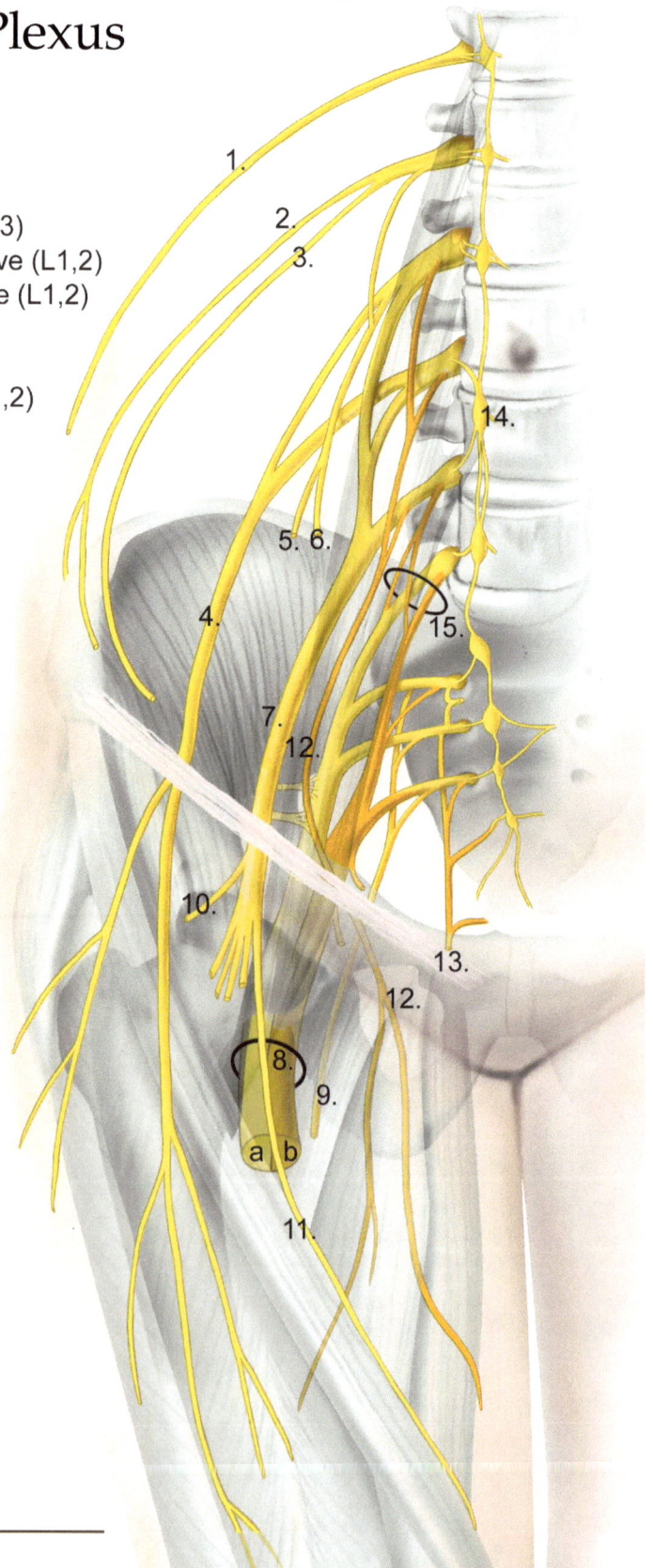

*Figure 8-1: The lumbosacral plexus.*

Please note:

The subcostal (1), ilioinguinal, and iliohypogastric nerves (2, 3) originate from the 12th thoracic (T12) and 1st lumbar (L1) vertebra, respectively.

The lateral cutaneous nerve of the thigh (4) and the genitofemoral nerve originate from the ventral rami of the 1st and 2nd lumbar vertebrae (L1 and L2), whereas the femoral nerve (7) stems from the dorsal rami of L2, L3, and L4.

The 5th lumbar spinal root also gives off a branch to the lumbosacral trunk (15) at the level of L5.

The anterior rami of L2 to L4 form the obturator nerve (12), while L5 and the first three sacral roots (S1, S2, and S3) form the sciatic nerve (8).

The pudendal nerve (13) also arises from these roots.

Ref:Capdevila X, Macaire P, Dadure C, et al.: Continuous psoas compartment block for postoperative analgesia after total hip arthroplasty: New landmarks, technical guidelines, and clinical evaluation. Anesth Analg 2002:94:1606-13.
• Hanna MH, Peat SJ, D'Costa F: Lumbar plexus block: an anatomical study. Anaesthesia 1993;48:675-8.

# The Posterior Retroperitoneal Space

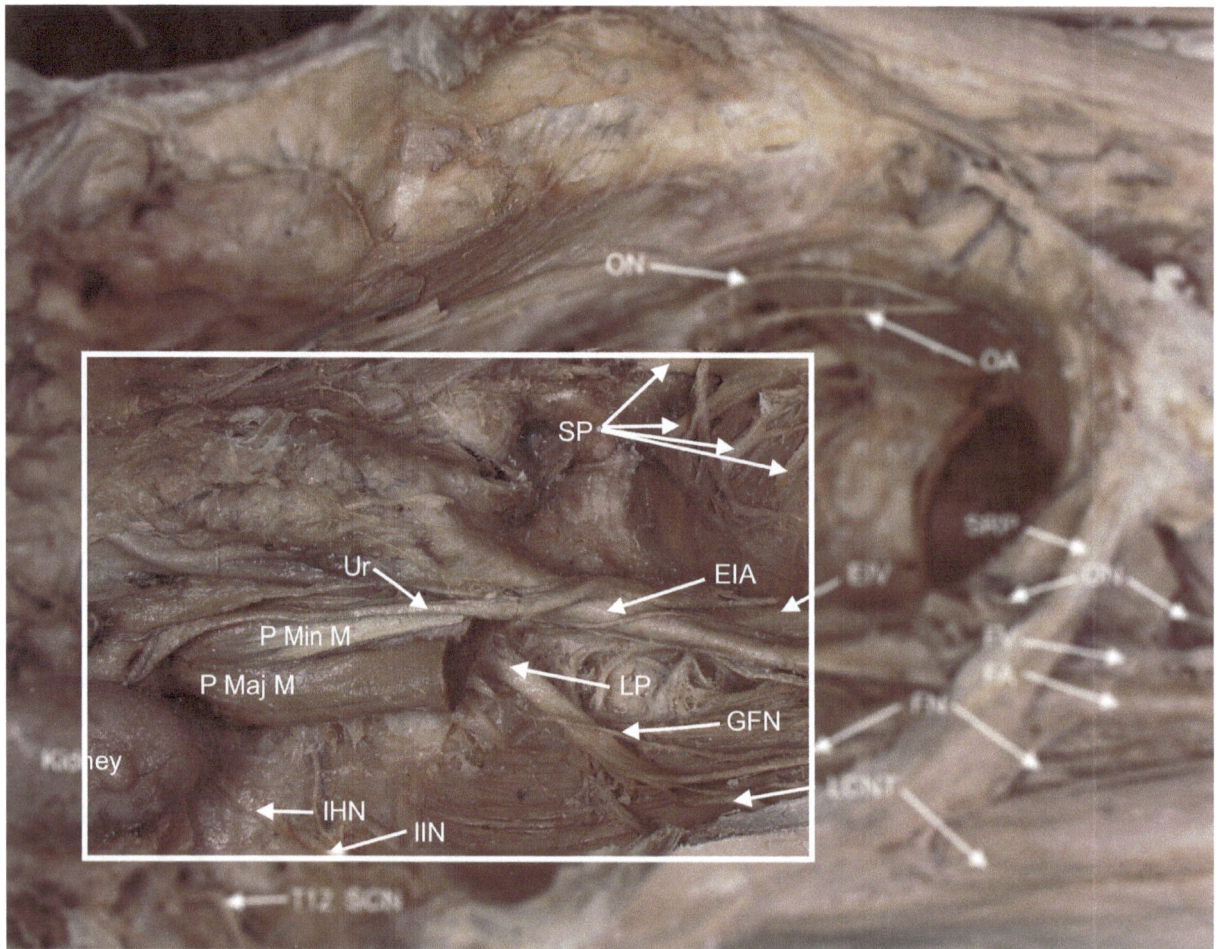

*Figure 8-2: Macroanatomy of the posterior retroperitoneal space.*

| | |
|---|---|
| EIA | External iliac artery |
| GFN | Genitofemoral nerve |
| IHN | Iliohypogastric nerve |
| IIN | Ilioinguinal nerve |
| LP | Lumbar plexus |
| ON | Obturator nerve |
| P Maj M | Psoas major muscle |
| P min M | Psoas minor muscle |
| SP | Sacral plexus |
| Ur | Ureter |

# Transection through the L4 Lumbar Area

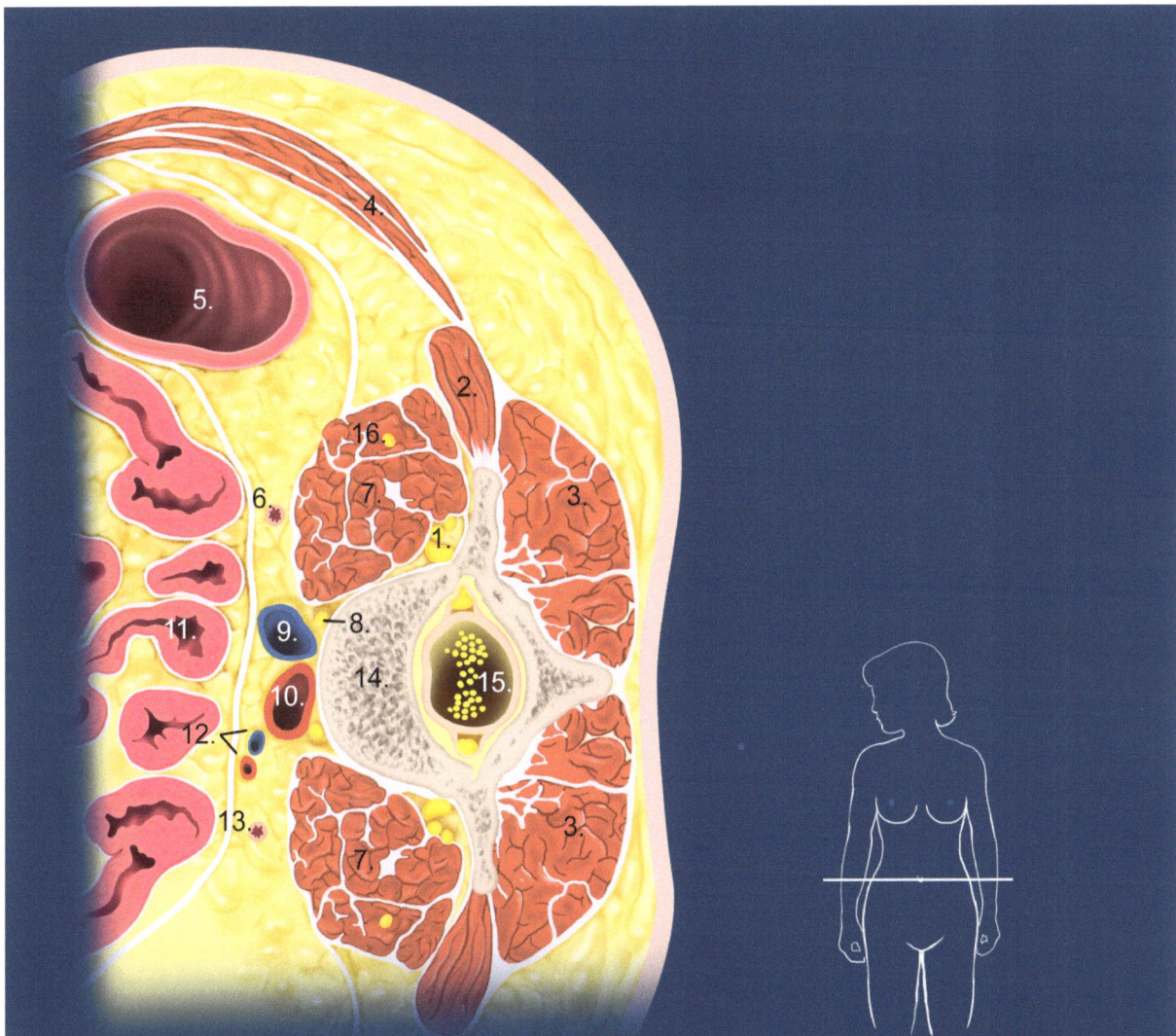

1. Lumbar plexus (ventral rami of L2-L4 becoming femoral and obturator nerves and L4 part of lumbosacral trunk)
2. Quadratus lumborum muscle
3. Erector spinae muscle
4. External and internal oblique muscles and Tranversus abdominis muscle
5. Ascending colon
6. Right ureter
7. Psoas major muscles
8. Sympathetic trunk
9. Inferior vena cava
10. Aortic bifurcation, common iliac arteries
11. Loops of small intestine
12. Inferior mesenteric artery and vein
13. Left ureter
14. Body of L4 vertebra
15. Cauda equina
16. Genitofemoral nerve

*Figure 8-3: Transection at L4 level: Relative positioning of lumbar plexus, genitofemoral nerve, and lumbar sympathetic chain at the level of the 4th lumbar vertebra.*

# Capdevila's Surface Landmarks for the Lumbar Paravertebral Block

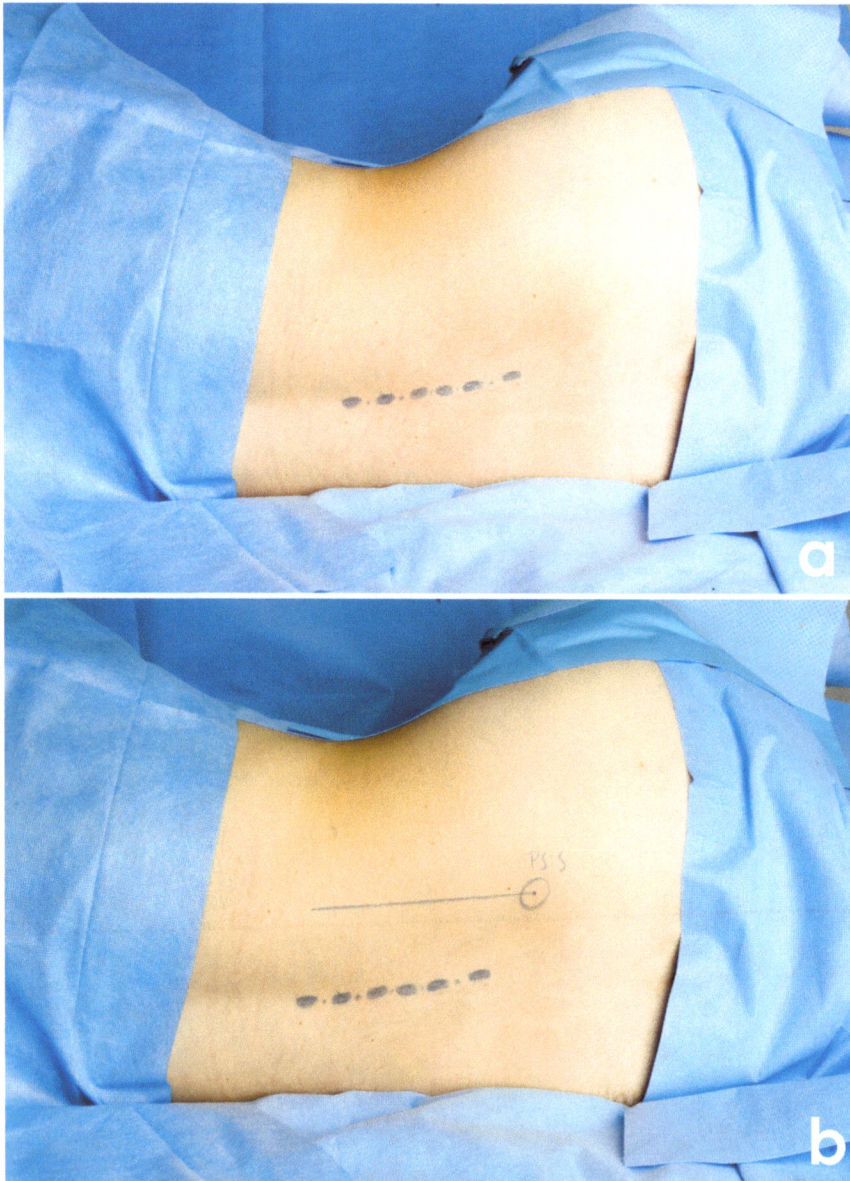

a. The patient is in the lateral (or sitting) position and a line is drawn to indicate the midline over the spinous processes of the lumbar vertebrae.

b. The posterior iliac spine (PSIS) is identified and a line parallel to the one in A is drawn from the PSIS.

*Figure 8-4: Capdevila Surface anatomy of the lumbar plexus.*

**Please refer to standard textbooks for indications for and techniques of performing any of the blocks referred to in this book.**

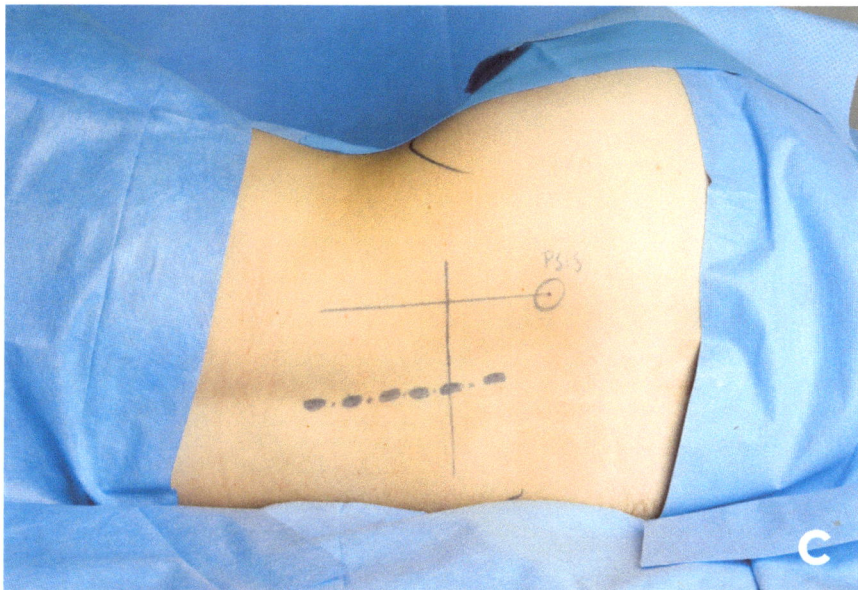

c. The line joining the left and right iliac crests is drawn; this is the so-called "Tuffier's line."

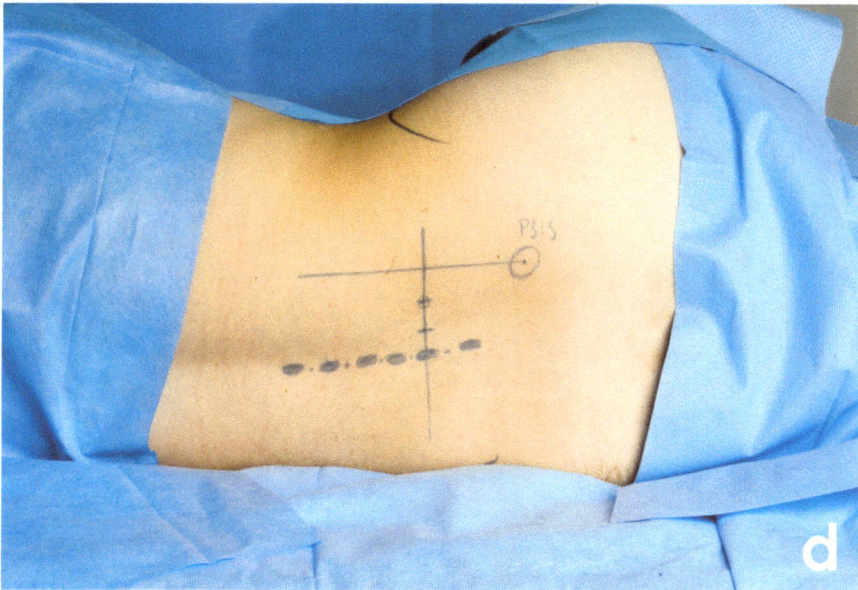

d. The distance from the lines in A and B is divided into three equal parts and needle entry is at the junction of the lateral and middle thirds – Capdevila's point.

Figure 8-5: Capdevila Surface anatomy of the lumbar plexus continued.

Ref: Capdevila X, Macaire P, Dadure C, et al.: Continuous psoas compartment block for postoperative analgesia after total hip arthroplasty: New landmarks, technical guidelines, and clinical evaluation. Anesth Analg 2002;94:1606-13.

# Needle Placement deep to Dura at Nerve Root Level

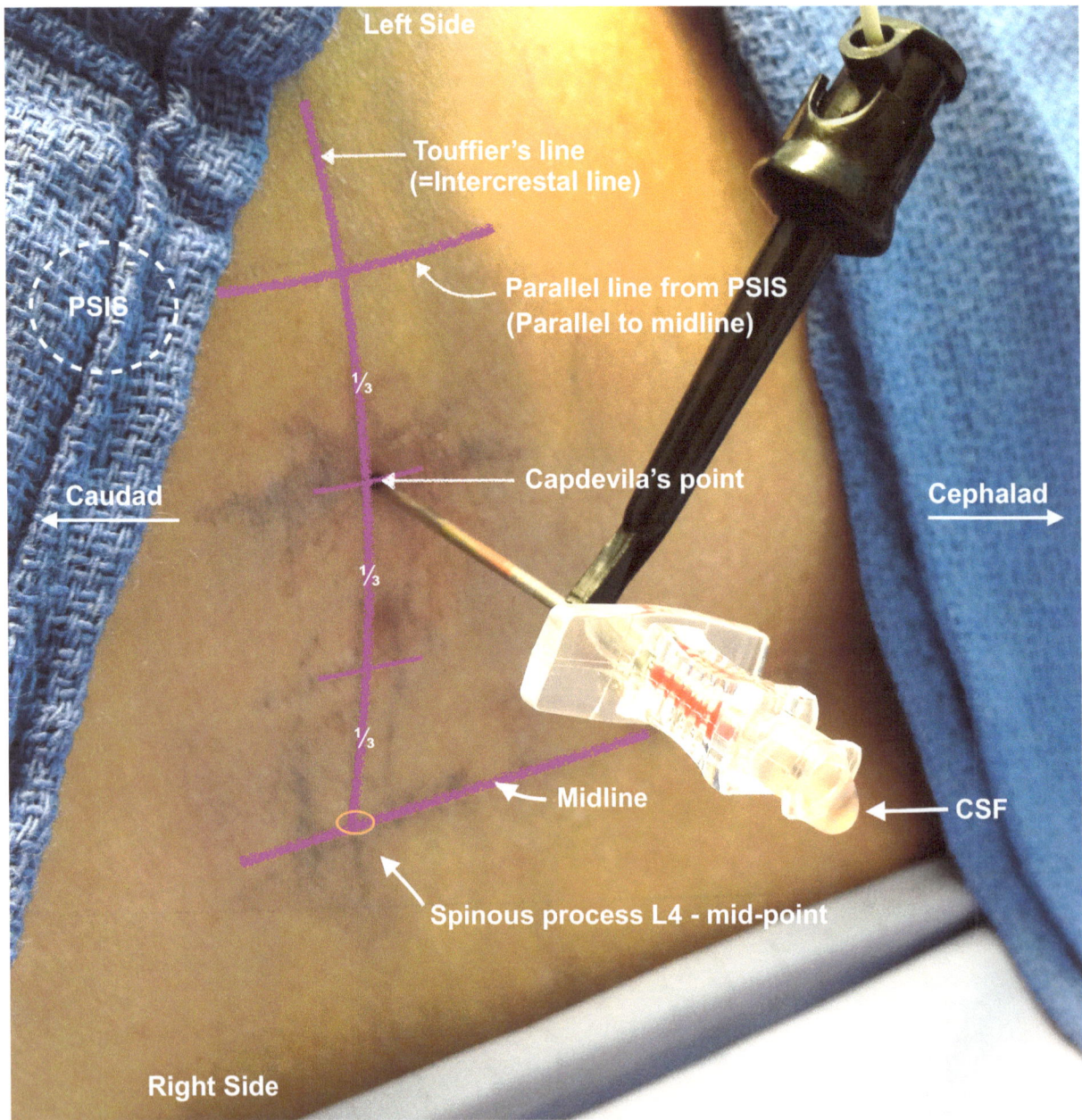

*Figure 8-6: Accidental dural puncture during attempted lumbar plexus block. Patient is in the right lateral decubitus position.*

**Please refer to pages 174-175 for more information regarding needle placement**

| | |
|---|---|
| CSF | Cerebrospinal fluid |
| L4 | 4th lumbar vertebra |
| PSIS | Posterior superior iliac spine |

Midline is a line on the spinous processes of vertebrae. Touffier's line connects the two iliac crests. Capdevila's point is two-thirds the distance from the parallel line from PSIS and midline

# Sonoanatomy

## Lateral Axial View of the Lumbar Plexus

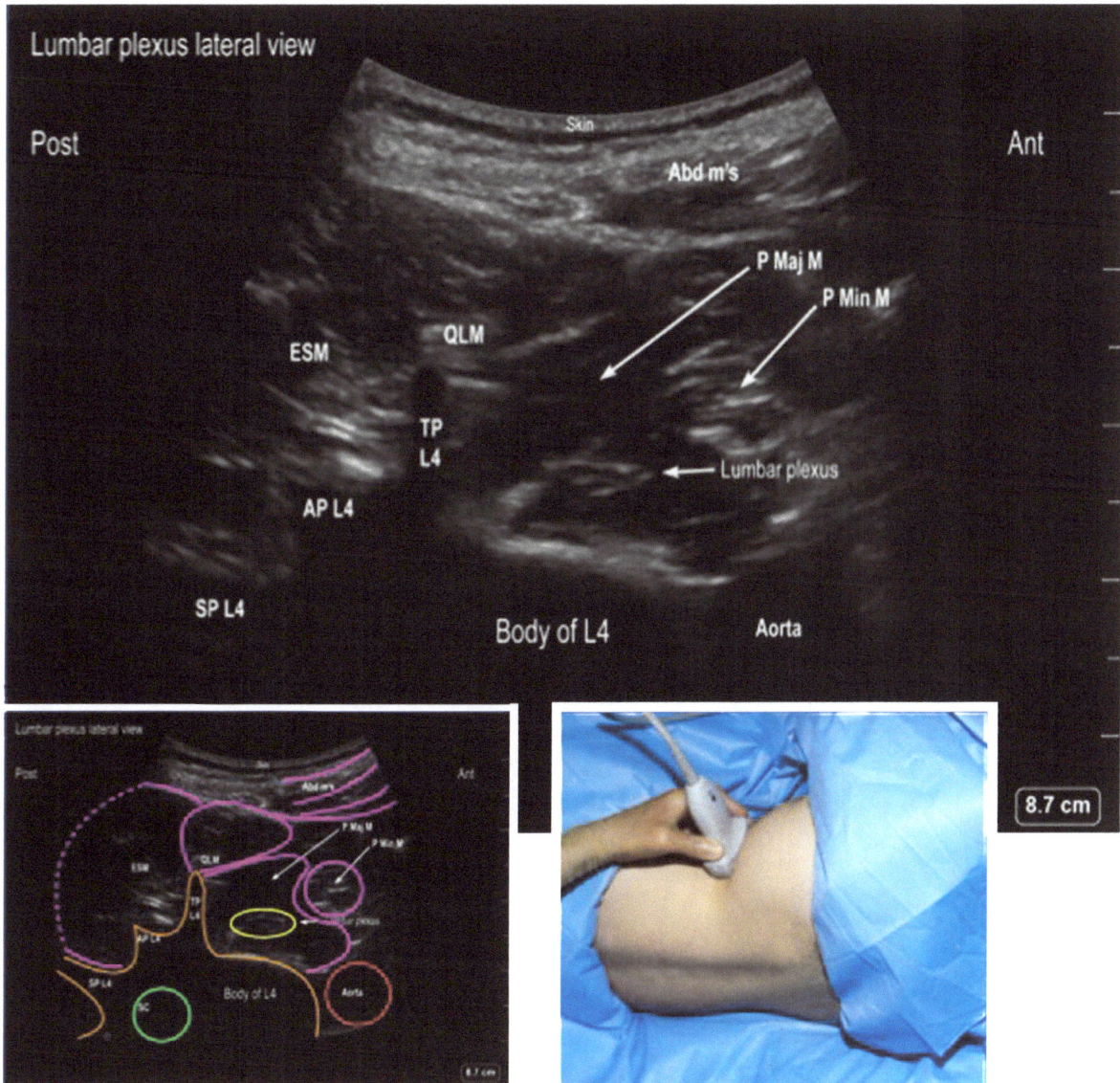

Figure 8-7: Sonoanatomy of the lumbar plexus as viewed laterally with the ultrasound probe in an axial plane.

| | | | | |
|---|---|---|---|---|
| Abd m's | Abdominal muscles | | Post | Posterior |
| Ant | Anterior | | QLM | Quadratus lumborum muscle |
| AP L4 | Articular process of the 4th lumbar vertebra | | SP L4 | Spinous process of the 4th lumbar vertebra |
| Body L4 | Body of the 4th lumbar vertebra | | TP L4 | Transverse process of the 4th lumbar vertebra |
| ESM | Erector spinae muscle | | | |
| P Maj M | Psoas major muscle | | 8.7 cm | Distance from ultrasound probe |
| P Min M | Psoas minor muscle | | | |

# Posterolateral Axial View of the Lumbar Plexus

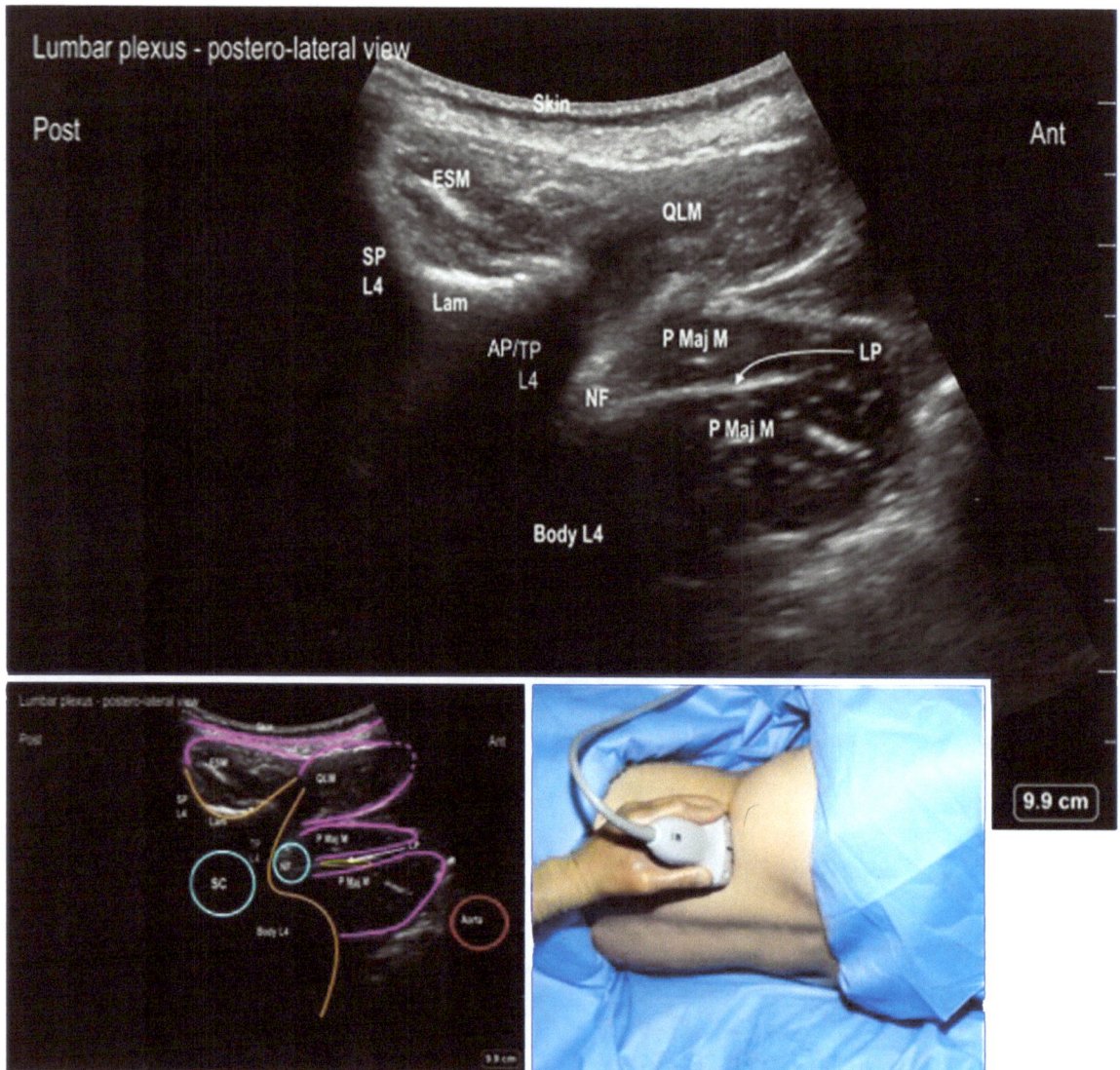

Figure 8-8: Sonoanatomy of the lumbar plexus from a posterolateral view with the ultrasound probe in an axial plane.

| | | | |
|---|---|---|---|
| Ant | Anterior | NF | Neuroforamen |
| AP/TP L4 | Transverse process to articular process transition area of the 4th lumbar vertebra | P Maj M | Psoas major muscle |
| | | Post | Posterior |
| | | QLM | Quadratus lumborum muscle |
| Body L4 | Body of the 4th lumbar vertebra. | SP L4 | Spinous process of the 4th lumbar vertebra |
| ESM | Erector spinae muscle | | |
| Lam | Lamina of the 4th lumbar vertebra | | |
| LP | Lumbar plexus | | |

# Posterior Sagittal View of the Lumbar Plexus

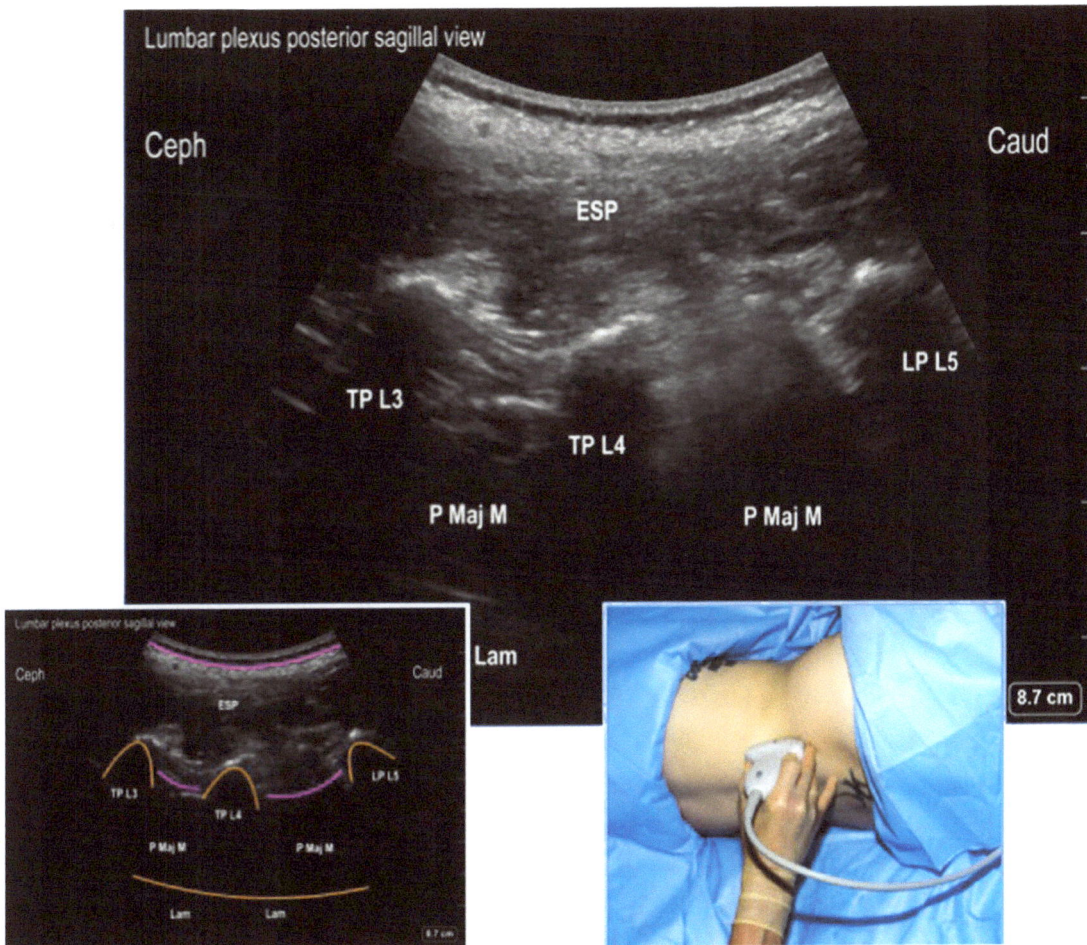

Figure 8-9: Sonoanatomy of the lumbar plexus viewed from a posterior position with the ultrasound probe in the paramedian sagittal plane.

| | |
|---|---|
| Ceph | Cephalad |
| ESP | Erector spinae muscle |
| Lam | Lamina of the 3rd lumbar vertebra |
| P Maj M | Psoas major muscle |
| TP L3 | Transverse process of the 3rd lumbar vertebra |
| TP L4 | Transverse process of the 4th lumbar vertebra |

| | |
|---|---|
| TP L5 | Transverse process of the 5th lumbar vertebra |

The distance from the skin or ultrasound probe is 8.7 cm

View Video at RAEducation.com
Acute Pain Medicine - Anatomy -
Sonoanatomy: Lumbar Plexus

# Chapter 9

# The Neuraxium

*Macroanatomy*
*Microanatomy*
*Sonoanatomy*

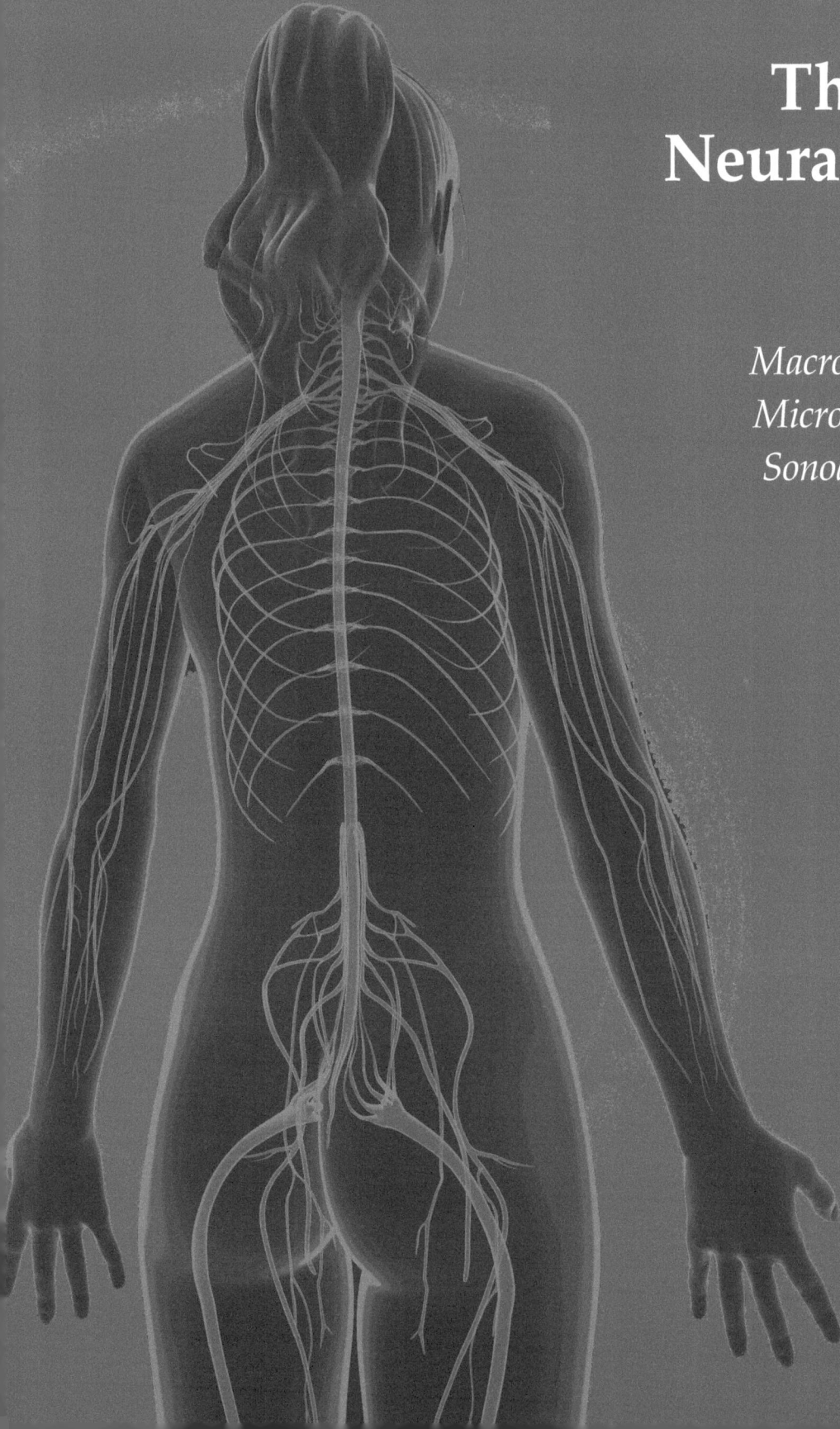

# Macroanatomy

## The Epidural Space

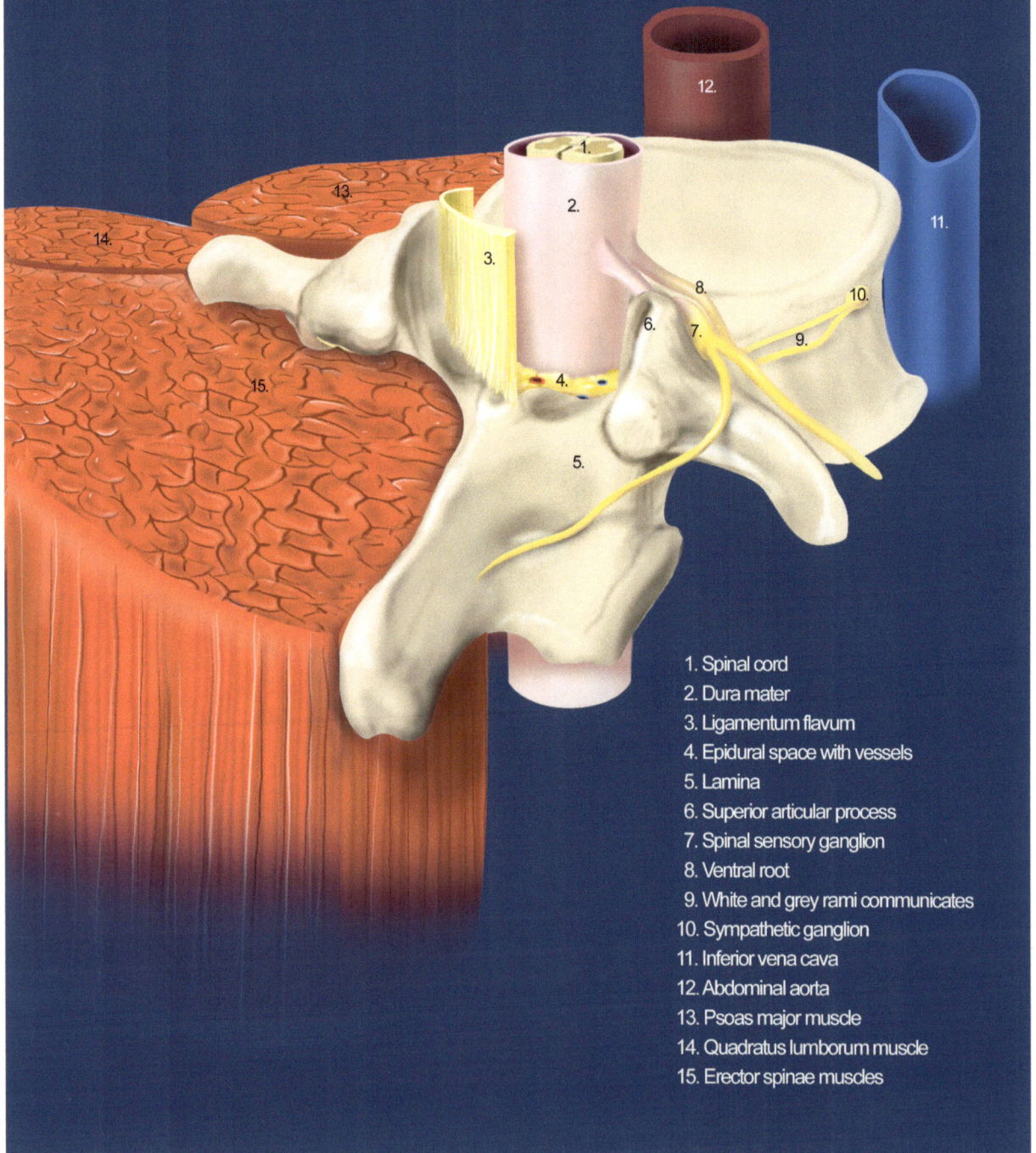

1. Spinal cord
2. Dura mater
3. Ligamentum flavum
4. Epidural space with vessels
5. Lamina
6. Superior articular process
7. Spinal sensory ganglion
8. Ventral root
9. White and grey rami communicates
10. Sympathetic ganglion
11. Inferior vena cava
12. Abdominal aorta
13. Psoas major muscle
14. Quadratus lumborum muscle
15. Erector spinae muscles

Figure 9-1: Schematic representation of the epidural space.

Ref: Netter FH. The Ciba Collection Of Medical Illustrations, Vol 1: Nervous system. New York, NY: Ciba, 1967; p 54.

# Ligamentum Flavum viewed from Anterior

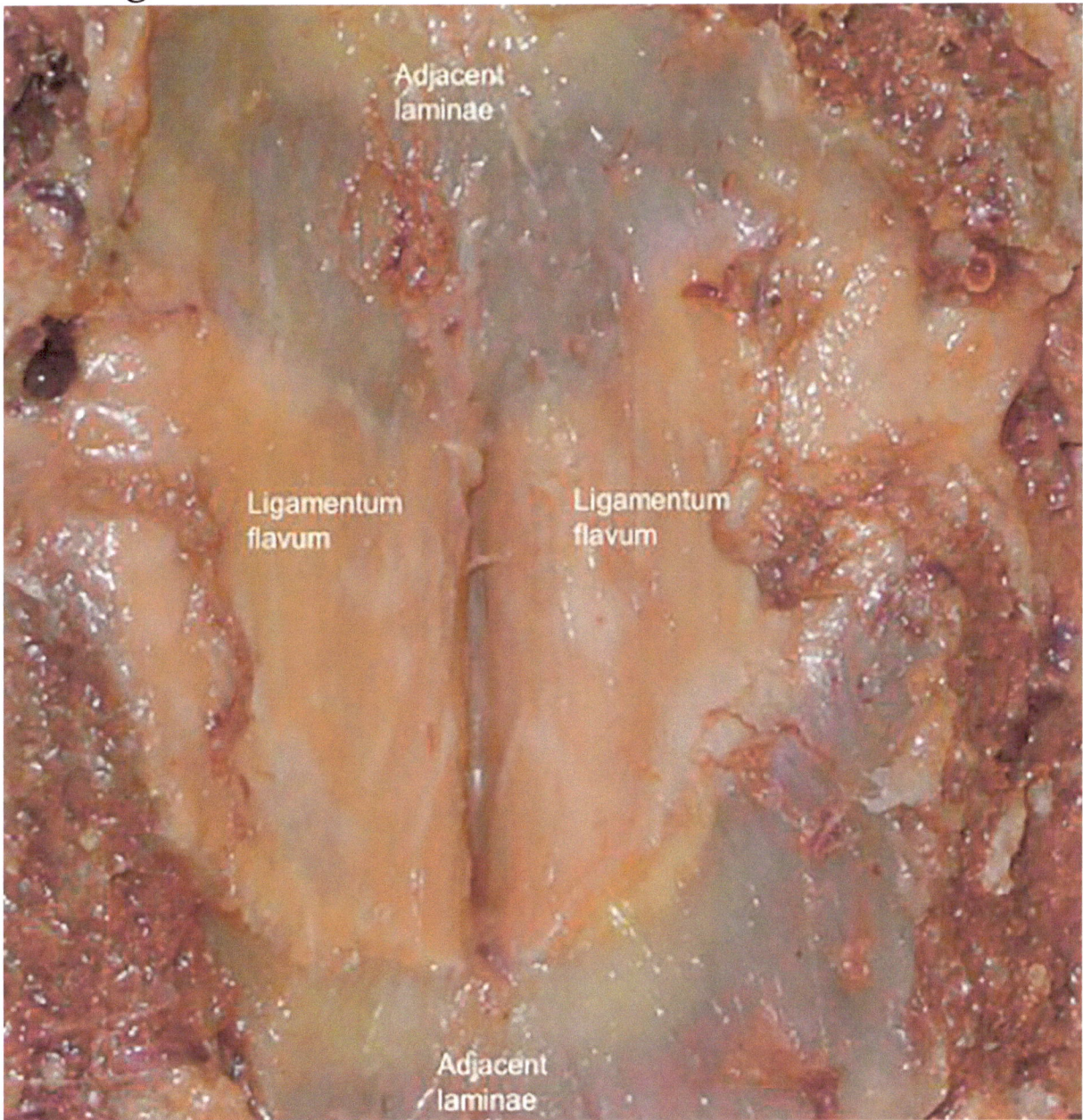

Figure 9-2: The ligamentum flavum as viewed from anterior.

It consists of a pair of disk-shaped halves that span two adjacent laminae. They loosely meet in the midline, often leaving a gap between the two dense and thick lateral parts. The epidural space is just deep (anterior) to this ligament.

Reprinted with permission from: Lirk P. The ligamentum flavum. In: Reina MA, Ed. Atlas of Functional Anatomy For Regional Anesthesia And Pain Medicine. New York: Springer, 2015; 640.

# Axial View of Ligamentum Flavum at L4 Level

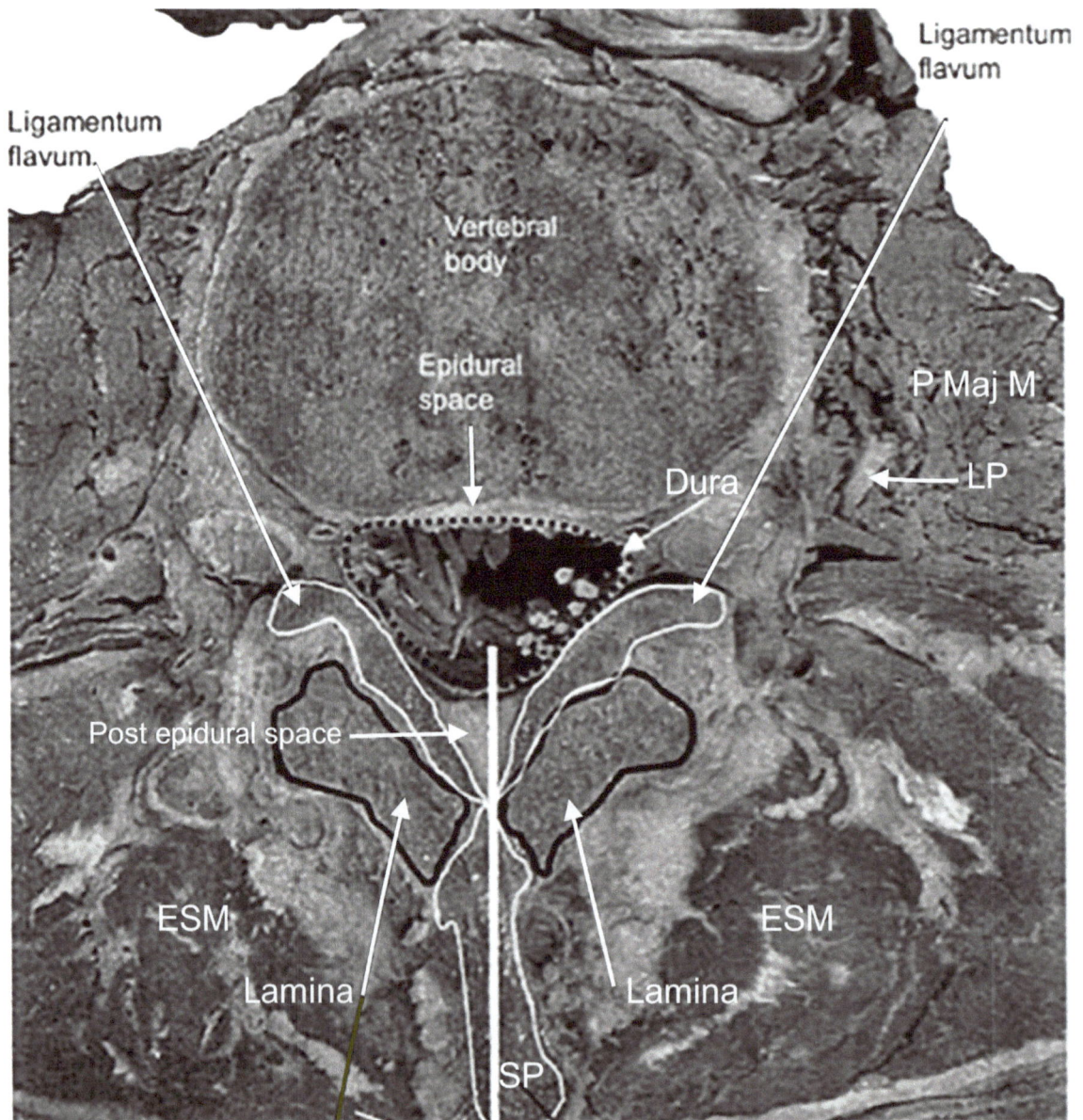

Figure 9-3: Transection through the 4th lumbar vertebra to illustrate the ligamentum flavum and its relationships with the epidural space, dura mater, and the laminae of the vertebra

In this case, there is a subtle midline gap.
ESM       Erector spinae muscle
Lamina  Lamina of 4th thoracic vertebra
LP         Lumbar plexus
P Maj M Psoas major muscle

Please note here the steep angles of the ligamentum flavum. Also note that it consists of two discs and the epidural space at the lumbar level is a triangular space. Midline approach to the epidural space will often not encounter the ligament, and therefore not any resistance.

*Reprinted with permission from: Lirk P. The ligamentum flavum. In: Reina MA, Ed. Atlas of Functional Anatomy For Regional Anesthesia And Pain Medicine. New York: Springer, 2015; 645*

# Ligamentum Flavum, Epipdural Space and Cauda Equina at L3 Level

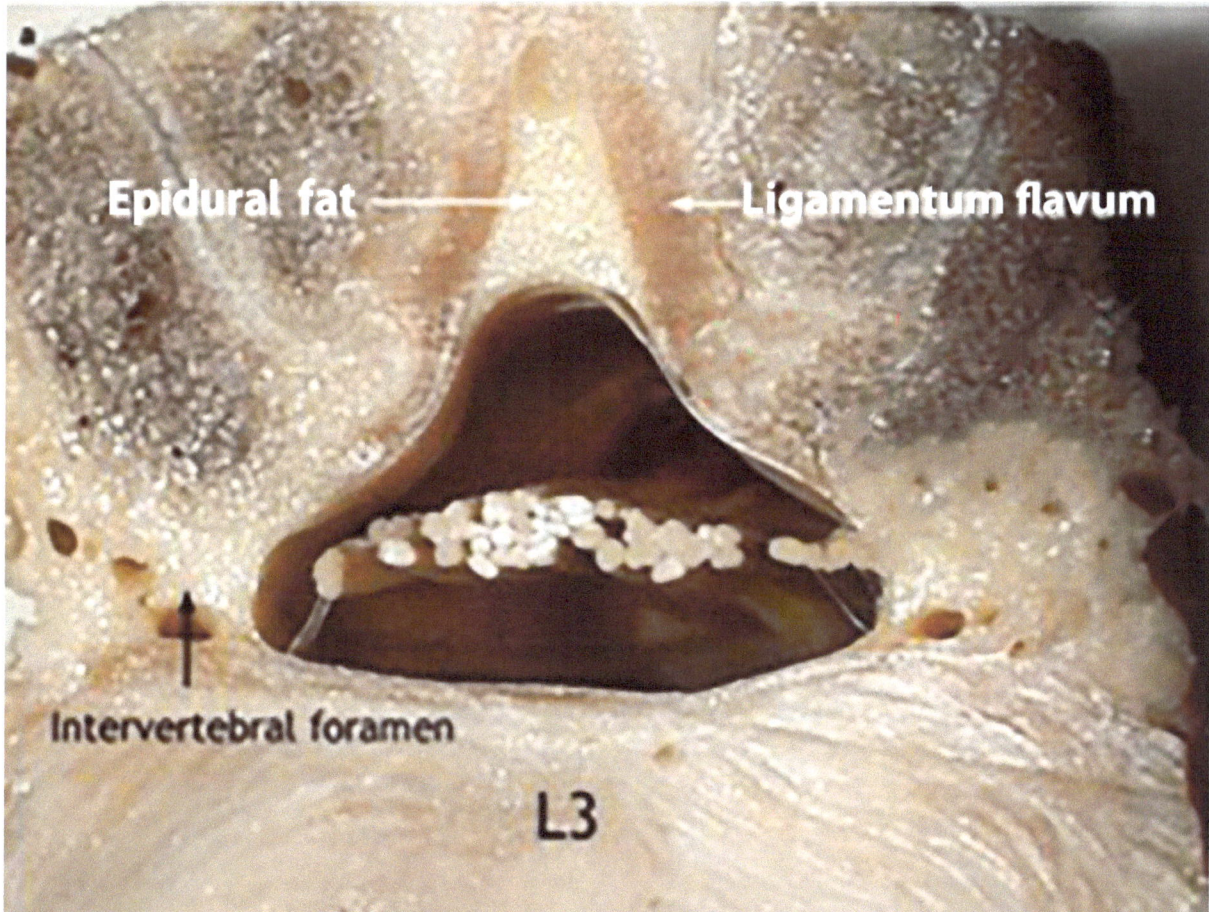

Epidural fat → ← Ligamentum flavum

Intervertebral foramen

L3

*Figure 9-4: Transverse section of the spinal canal at the level of L3 showing ligamentum flavum*

Please note here again the steep angles of the two discs of the lligamentum flavum and the triangular epidural space. Also note that the cauda equina spinal roots are all bundled together. This may be important for spinal anesthesia. Further caudad the spinal roots scatter.

Please also keep in mind that the spinal roots of the cauda equina cannot stretch, so flexing the spine convex outward ("mad cat") moves these spinal roots more anteriorly and out of the way of the spinal needle

*Reprinted with permission from: Lirk P. The ligamentum flavum. In: Reina MA, Ed. Atlas of Functional Anatomy For Regional Anesthesia And Pain Medicine. New York: Springer, 2015; 669.*

# CT Scan of Epidural Space showing Epidural Septum and Resulting Hemi-Epidural Block

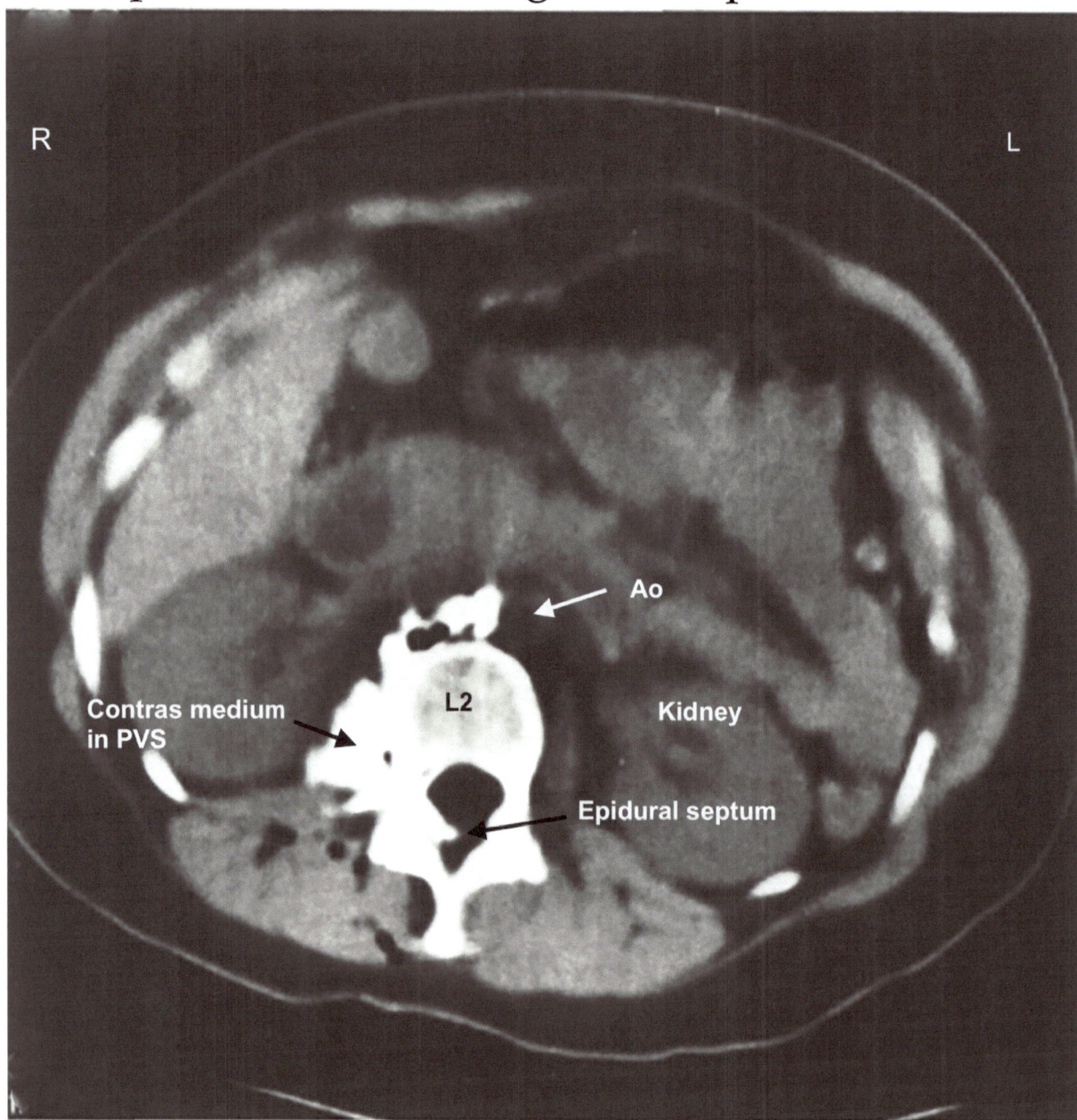

*Figure 9-5: Computerized axial temo-epidurographic (CAT scan) documentation following unilateral epidural block due to congenital epidural septum.*

| | | | |
|---|---|---|---|
| Ao | Abdominal aorta | PVS | Paravertebral space |
| L | Left | R | Right |
| L2 | Body of 2nd lumbar vertebra | | |

*Ref: Boezaart AP. Computerized axial temo-epidurographic and radiologic documentation of unilateral epidural analgesia. Can J Anaesth 1989;36:697-700.*

# Axial Sections outlining Level Differences

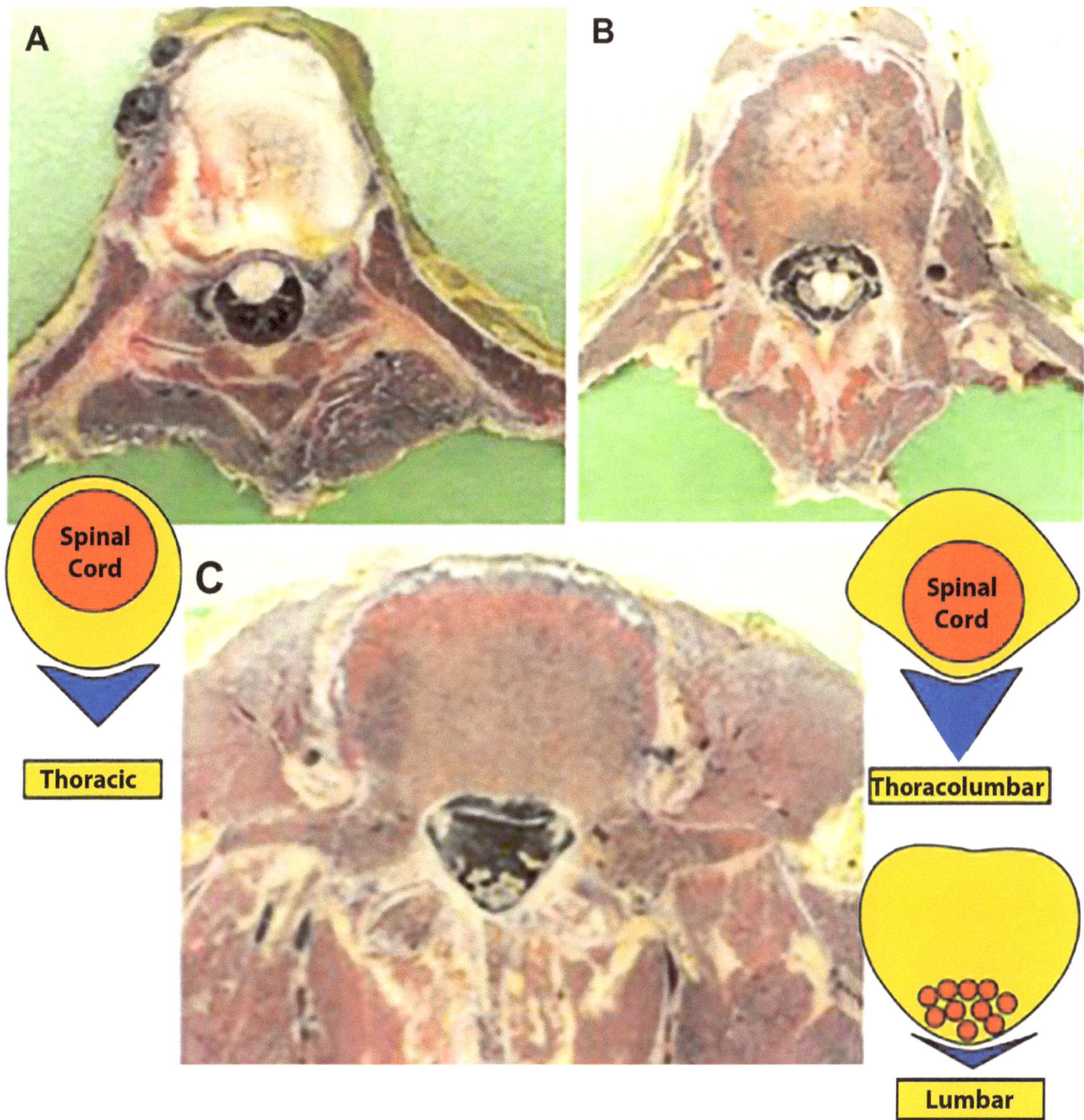

Figure 9-6: Anatomic axial sections at the (A) mid-thoracic region, (B) thoracolumbar region, and (C) lower lumbar regions, showing the respective relationships in the spinal canal.

| | | | |
|---|---|---|---|
| Blue | Epidural space | Yellow | Subarachnoid space |
| Red | Spinal cord or cauda equina | | The triangular blue epidural space is posterior |

Reprinted with permission from: Lataster LMA, van Zundert AAJ. Anatomy of the thoracic spinal canal in different postures: An MRI investigation. In: Reina MA, Ed. Atlas of Functional Anatomy For Regional Anesthesia And Pain Medicine. New York: Springer, 2015; 696.

# Sonoanatomy
## Axial Midline of Thoracic Epidural Space

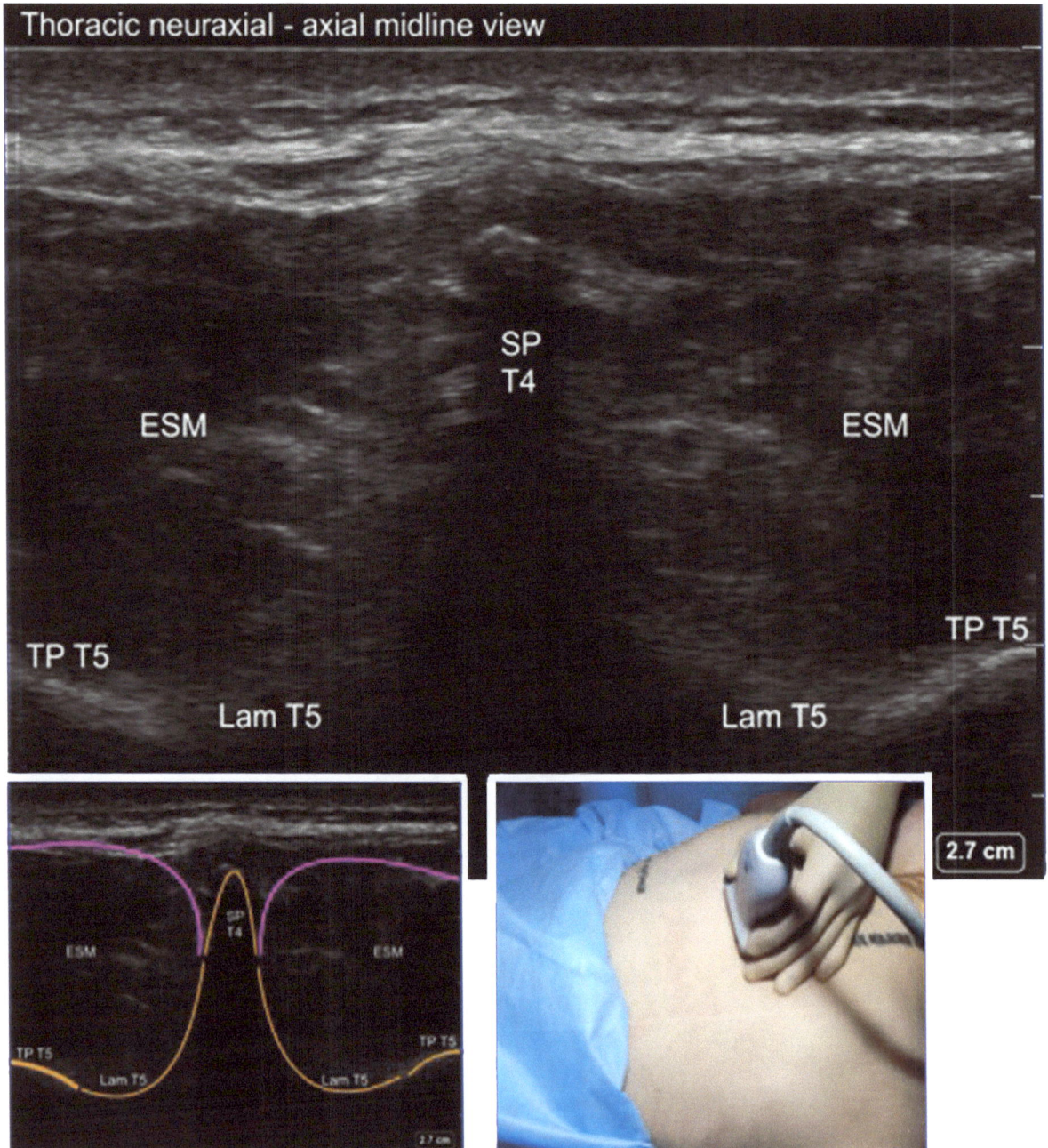

Figure 9-7: Sonoanatomy of the 5th thoracic vertebra as seen in the axial view. The left side of the image is the left side of the model.

ESM     Erector spinae muscle

Lam L5    Lamina of the 5th thoracic vertebra

SP T4    Spinous process of the 4th thoracic vertebra

TP L5    Transverse process of the 5th thoracic vertebra

# Sagittal Para-Spinal View of Thoracic Epidural Space

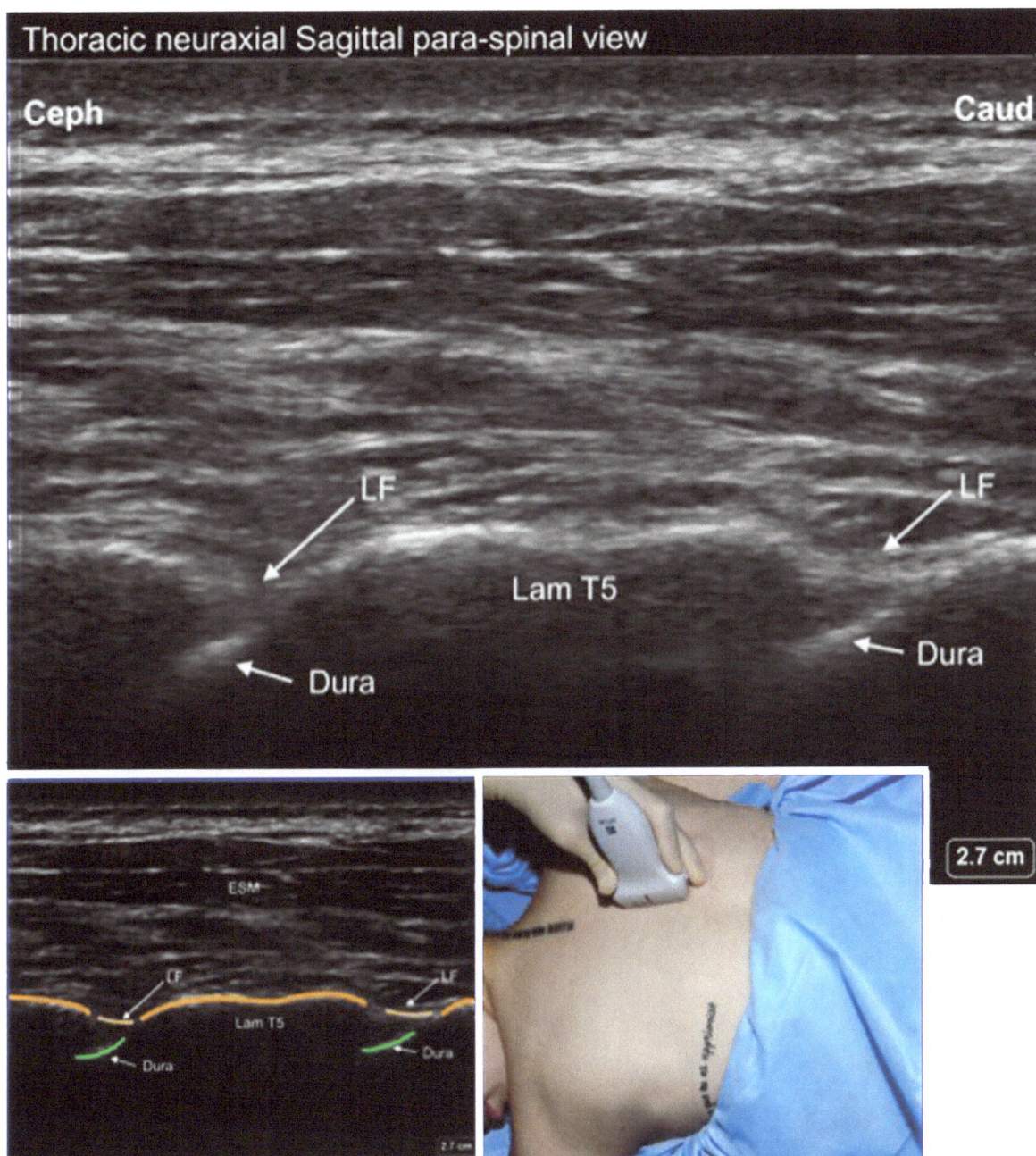

*Figure 9-8: Sonoanatomy of the 5th thoracic vertebra as seen in the paramedian sagittal plane.*

Ceph     Cephalad
Caud     Caudad
dura     Dura mater
Lam T5   Lamina of the 5th thoracic vertebra
LF       Ligamentum flavum

# Axial Midline View of the Lumbar Epidural Space

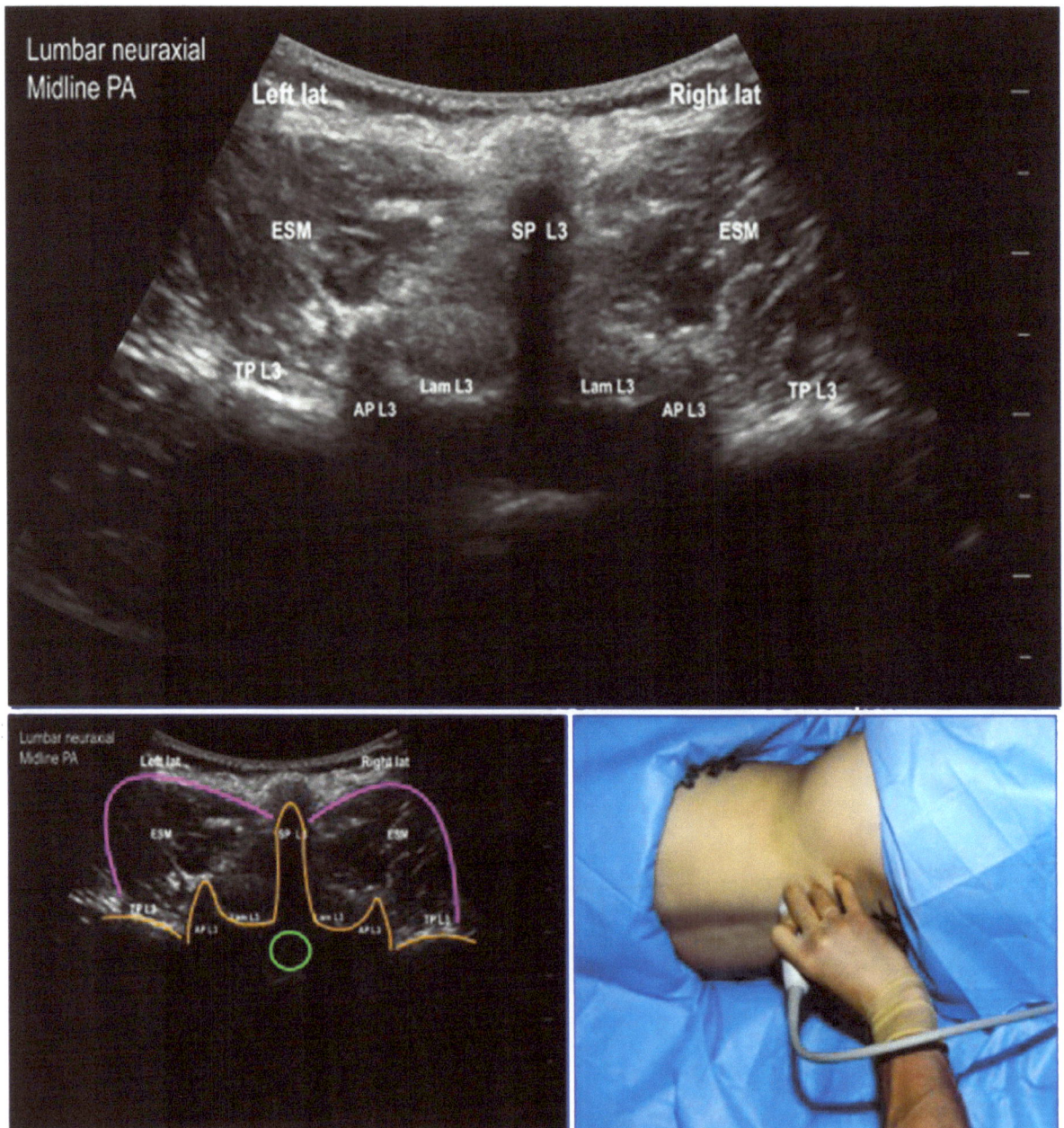

*Figure 9-9: Sonoanatomy of the 4th lumbar vertebra as viewed in the axial plane.*

| | | | |
|---|---|---|---|
| AP L3 | Articular process of the 3rd lumbar vertebra | Left lat | Left lateral |
| ESM | Erector spinae muscle | Right lat | Right lateral |
| Lam L3 | Lamina of the 3rd lumbar vertebra | SP L3 | Spinous process of the 3rd lumbar vertebra |
| | | TP L3 | Transverse process of the 3rd lumbar vertebra |

# Sagittal Para-Spinal View of Lumbar Epidural Space

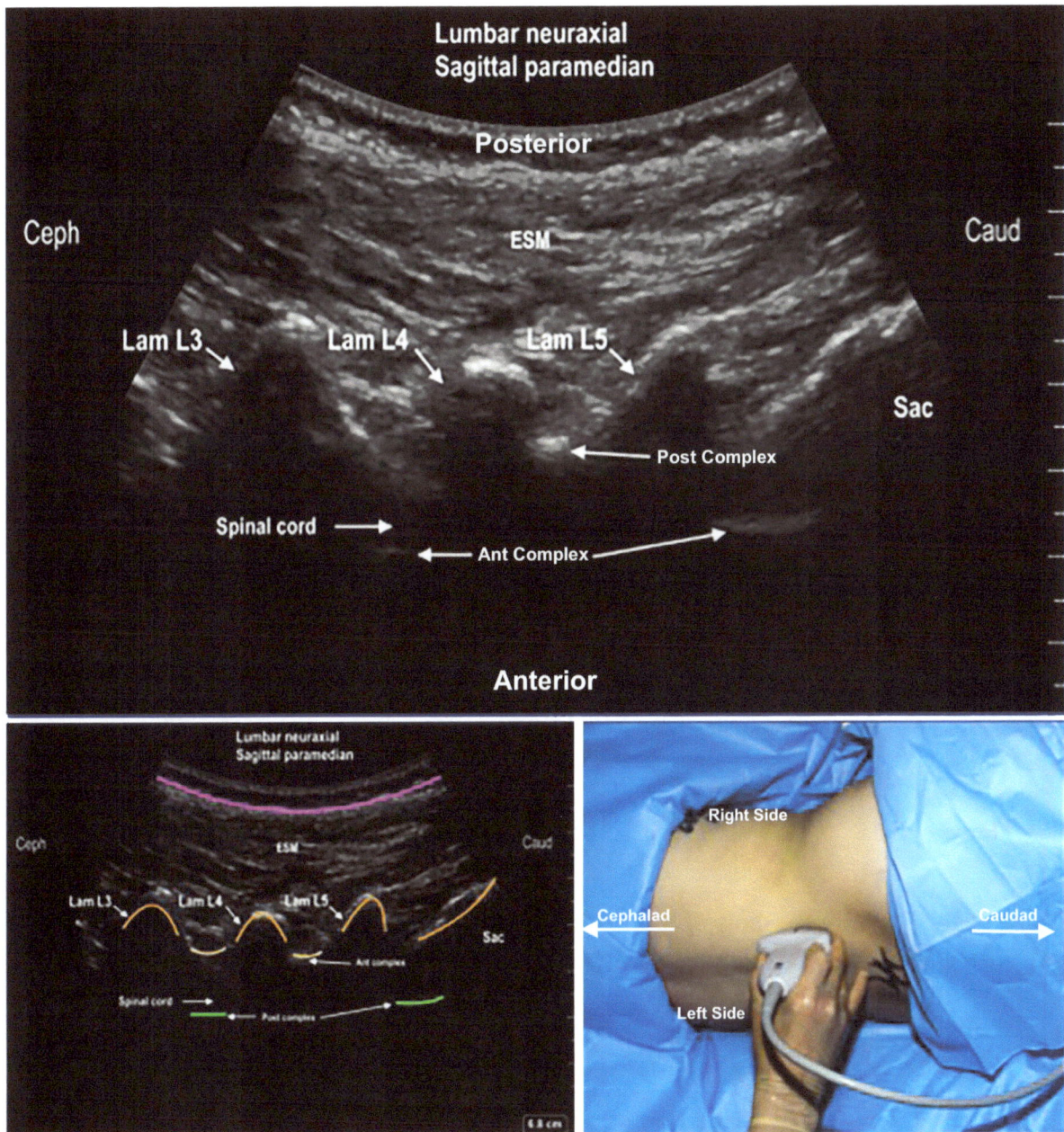

Figure 9-10: Sonoanatomy of the 3rd, 4th, and 5th lumbar vertebrae as viewed in the sagittal plane.

| | |
|---|---|
| Caud | Caudad |
| Ceph | Cephalad |
| ESM | Erector spinae muscle |
| Lam | Laminae of 3rd, 4th, and 5th lumbar vertebrae |
| Sac | Sacrum |

# As Yet Not Described Fibrous Antero-Laminar Body

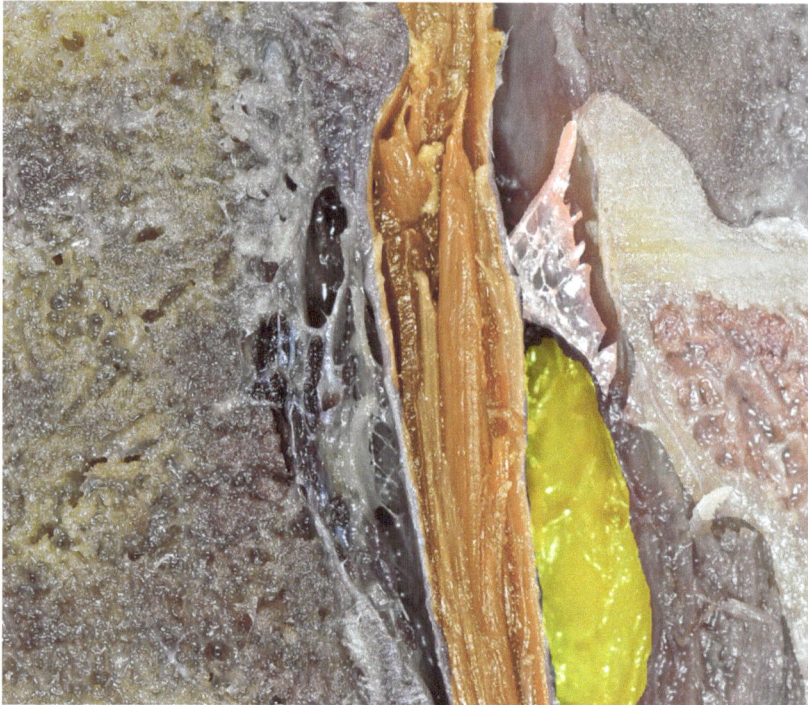

*Figure 9-11: Antero-laminar fibrous body*

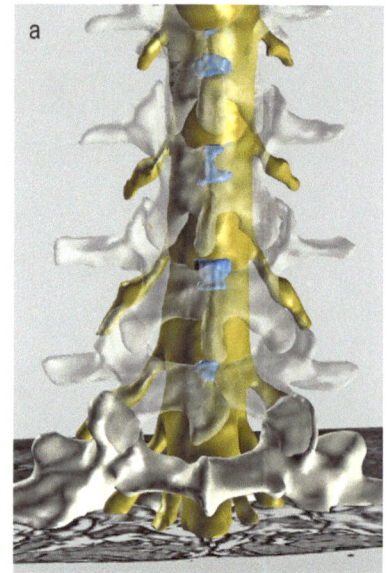

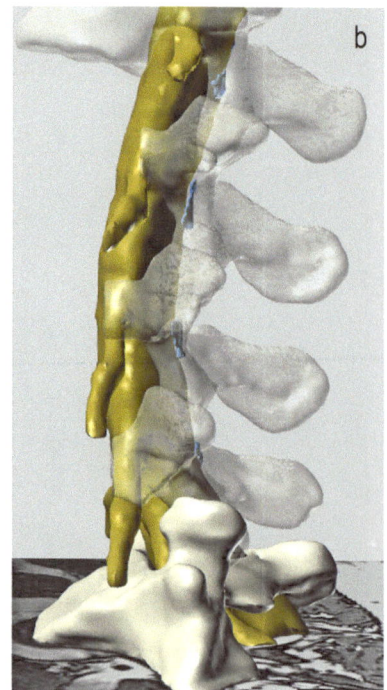

Please note: This fibrous body has not yet been described, and Nin, Prats-Galino and Reina recently discovered this body. Its function is not yet determined. They also discovered that the epidural fat pad is not continuous but interrupted by this fibrous body. The fat pad is anterior to the ligamentum flavum only.

# Chapter 10

## The Abdominal and Pelvic Sympathetic Ganglia

*Macroanatomy*
*Flouroscopic Anatomy*

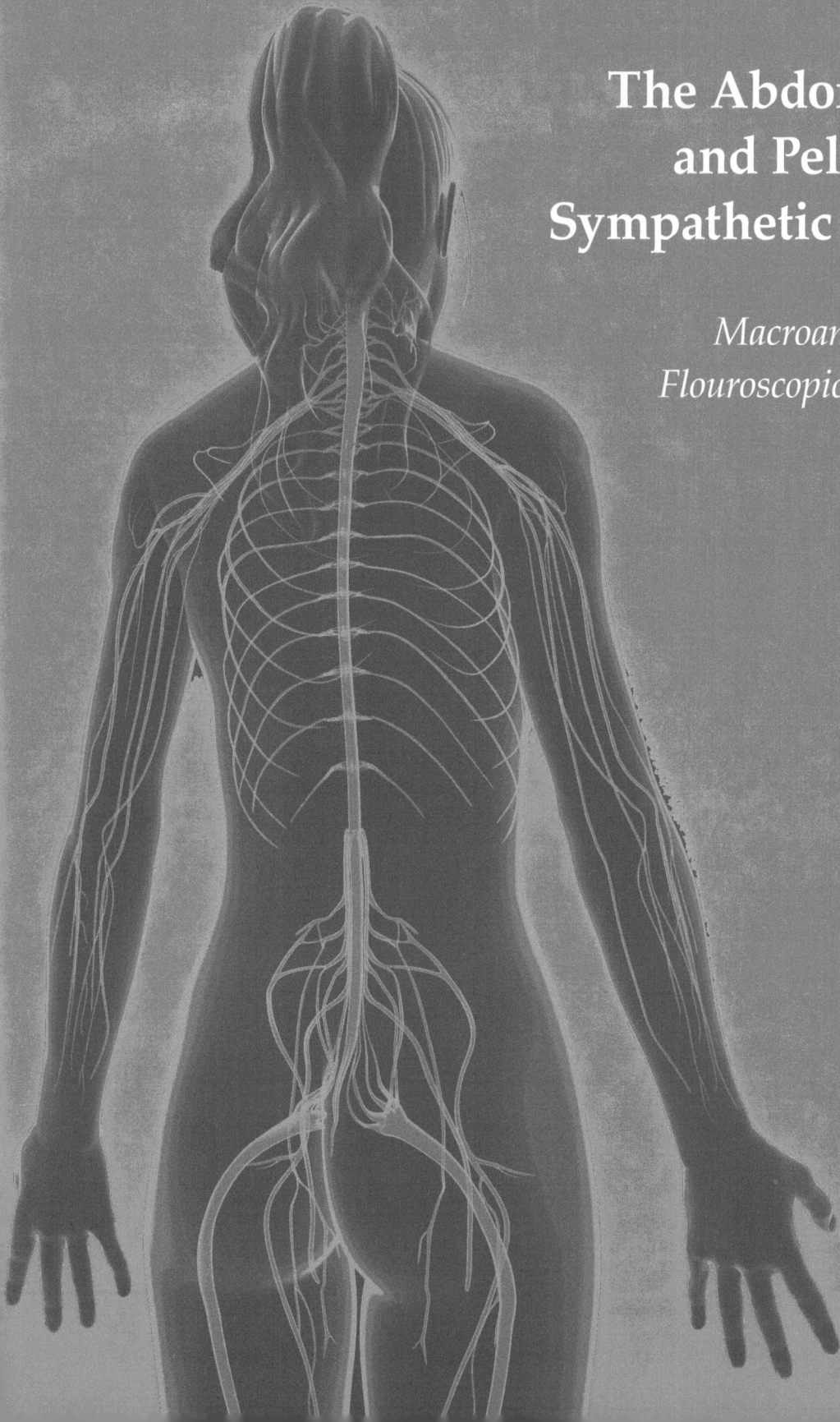

# Macronanatomy
## The Abdominal and Pelvic Sympathetic Ganglia

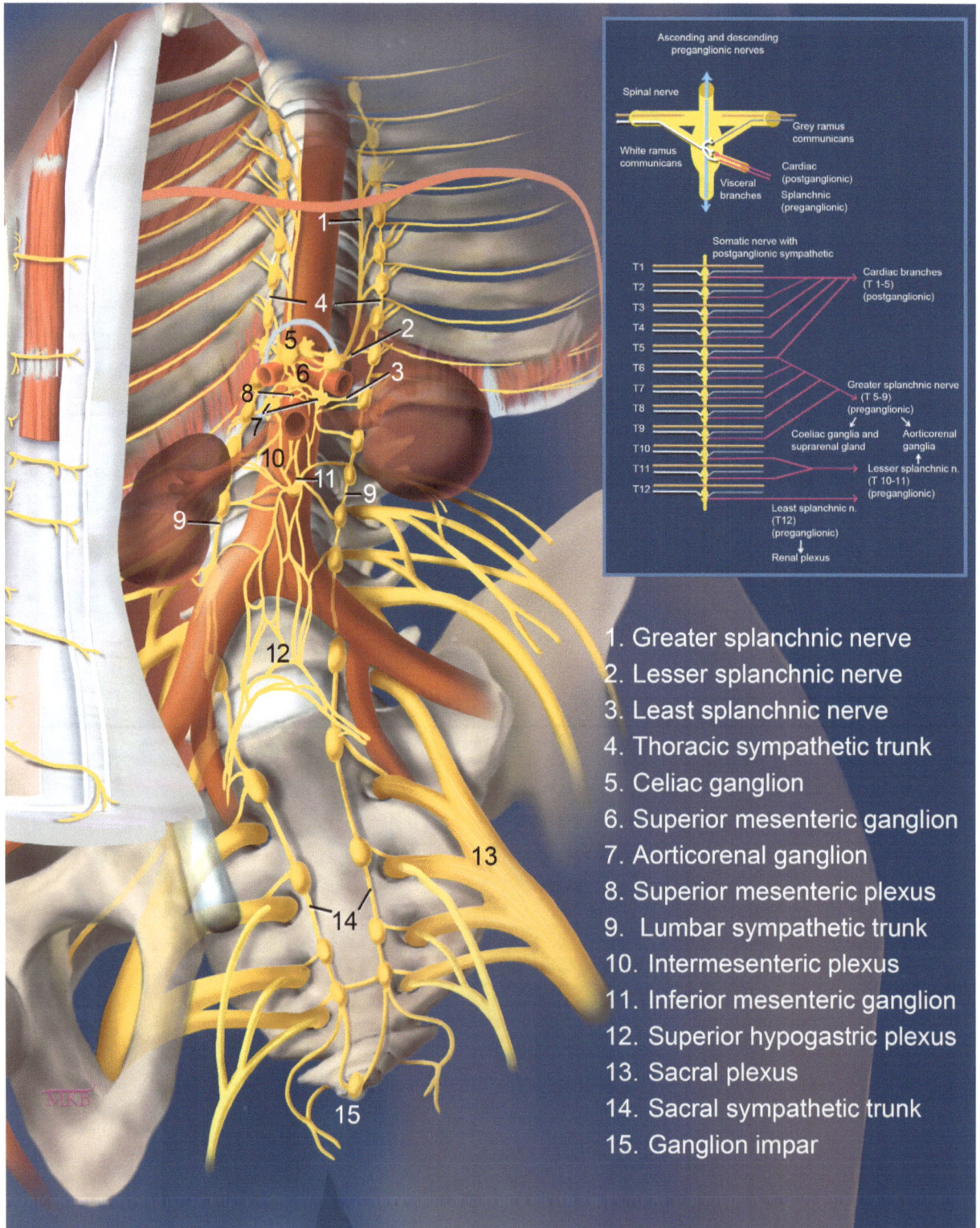

Ascending and descending
preganglionic nerves

Spinal nerve

Grey ramus
communicans

White ramus
communicans

Cardiac
(postganglionic)

Visceral
branches

Splanchnic
(preganglionic)

Somatic nerve with
postganglionic sympathetic

| | |
|---|---|
| T1 | Cardiac branches (T 1-5) (postganglionic) |
| T2 | |
| T3 | |
| T4 | |
| T5 | |
| T6 | |
| T7 | Greater splanchnic nerve (T 5-9) (preganglionic) |
| T8 | |
| T9 | |
| T10 | Coeliac ganglia and suprarenal gland / Aorticorenal ganglia |
| T11 | Lesser splanchnic n. (T 10-11) (preganglionic) |
| T12 | |

Least splanchnic n.
(T12)
(preganglionic)

Renal plexus

1. Greater splanchnic nerve
2. Lesser splanchnic nerve
3. Least splanchnic nerve
4. Thoracic sympathetic trunk
5. Celiac ganglion
6. Superior mesenteric ganglion
7. Aorticorenal ganglion
8. Superior mesenteric plexus
9. Lumbar sympathetic trunk
10. Intermesenteric plexus
11. Inferior mesenteric ganglion
12. Superior hypogastric plexus
13. Sacral plexus
14. Sacral sympathetic trunk
15. Ganglion impar

*Figure 10-1: Antero-superior view of the abdominal & pelvic sympathetic chains, ganglia, & plexus.*

# Positioning for a Ganglion Impar Block

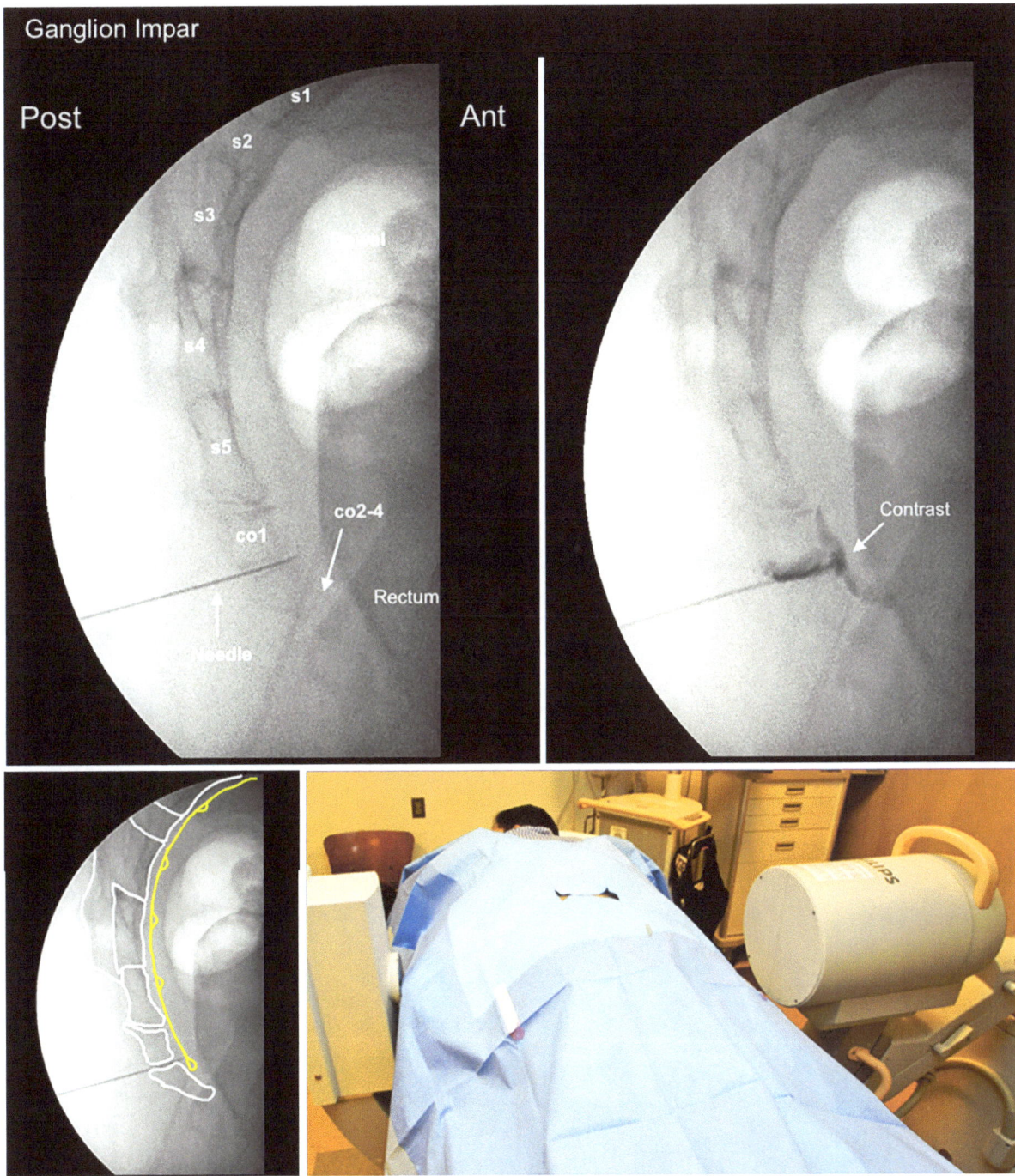

*Figure 10-2: Fluoroscopic anatomy of the transverse view showing placement of a needle and dye extension onto the ganglion impar.*

In the transverse view, the sacral vertebrae (s1-s5) and coccygeal vertebrae (co1, co2-4) are identified. A needle passes through the inter-coccygeal joint space between the first (co1) and 2nd (co2) coccygeal vertebrae, with radiocontrast dye extending in a cranio-caudal direction in the region of the ganglion impar (yellow line).

**Please refer to standard textbooks for indications for and techniques of performing any of the blocks referred to in this book.**

# Positioning for a Coeliac Plexus Block

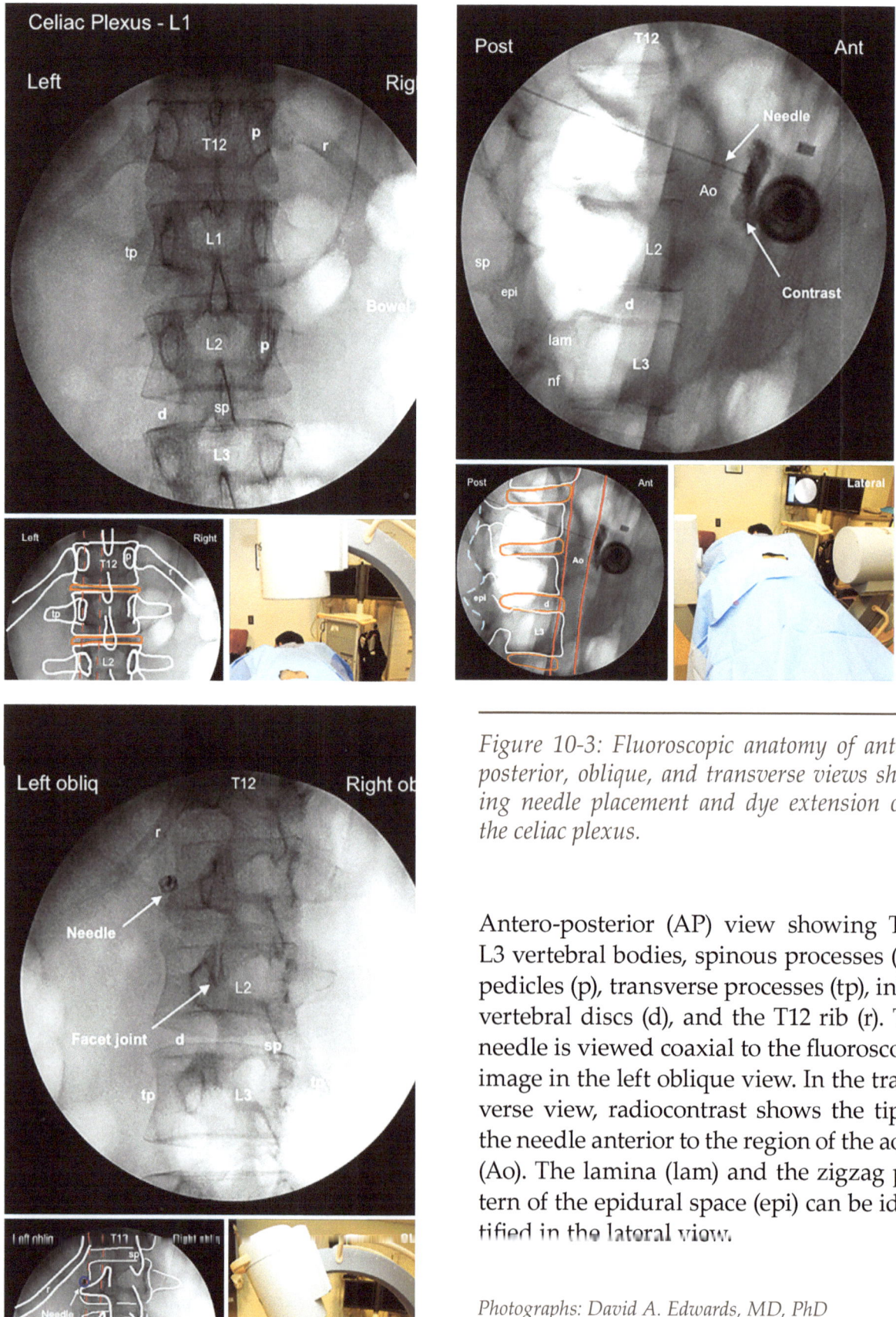

Figure 10-3: *Fluoroscopic anatomy of antero-posterior, oblique, and transverse views showing needle placement and dye extension onto the celiac plexus.*

Antero-posterior (AP) view showing T12-L3 vertebral bodies, spinous processes (sp), pedicles (p), transverse processes (tp), inter-vertebral discs (d), and the T12 rib (r). The needle is viewed coaxial to the fluoroscopic image in the left oblique view. In the transverse view, radiocontrast shows the tip of the needle anterior to the region of the aorta (Ao). The lamina (lam) and the zigzag pattern of the epidural space (epi) can be identified in the lateral view.

*Photographs: David A. Edwards, MD, PhD*

# Positioning for a Lumbar Sympathetic Chain Block

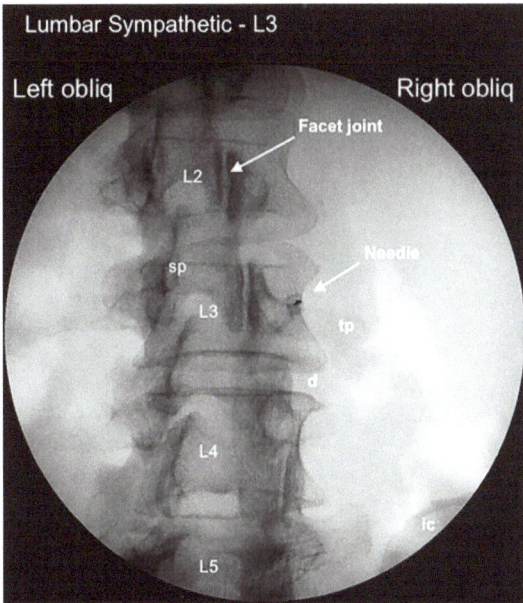

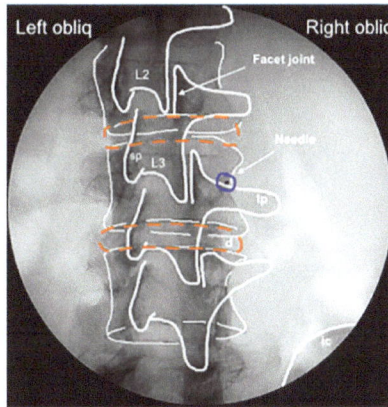

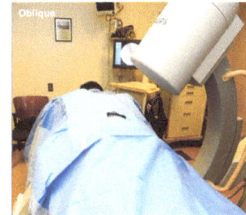

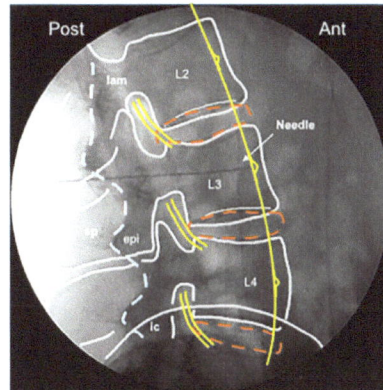

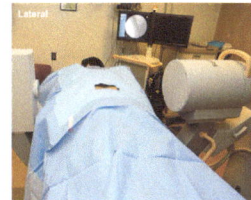

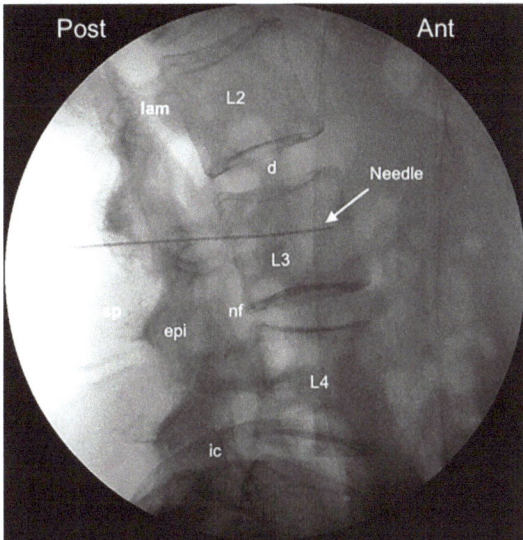

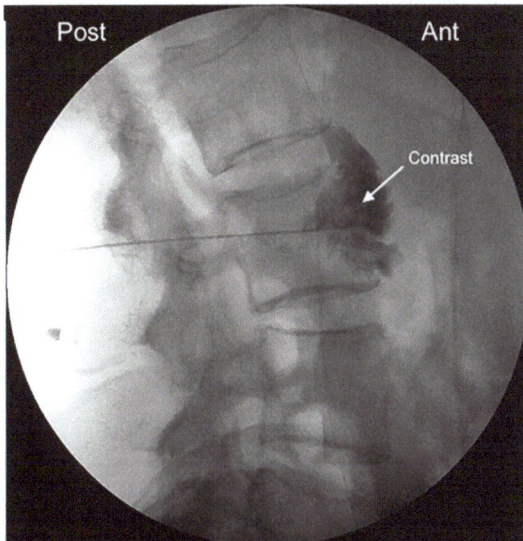

*Figure 10-4: Fluoroscopic anatomy of oblique & transverse views showing placement of a needle & dye extension onto the lumbar sympathetic chain.*

In the right oblique view at the level of the lumbar vertebrae (L2-L5), the facet joints are seen coaxial to the fluoroscopic image. The needle is viewed coaxial to the fluoroscopic image cranial to the right transverse process (tp) of L3. The intervertebral discs (d) and spinous processes (sp) are identified. In the lateral view, the lamina (lam), zigzag pattern of the epidural space (epi), neuroforamen (nf), and the iliac crest (ic) are identified. Radiocontrast dye can be seen spreading in a cranial-caudal direction along the anterolateral aspect of the vertebral bodies, which is the region of the sympathetic trunk (yellow line)

*Photographs: David A. Edwards, MD, PhD*

# Chapter 11

# The Pterygopalatine Ganglion

*Macroanatomy*
*Microanatomy*
*Sonoanatomy*
*Surface Anatomy*

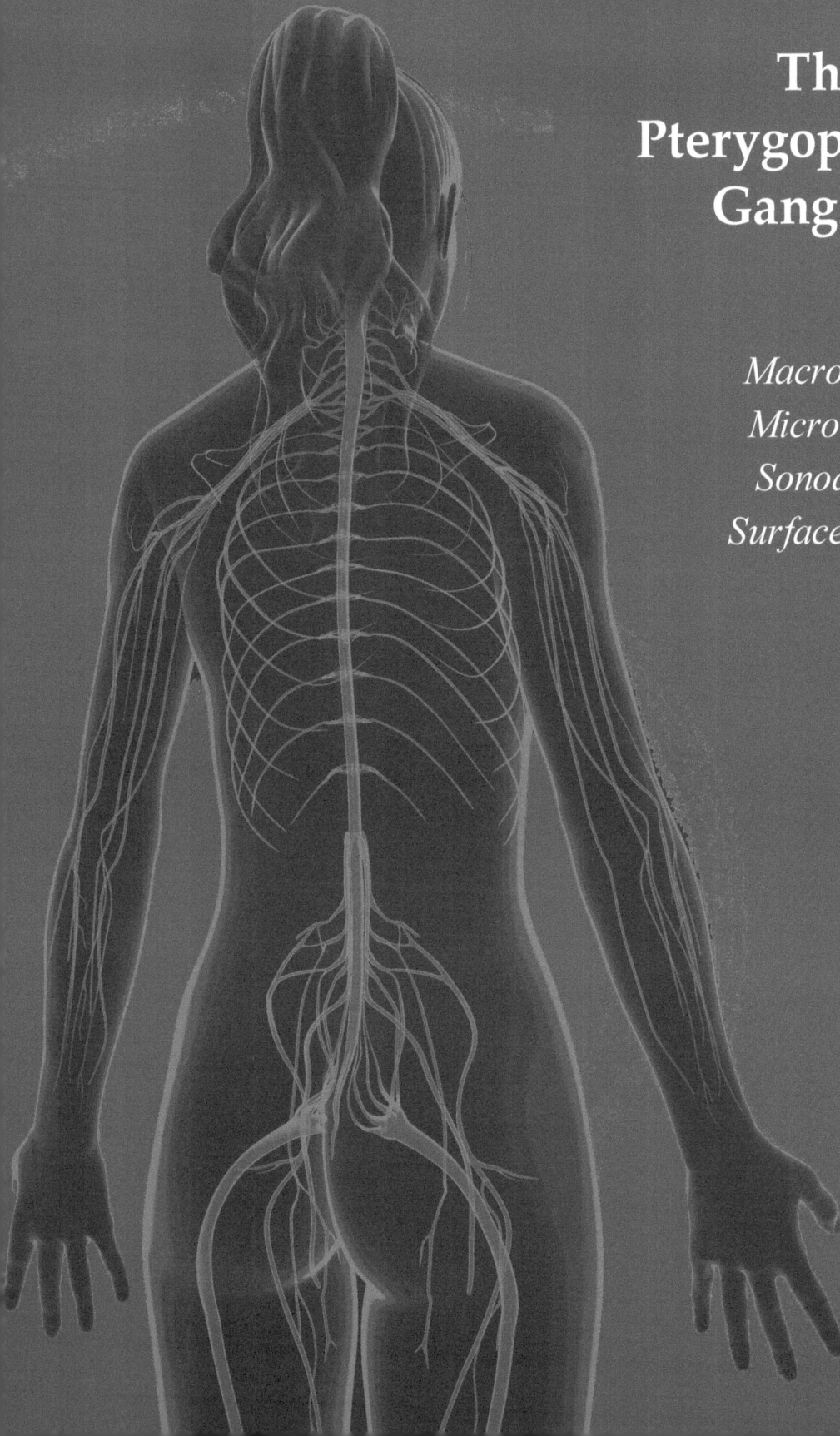

# Macroanatomy

## The Pterygopalatine Ganglion

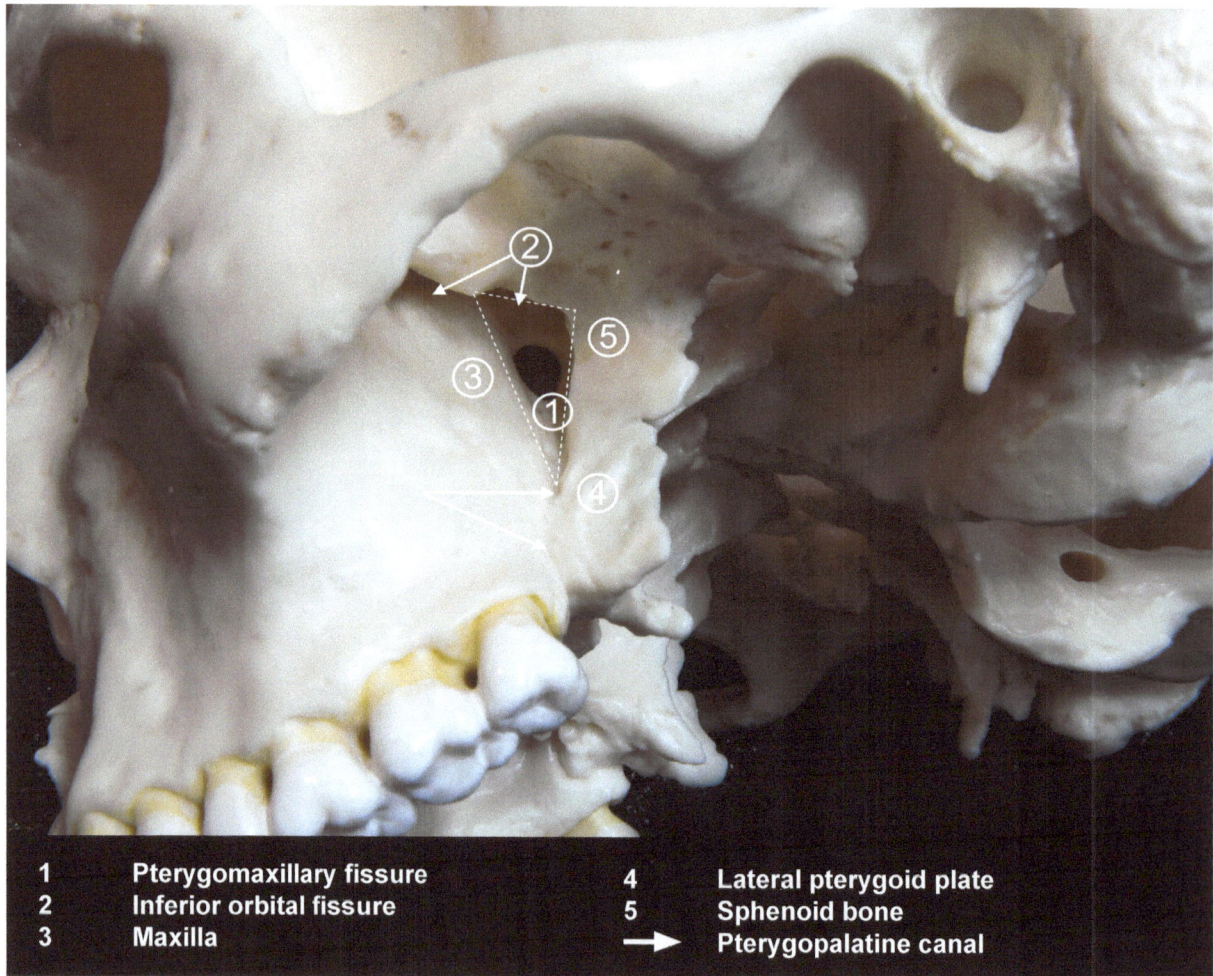

| 1 | Pterygomaxillary fissure | 4 | Lateral pterygoid plate |
|---|--------------------------|---|-------------------------|
| 2 | Inferior orbital fissure | 5 | Sphenoid bone |
| 3 | Maxilla | → | Pterygopalatine canal |

*Figure 11-1: The pterygopalatine fissure.*

The pterygomaxillary fissure (1) is a triangular space located in the pterygomaxillary fossa, situated between the intratemporal or posterior aspect of the maxilla (3), which contains the maxillary sinus. The posterior wall of the fissure is formed by the lateral pterygoid plate (4). Superiorly, the fissure is situated anterior to the infratemporal surface of the greater wing of the sphenoid bone (5). At its superior wider base is the inferior orbital fissure (2). Inferiorly, at the apex of the triangular space the pterygopalatine canal is found (indicated by the arrow). This pterygomaxillary fissure leads into the pterygopalatine fossa, which houses the pterygopalatine ganglion.

# Lateral View of the Maxillary Nerve

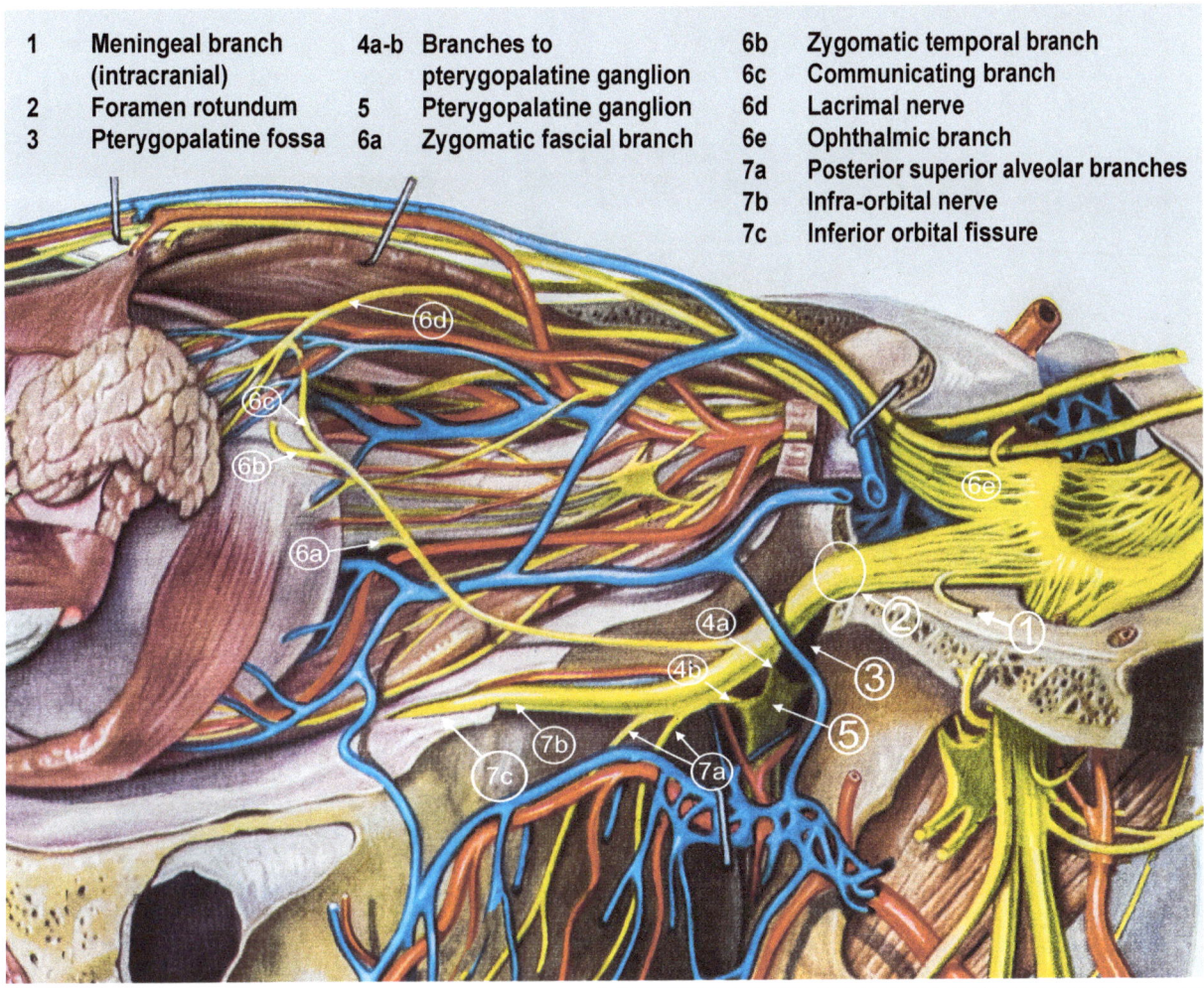

| | | | |
|---|---|---|---|
| 1 | Meningeal branch (intracranial) | 4a-b | Branches to pterygopalatine ganglion |
| 2 | Foramen rotundum | 5 | Pterygopalatine ganglion |
| 3 | Pterygopalatine fossa | 6a | Zygomatic fascial branch |

| 6b | Zygomatic temporal branch |
|---|---|
| 6c | Communicating branch |
| 6d | Lacrimal nerve |
| 6e | Ophthalmic branch |
| 7a | Posterior superior alveolar branches |
| 7b | Infra-orbital nerve |
| 7c | Inferior orbital fissure |

*Figure 11-2: Lateral view of the orbit, middle cranial fossa and the pterygopalatine fissure.*

The maxillary nerve is the second division of the trigeminal nerve (Vth cranial nerve) or trigeminal (Gasserian) ganglion. While still intracranial, the maxillary nerve gives off the 1st of its six branches, the dural or meningeal branch (Fig 11-2, 1). It then passes through the foramen rotundum (Fig 11-2, 2) to enter the pterygopalatine fossa (Fig 11-2, 3) near the inferior orbital fissure, which connects the pterygopalatine fossa with the orbit. Here it gives off two branches (Fig 11-2, 4a-4b) to the pterygopalatine ganglion (Fig 11-2, 5), which is also called the sphenopalatine ganglion or Meckel's ganglion or the nasal ganglion. It continues further anterior in the pterygopalatine fossa and gives of a zygomatic branch, which then enters the orbit and splits into three branches:

1. Zygomatic facial branch (Fig 11-2, 6a)
2. Zygomatic temporal branch (Fig 11-2, 6b)
3. A communicating branch (Fig 11-2, 6c) to the lacrimal branch (Fig 11-2, 6d) of the ophthalmic nerve (Fig 11-2, 6e)

This communicating branch is a parasympathetic secreto-motor nerve that originates from the pterygopalatine ganglion.

# Branches of the Pterygopalatine Ganglion

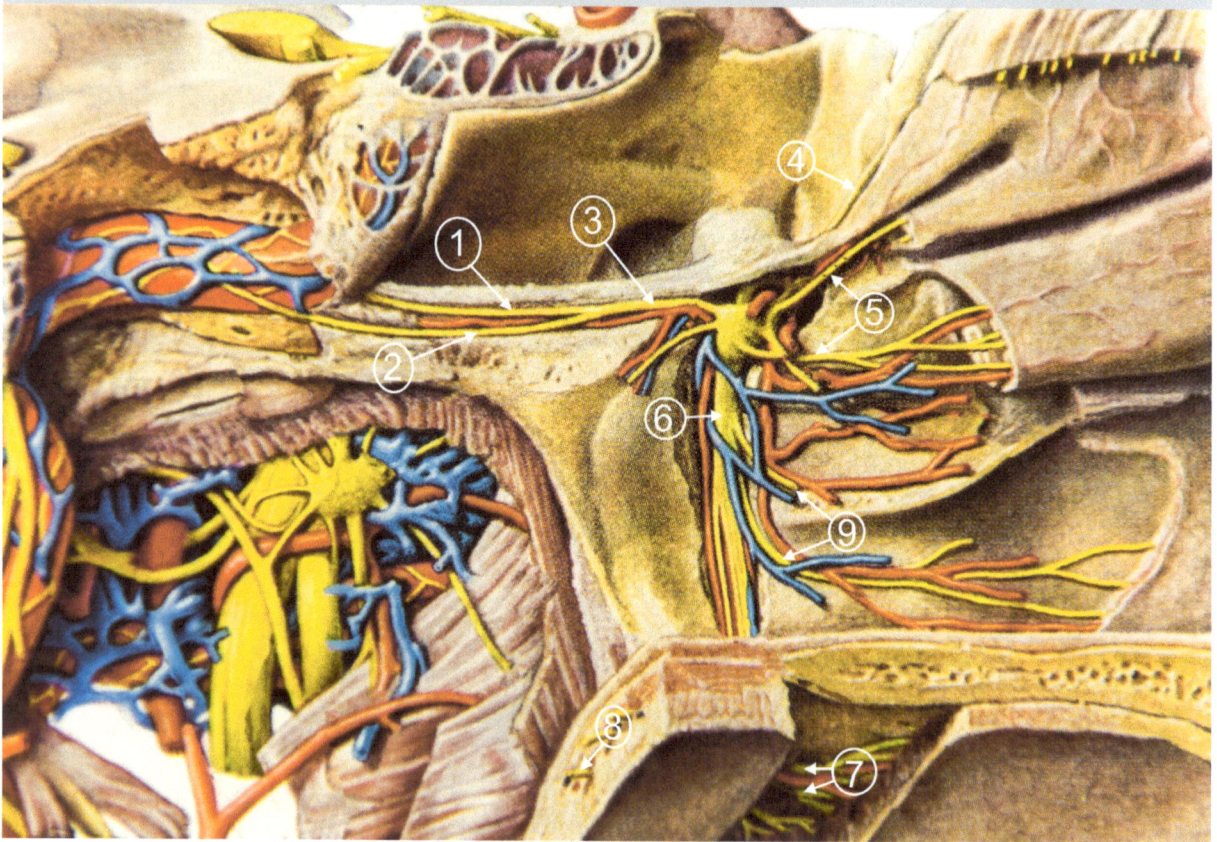

| | | | | | |
|---|---|---|---|---|---|
| 1 | Greater petrosus nerve | 4 | Orbital branches | 7 | Greater palatine nerve branches |
| 2 | Deep petrosus nerve | 5 | Nasal branches | 8 | Lesser palatine nerve branches |
| 3 | Vidian nerve | 6 | Palatine nerve | 9 | Nasal branches of palatine nerve |

*Figure 11-3: Lateral view of branches to the pterygopalatine ganglion.*

Further anterior, still in the pterygopalatine fossa, the maxillary nerve gives of one or two posterior superior alveolar branches, which innervates the three upper molar teeth. The maxillary nerve then continues further anterior as the infra-orbital nerve (Fig 11-2, 7b).

The infra-orbital nerve (Fig 11-2, 7b) enters the orbit through the inferior orbital fissure (Fig 11-2, 7c) and runs anterior in the infra-orbital groove in the floor of the orbit where it gives off the middle superior al-veolar branch that innervate the premolar teeth. It then enters the infra-orbital canal to exit from the inferior orbital foramen just inferior to the infra-orbital ridge. Here the infra-orbital nerve splits into three terminal branches, the inferior palpebral branch that innervates the lower eyelid, the nasal branch and the superior labral branch.

The pterygopalatine ganglion not only receives sensory fibers from the maxillary nerve, it also receives preganglionic para-sympathetic fibers from the superior salivatory nucleus in the medulla. These fibers, pass via the geniculum of the facial nerve to become the greater petrosal nerve (Fig 11-3, 1). The greater petrosal nerve then enters the pterygopalatine canal where it joins the deep petrosal nerve (Fig 11-3, 2), which is a purely sympathetic nerve to form the Vidian nerve (Fig 11-3, 3).

The pregangionic parasympathetic nerves form synapses in the pterygopalatine ganglion and the then postganglionic parasympathetic nerves are secreto-motor nerves. The sympathetic nerves originate from the superior cervical ganglion, and are thus postganglionic nerves that pass with the internal carotid artery and are purely vasomotor nerves. All the indirect maxillary nerve branches – the branches that go through the ganglion, are all postganglionic and contain sympathetic vaso-motor fibers, parasympathetic secreto-motor fibers, and somatic touch, pain and temperature fibers.

The maxillary nerve has five indirect branches that all go through the pterygopalatine ganglion and pick up sympathetic and parasympathetic fibers on their way through it.

These are:
1. Orbital branches (Fig 11-3, 4) that innervate the orbital periosteum, and the sphenoidal sinus mucosa.
2. Nasal branches (Fig 11-3, 5): Posterior superior nasal branches, which splits into medial and lateral branches. One of the medial (septal) branches continue to enter through the anterior incisive fossa of the palate as the nasopalatine nerve.
3. Palatine nerve (Fig 11-3, 6), which courses inferiorly through the pterygopalatine canal where it splits into anterior (Fig 11-3, 7) and posterior branches (Fig 11-3, 8); the greater (anterior) and lesser palatine (posterior) nerves. The greater palatine nerve innervates the hard palate. The lesser palatine nerve innervates the soft palate and the tonsils. The greater palatine nerve also gives off at least 2 nasal branches (Fig 11-3, 9) on its way through the pterygopalatine canal.

(Interestingly, taste fibers that originate from the solitary tract and nucleus in the lower medulla oblongata, tract via the facial nerve and split off to join the great petrosal nerve and the Vidian nerve to join the lesser palatine nerve and supply it with taste fibers, or taste buds in the soft palate).

All the direct and indirect branches of the maxillary nerve are blocked with a pterygopalatine block.

# The Shenopalatine Foramen – Ventral View

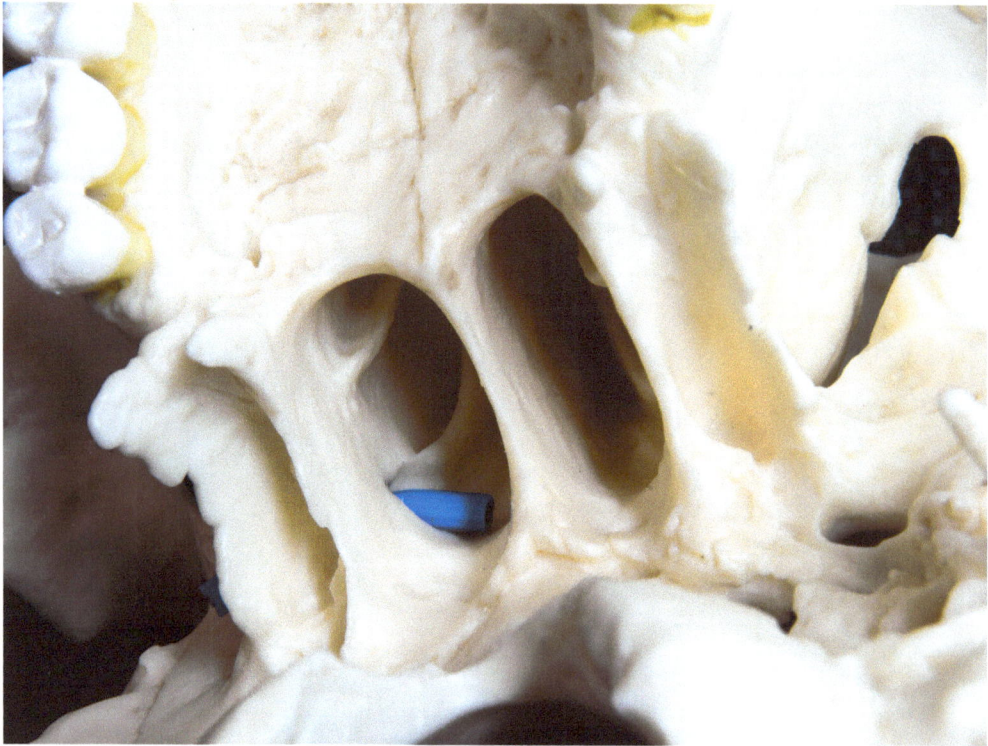

## Postero-Ventral View

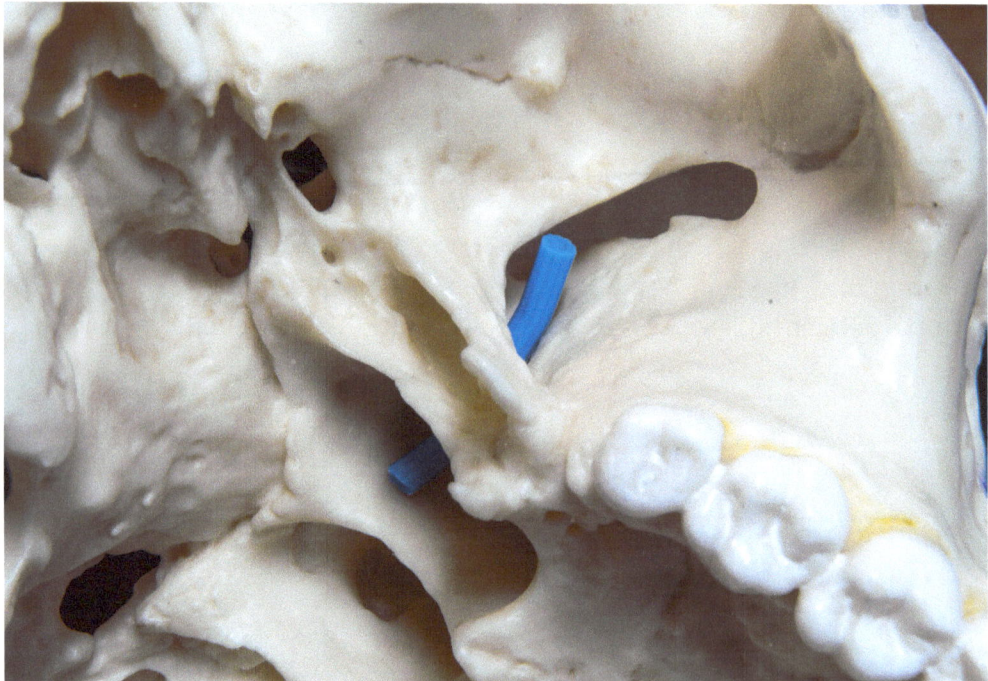

*Figure 11-4 (top): A 45-degree ventral view of the bony naso pharynx. The blue marker indicates the nasal side of the sphenopalatine foramen in the posterior aspect of the lateral wall of the nose.*
*Figure 11-5 (bottom): A postero-ventral view of the nasopharynx, pterygoid plates and posterior maxilla: The blue marker indicates the exit of the sphenopalatine foramen into the pterygopalatine fossa.*

# The Pterygopalatine Fossa

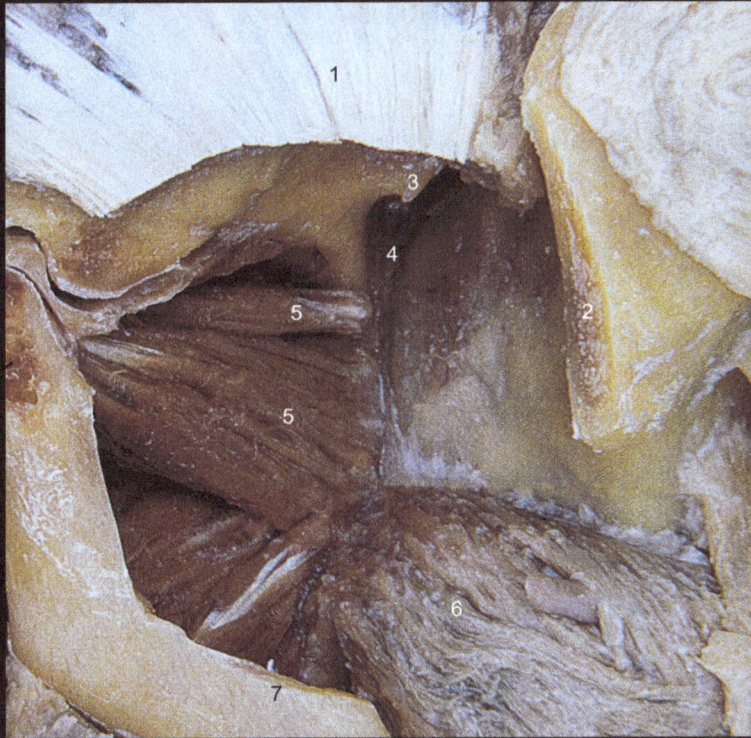

**The Temporalis Muscle & Zygomatic Arch have been removed**

1 Temporalis muscle (cut)

2 Zygomatic arch (cut)

3 Infratemporal crest

4 Pterygopalatine fossa

5 Lateral pterygoid muscle (upper and lower head)

6 Buccinator muscle

7 Coronoid process (cut away)

# Coronal Section through Pterygopalatine Fossa

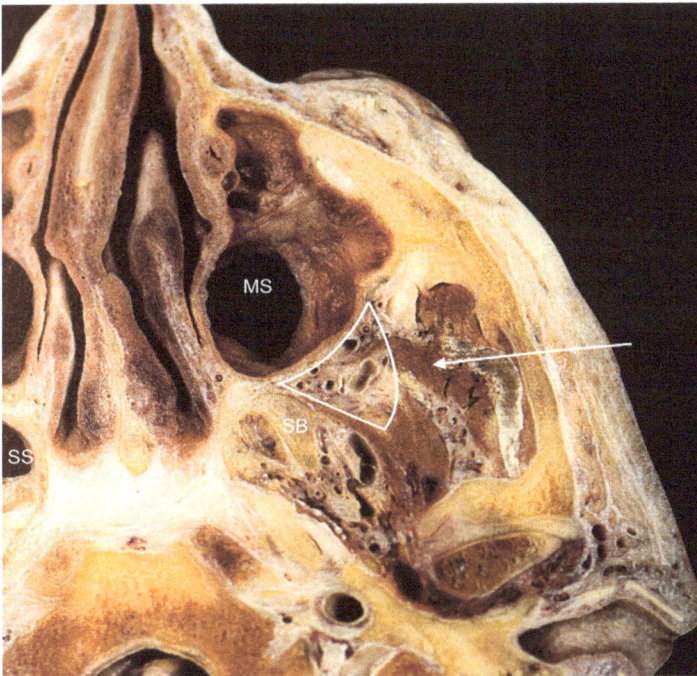

▲ Pterygopalatine fossa with content

→ Temporalis muscle

MS Maxillary sinus

SB Sphenoid bone

SS Sphenoid sinus

*Figure 11-6 (top): Anatomy of the pterygopalatine fossa after removal of temporalis muscle and zygomatic arch. Figure 11-7 (bottom): Coronal section through pterygopalatine fossa (triangular space) immediately deep to the temporalis muscle*

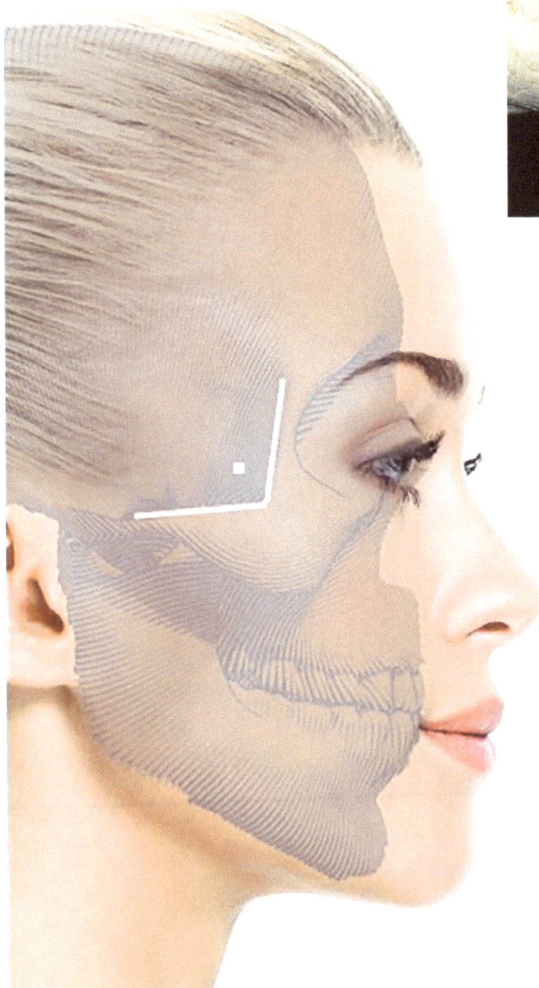

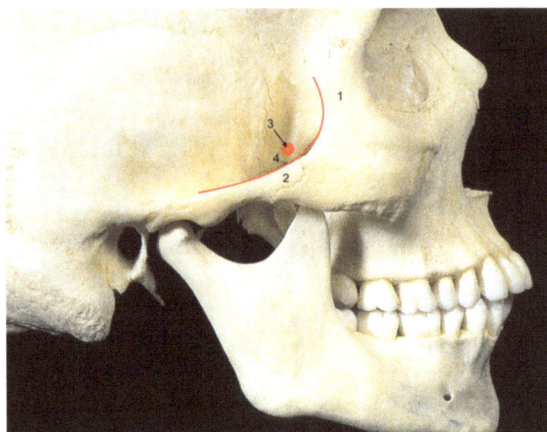

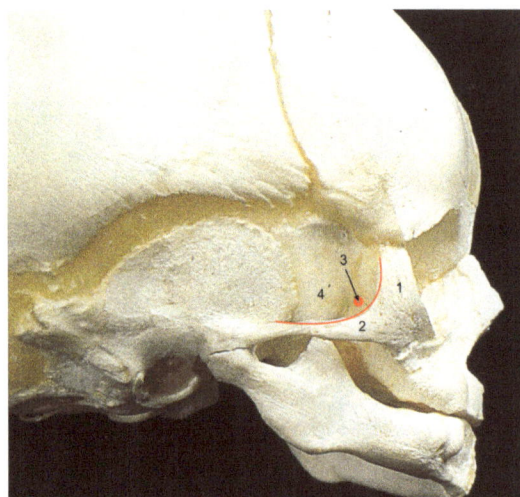

**Redline indicates Fronto-Zygomatic angle**
1    **Zygomatic bone**
2    **Zygomatic arch**
3    **Position of Needle Entry**
4    **Sphenoid Bone**

*Left, Figure 11-8:  Surface landmarks for performing a pterygopalatine ganglion block.
Top Right, Figure 11-9: Surface Landmarks for performing a pterygopalatine ganglion block on adult.  Bottom Right, Figure 11-10:  Surface Landmarks for performing a pterygopalatine block on an infant.*

The zygomatic arch is palpated on the side of the face.  This is a horizontal bony structure on the level of the inferior orbital brim.  At almost 90 degrees to it, we can palpate the frontal process of the zygoma or the posterior orbital rim.  Needle entry is in the corner formed by these two lines (illustrated by the white dot).

# Microanatomy

## The Pterygopalatine Ganglion and the Pterygopalatine Trigeminovascular System (PPTVS)

In a microanatomic dissection study,* Rusu set out to define as positive or negative the presence of a pterygopalatine trigemino-vascular system. He micro-dissected 18 pterygopalatine fossae (PPF) of 9 cadaver specimens with 4.5x magnification. The content of the PPF was embedded in a consistent pterygopalatine adipose body that continued superior into the orbital apex and extended further as parasellar adipose body; inferior and distinctive from the orbital adipose tissue. Distal to the foramen rotundum, the maxillary nerve contributes fibers directly to the maxillary arterial plexus and its anterior trigeminal branches. It also contributed to the trigeminal-autonomic plexus located in the upper lateral quadrant of the pterygopalatine "cross", underneath the roof of the fossa. These are anastomotic branches between the PPG and the trigeminal ganglion.

The study convincingly provided evidence of the existence of an anatomically defined pterygopalatine trigemino-vascular system. This would comfortably explain why a pterygopalatine ganglion block would block the parasympathetic nerves to the cerebral, pia mater and dura mater vasculature and reverse the effects of noxious vasodilatation and sterile vascular inflammation (vasculitis) as evident in trigeminal autonomic cephalgias. The anastomoses involving autonomic and trigeminal fibers, located in the PPF passage to the orbital apex, support the complex and polymorphous neural input to the orbit, while the evidence of a pterygopalatine trigeminovascular scaffold offers a substrate for a better understanding of various facial algias.

*This section is basically a summary of the original article by M. C. Rusu MD, PhD of the Department of Anatomy and Embryology of the University of Medicine and Pharmacy, Bucharest, Romania.

# Sonoanatomy

## Temporo Mandibular Joint & Coronal Process of Mandible

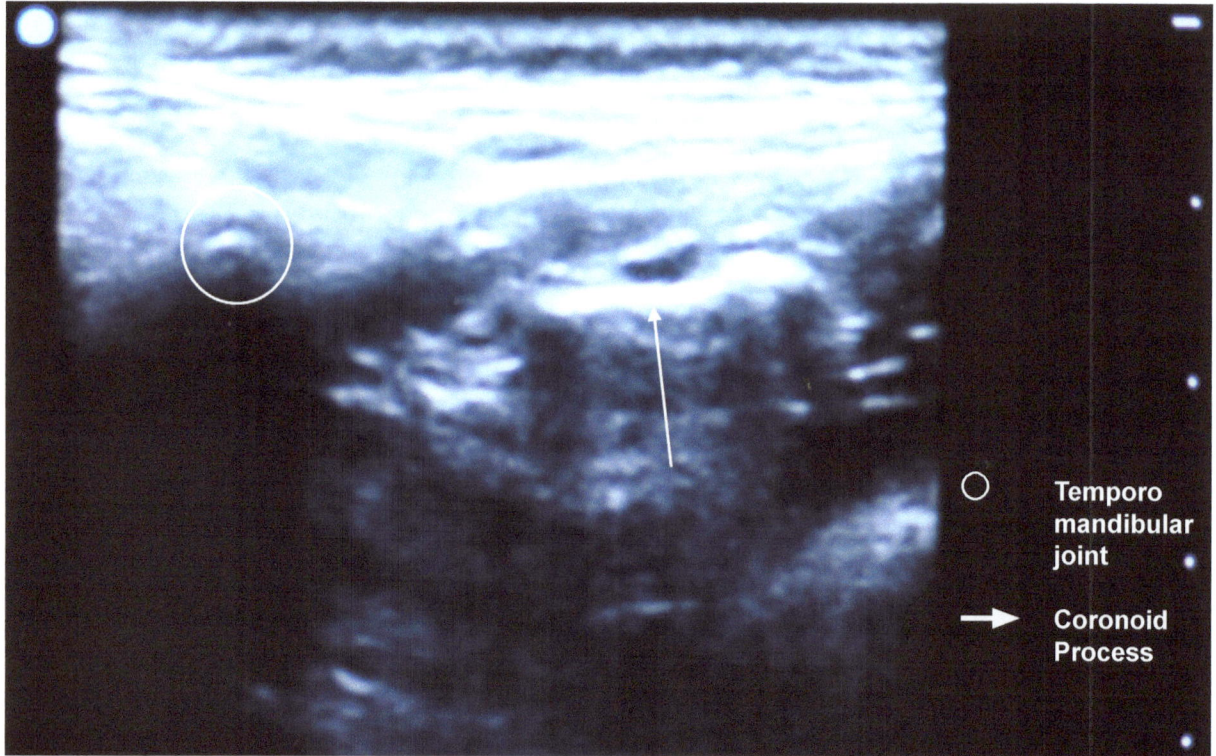

Temporo mandibular joint

Coronoid Process

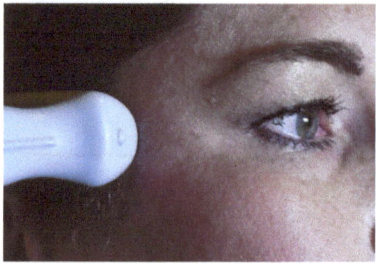

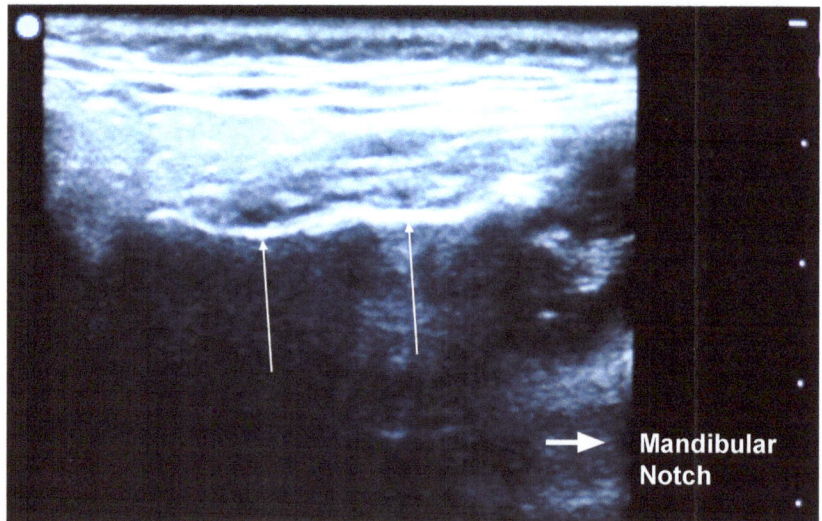

Mandibular Notch

*Left, Figure 11-11: Lateral view of face and placement of probe. Top, Figure 11-12: Ultrasound View with probe placement shown in Figure 11-11. Right, Figure 11-13: The mandibular notch appears as one flat bony structure as probe is moved down.*

# Move Probe More Anterior on Zygomatic Arch

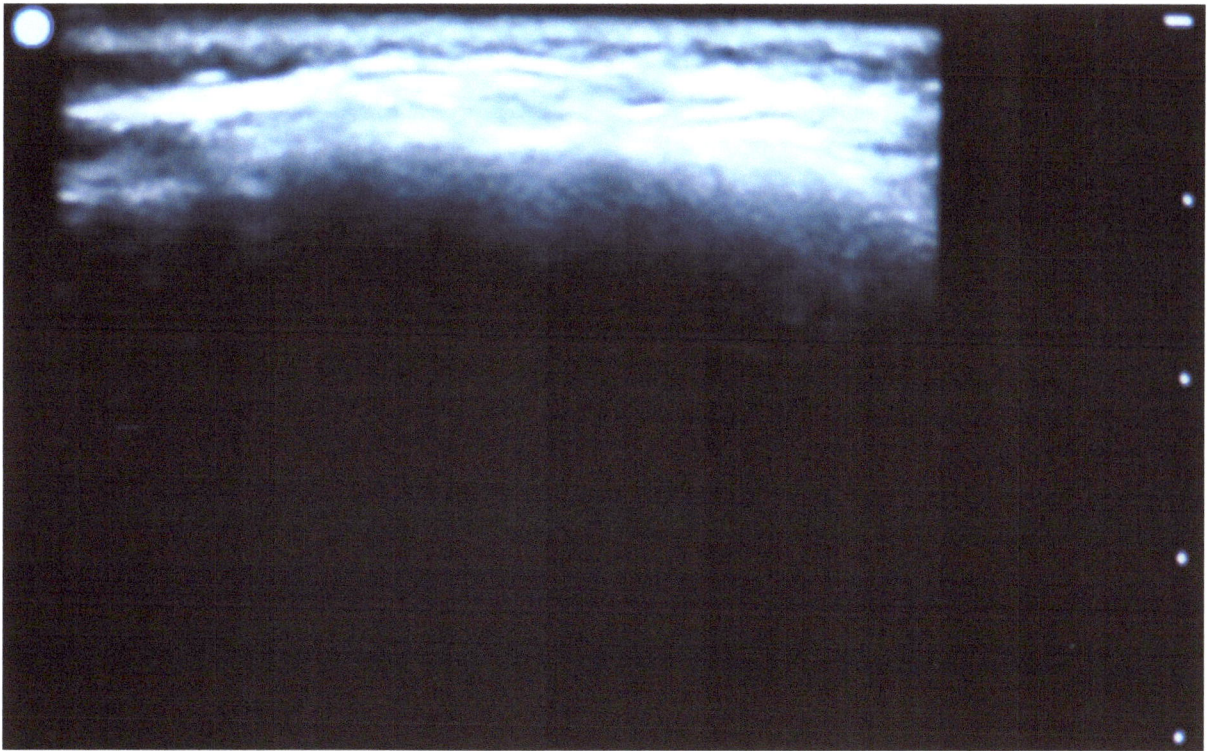

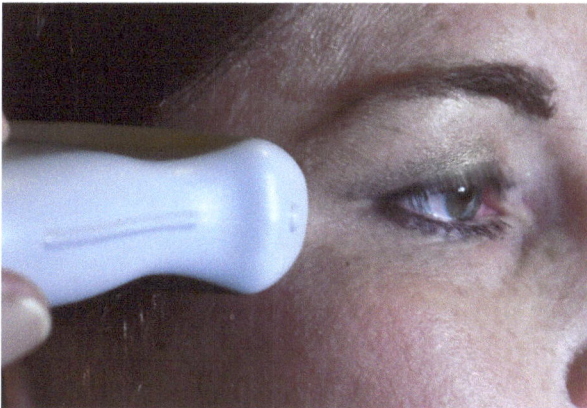

*Left, Figure 11-14: Placement of the probe having moved it anteriorly on the zygomatic arch. Top, Figure 11-15: Continuing anteriorly, the Zygomatic arch appears.*

# The Pterygopalatine Fossa

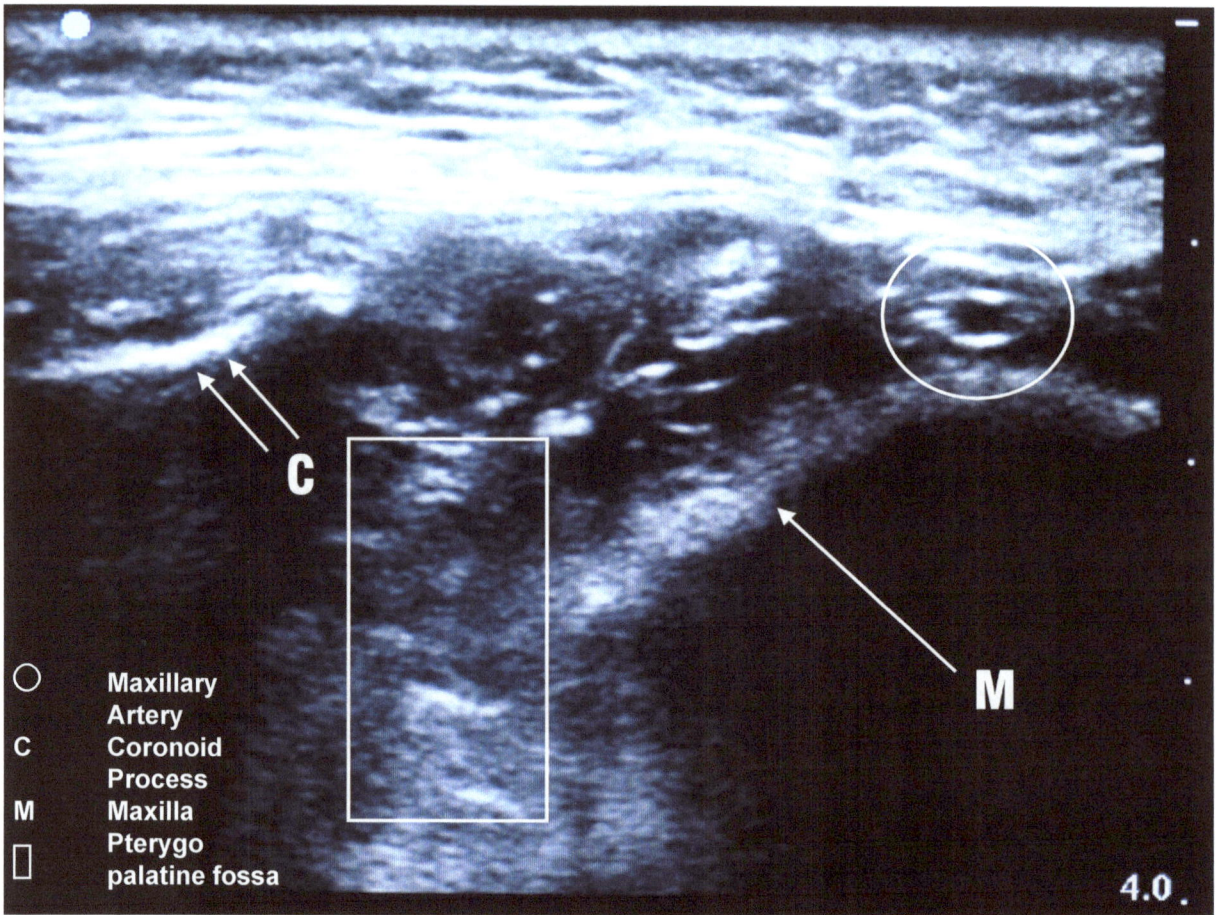

Maxillary
Artery

C Coronoid
Process

M Maxilla

▯ Pterygo
palatine fossa

4.0

---

*Right, Figure 11-16: Lateral view of the right side of the face and placement of the probe.*
*Top, Figure 11-17: View on the ultrasound screen with probe placement shown in Figure 11-16.*

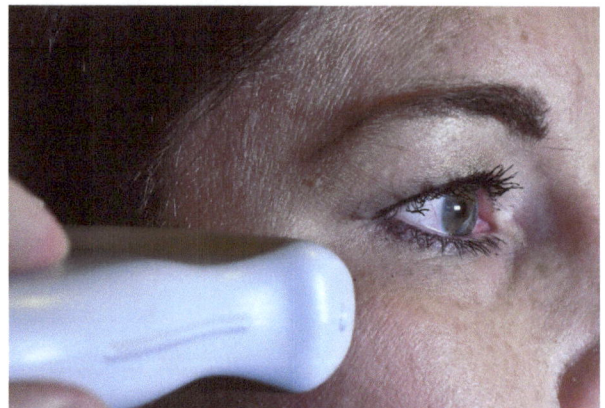

Moving the probe caudad, "slipping off" the zygomatic arch, shows the pterygopalatine fossa with its content, the maxilla and the coronoid process of the mandible. When the mouth is opened the coronoid process moves out of the field and the greater wing of the sphenoid bone comes into view.

Note the arch formed by the maxilla on the right-hand side. Also note the branch of the maxillary artery, which can be seen pulsating. The coronoid process of the mandible and, sometimes, in babies and young chil-

dren, the sphenoid sinus can also be seen. This is almost never possible in older children adolescents or adults, due to the relative thickness of the infra-temporal surface of the greater wing of the sphenoid bone (not seen). The pterygopalatine fossa, which houses the pterygopalatine ganglion is indicated by the rectangle in Figure 11-17.

# Self-study plan

**Study the figures and their legends in this booklet.**

View the movies on https://www.RAEducation.com/ebook
Answer 10 of these questions per day.
Answers to questions that cannot be found in The Primer can be found on https://www.RAEducation.com.
Specifically view the "Must-know Anatomy" section's pdf's and lectures.

# Week 1 - Upper Limb

## Day 1: Anatomy of the roots and trunks of the brachial plexus (Chap 1).

Questions:
1. How many roots form the brachial plexus, and what peripheral nerves originate from each root?
2. What parts of the roots contain sensory nerve fibers, and which part contains motor fibers?
3. Name the membrane(s) surrounding the roots of the brachial plexus.
4. Describe proximal and distal attachments of the anterior, middle and posterior scalene muscles, and name the 5 scalene muscles.
5. Describe the difference between an interscalene and a cervical paravertebral block in anatomical terms?
6. How many trunks form the brachial plexus, name them and name the nerves that originate from each trunk.
7. What roots form the superior, middle and inferior trunks respectively?
8. What is the origin of the Phrenic Nerve?
9. What are the origin, motor response and importance of the dorsal scapular and long thoracic nerves?
10. What structures form the boundaries of the posterior triangle of the neck and the supraclavicular space?

## Day 2: Anatomy of the divisions & cords of brachial plexus ( Chap 1 &2).

Questions:
1. How many divisions form the brachial plexus and what are their origins from the trunks?
2. What is the relationships of the brachial plexus as it crosses the first rib?What is the relationship of each of the brachial plexus cords to the Subclavian Artery? Describe these in the proximal and distal subclavian fossa.
3. Describe the origin of the Middle and Lateral Pectoral Nerves, and name the nerve connecting them, and what is the importance of this nerve?
4. Name the 5 nerves originating from the posterior cord.
5. Name the 5 nerves originating from the Medial Cord.
6. Name the 2 nerves originating from the Lateral cord.
7. What motor response do you expect when you stimulate each of the 3 cords?
8. Describe the supraclavicular surface and sono-anatomy.
9. Describe the infraclavicular surface and sono-anatomy.

## Day 3: Neuro-anatomy of the axilla (Chap 2).

Questions:
1. Describe the relationship of the Musculocutaneous and Axillary Nerves to the humerus.
2. What muscles are innervated by the Axillary nerve, and what motor response to you expect when stimulating this nerve? What sensory area is innervated by this nerve?
3. What muscles are innervated by the Musculocutaneous nerve, what motor response to you expect when stimulating this nerve, and what sensory area is innervated by this nerve?
4. What muscles are innervated by the Radial nerve, what motor response to you expect when stimulating this nerve, and what sensory area is innervated by this nerve?
5. What muscles are innervated by the Ulnar nerve, what motor response to you expect when stimulating this nerve, and what sensory area is innervated by this nerve?
6. What muscles are innervated by the Median nerve, what motor response to you expect when stimulating this nerve, and what sensory area is innervated by this nerve?
7. Describe the relationship between the above nerves and the Brachial Artery and Veins and the Basilic Vein.
8. Describe the surface and sono-anatomy of the nerves in the axilla.
9. Describe the innervation of the scapula.
10. Describe the innervation of the shoulder joint and clavicle.

## Day 4: Nerves around the elbow (Chap 2).

Questions:
1. Describe the surface and sono-anatomy of the Ulnar Nerve.
2. Describe the surface and sono-anatomy of the Radial Nerve.
3. Describe the surface and sono-anatomy of the Median Nerve.
4. Describe the surface and sono-anatomy of the Musculocutaneous Nerve.
5. Describe the motor response when stimulating the Ulnar Nerve.
6. Describe the motor response when stimulating the Radial Nerve.
7. Describe the motor response when stimulating the Median Nerve.
8. Describe the motor response when stimulating the Musculocutaneous Nerve at the elbow.
9. Describe the sensory innervation of the elbow joint.
10. What nerves innervate the medial parts of the arm and forearm?

## Day 5: Anatomy of the epidural space (Chap 9)

Questions:
1. How do the epidural spaces of the cervical thoracic, lumbar and sacral areas differ from each other?
2. What is the content of the epidural space, and why are epidural blocks segmental?
3. What is your understanding of the subdural extra-arachnoid space? And how does a subdural (extra-arachnoid) block differ from an epidural and a subarachnoid block?
4. In the midline of the lumbar areas, what structures do you penetrate before reaching the subdural space – starting at the skin.
5. Sympathetic ganglia originating from which spinal nerves innervate the heart?
6. Which sympathetic spinal nerves innervate the adrenals?
7. Sympathetic ganglia originating from which spinal nerves innervate the Celiac Ganglion and via which nerve?
8. What is the difference in the hypotension associated by high thoracic, low thoracic and lumbar epidural block in anatomical terms?
9. Describe the circulation of cerebrospinal fluid.
10. What is the significance of the dural sleeve surrounding all the nerve roots as they leave the spine or cranium?

# Week 2 - Lower Limb

## Day 1: Anatomy of the lumbosacral plexus (Chap 3 & 4).

Questions:
1. What is the origin of the Lumbar Plexus?
2. What is the origin of the Sacral Plexus?
3. What do you understand from the term Lumbosacral trunk?
4. Where does the Femoral Nerve originate from?
5. Where does the Lateral Cutaneous Nerve of the Thigh (LCNT) originate from?
6. Where does the obturator nerve originate from?
7. What nerve(s) originate from T12 & L1?
8. What is the origin of the Sciatic Nerve?
9. What connects the spinal roots of the Lumbosacral plexus to the Sympathetic trunk?
10. Describe the "Capdevila" surface landmarks of lumbar plexus block.

## Day 2: Anatomy of the nerves in the groin area (Chap 3).

Questions
1. Describe the surface anatomy of the Femoral Nerve
2. Describe the surface and sono-anatomy of the LCNT
3. Describe the surface and sono-anatomy of the Obturator Nerve
4. What are the branches of the Femoral Nerve?
5. What are the branches of the Obturator Nerve?
6. Describe the motor innervation of the Femoral Nerve. Describe the motor responses you get when stimulating the Femoral, Nerve to Sartorius and Obturator Nerves.
7. Describe the sensory areas innervated by the femoral nerve.
8. Describe the sensory areas innervated by the Obturator and LFCT nerves.
9. Describe the fascia relationships of the Femoral Nerve, Femoral Artery and Femoral Vein.
10. Describe the tissue layers (micro-anatomy) surrounding the femoral nerve.

## Day 3:  Anatomy of the proximal Sciatic Nerve (Chap 4).

Questions:
1.  Describe the surface anatomy of the Sciatic Nerve in the parasacral, transgluteal (Labat & Winnie), and subgluteal areas.
2.  What is the relationship of the Sciatic Nerve to the Posterior Cutaneous Nerve of the Thigh?
3.  What is the relationship of the Piriformis Muscle to the Sciatic Nerve?
4.  Describe the sensory innervation of the hip joint.
5.  Describe the sensory innervation of the knee joint.
6.  Describe the motor innervation of the Sciatic Nerve.  Describe the motor responses of Sciatic Nerve stimulation.
7.  Describe the sensory areas innervated by the Sciatic Nerve
8.  Where does the innervation of the hamstrings originate, and if, while doing a subgluteal nerve block, you get a hamstring motor response, in which direction must you move the needle tip.
9.  Describe the sono-anatomy of the subgluteal Sciatic Nerve.
10. Name the 2 muscles forming the groove through which a subgluteal Sciatic Nerve block is typically done.

## Day 4:  Anatomy of the popliteal fossa (Chap 4).

Questions:
1.  What muscles form the popliteal triangle?
2.  At what level does the Sciatic Nerve usually split in the popliteal area?
3.  Name five nerves that originate from the Sciatic Nerve in the popliteal area.
4.  Describe the surface anatomy of the Sciatic Nerve in the popliteal area.
5.  What is the relationship of the Tibial Nerve to the Popliteal Artery and Vein?
6.  Describe the sono-anatomy of the Sciatic Nerve in the popliteal area.
7.  Describe the sensory area innervated by the Common Peroneal Nerve.  What is another name that this nerve also goes by?
8.  Describe the motor response you get when stimulating the Common Peroneal Nerve.
9.  Describe the sensory area innervated by the Tibial Nerve.
10. What is the motor response upon stimulation of the Tibial nerve?

Questions:
1. Name the 5 nerves that innervate the foot.
2. Describe the relationship or these nerves to the fascia around the ankle joint.
3. What is the motor response when stimulating each of these nerves?
4. What part of the foot does the Posterior Tibial Nerve innervate?
5. What part of the foot does the Deep Peroneal Nerve innervate?
6. What part of the foot does the Saphanous Nerve innervate?
7. What part of the foot does the Superficial Peroneal Nerve innervate?
8. What part of the foot does the Sural Nerve innervate?
9. Describe the innervation of the ankle joint?
10. Describe the Surface anatomy of each of the 5 nerves around the ankle.

For ABA practice questions on anatomy and regional anesthesia,

Visit RAEducation.com

Other resources for further self-study are:

http://www.asahq.org/education/online-learning/ace-program

http://www.truelearn.com/anesthesiology/

https://m5boardreview.com